Tumors of the Spinal Canal

Surgical Approaches and Future Therapies

Ankit I. Mehta, MD, FAANS, FACS
Neurosurgeon
Associate Professor
Director of Spinal Oncology
Associate Program Director
Neurosurgical Residency Program
Department of Neurosurgery;
Adjunct Professor of Chemical Engineering and
Orthopedic Surgery
University of Illinois at Chicago
Chicago, Illinois,
USA

249 Illustrations

Thieme
New York • Stuttgart • Delhi • Rio de Janeiro

Library of Congress Cataloging-in-Publication Data is available from the publisher.

Important note: Medicine is an ever-changing science undergoing continual development. Research and clinical experience are continually expanding our knowledge, in particular our knowledge of proper treatment and drug therapy. Insofar as this book mentions any dosage or application, readers may rest assured that the authors, editors, and publishers have made every effort to ensure that such references are in accordance with **the state of knowledge at the time of production of the book.**

Nevertheless, this does not involve, imply, or express any guarantee or responsibility on the part of the publishers in respect to any dosage instructions and forms of applications stated in the book. **Every user is requested to examine carefully** the manufacturers' leaflets accompanying each drug and to check, if necessary in consultation with a physician or specialist, whether the dosage schedules mentioned therein or the contraindications stated by the manufacturers differ from the statements made in the present book. Such examination is particularly important with drugs that are either rarely used or have been newly released on the market. Every dosage schedule or every form of application used is entirely at the user's own risk and responsibility. The authors and publishers request every user to report to the publishers any discrepancies or inaccuracies noticed. If errors in this work are found after publication, errata will be posted at www.thieme.com on the product description page.

Some of the product names, patents, and registered designs referred to in this book are in fact registered trademarks or proprietary names even though specific reference to this fact is not always made in the text. Therefore, the appearance of a name without designation as proprietary is not to be construed as a representation by the publisher that it is in the public domain.

Thieme addresses people of all gender identities equally. We encourage our authors to use gender-neutral or gender-equal expressions wherever the context allows.

Thieme Publishers New York
333 Seventh Avenue, New York, NY 10001 USA
+1 800 782 3488, customerservice@thieme.com

Cover design: © Thieme
Cover illustration: Victoria Zakrzewski
Typesetting by TNQ Technologies, India

Printed in Germany by Beltz Grafische Betriebe   5 4 3 2 1

ISBN 978-1-62623-931-9

Also available as an e-book:
eISBN: 978-1-62623-932-6
eISBN (epub): 978-1-63853-586-7

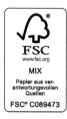

FSC
www.fsc.org
MIX
Papier aus ver-
antwortungsvollen
Quellen
FSC® C089473

Dedicated to the teachers, surgeons, researchers, and healers who drive care and innovation to provide hope to our patients. In addition, I would like to thank our patients who place their ultimate trust in the medical community and give selflessly their knowledge.

Special thanks to my wife (Mona), daughter (Amaya), parents (Indravadan and Darshana), and sister (Arpita).

Contents

Section I: Intramedullary Spinal Tumors

13 Peripheral Nerve and Paraspinal Tumors: Future Directions of Therapy 123

Clayton L. Rosinski, Rown Parola, Srjan Sreepathy, Anisse N. Chaker, and Ankit I. Mehta

Preface

Tumors of the Spinal Canal provides a comprehensive review of the natural history, approach for treatment, advanced surgical techniques, and future therapies for intradural tumors. This book provides the reader with mastery in the management of these clinically difficult tumors, both from a medical and surgical standpoint. In addition, it focuses on the research innovations associated with tumors of the spinal canal, with an emphasis on imaging, drug delivery, and electrophysiological monitoring.

Ankit I. Mehta, MD, FAANS, FACS

Contributors

Hussam Abou-Al-Shaar, MD
Department of Neurological Surgery
University of Pittsburgh Medical Center
Pittsburgh, Pennsylvania, USA

Abdullah M. Abunimer, MD
Postdoctoral Research Fellow
Department of Neurosurgery
Brigham and Women's Hospital
Harvard Medical School
Boston, Massachusetts, USA

Owoicho Adogwa, MD, MPH
Assistant Professor
Department of Neurological Surgery;
Chief of Neurological Surgery
North Dallas Veterans Affairs Hospital
University of Texas Southwestern Medical School
Dallas, Texas, USA

Tania M. Aguilar, BSc
Department of Neurosurgery
University of Illinois at Chicago
Chicago, Illinois, USA

Amanda Allen, DO
Department of Radiology
College of Medicine
University of Illinois at Chicago
Chicago, Illinois, USA

Sean M. Barber, MD
Department of Neurosurgery
Houston Methodist Neurological Institute
Houston, Texas, USA

Nikki M. Barrington, MPH
Department of Neurosurgery
University of Illinois at Chicago
Chicago, Illinois, USA
Rosalind Franklin University of Medicine and Science
North Chicago, Illinois, USA

Cameron Brimley, MD
Department of Neurosurgery
Geisinger Neuroscience Institute
Danville, Pennsylvania, USA

Anisse N. Chaker, MD
Department of Neurosurgery
Henry Ford Health System
Detroit, Michigan, USA

William Clifton III, MD
Department of Orthopedic Surgery
Columbia University Medical Center
New York, New York, USA

Douglas A. Cotanche, PhD
Associate Professor of Anatomical Sciences
Department of Medical Foundations
Ross University School of Medicine
Bridgetown, Barbados

John E. Donahue, MD
Department of Pathology and Laboratory Medicine
The Warren Alpert Medical School of Brown University
Providence, Rhode Island, USA

Hamidou Drammeh, BS
Department of Neurosurgery
University of Illinois at Chicago
Chicago, Illinois, USA

Anteneh M. Feyissa, MD
Mayo Clinic, Department of Neurology
Jacksonville, Florida, USA

Christopher Florido, MD
Department of Radiology
College of Medicine, University of Illinois at Chicago
Chicago, Illinois, USA

Jared S. Fridley, MD
Department of Neurosurgery
The Warren Alpert Medical
School of Brown University
Providence, Rhode Island, USA

Shashank V. Gandhi, MD
Texas Back Institute
Plano, Texas, USA

Anand V. Germanwala, MD
Associate Professor and Residency Program Director
Department of Neurological Surgery
Loyola University Stritch School of Medicine
Maywood, Illinois, USA

Ziya L. Gokaslan, MD, FAANS, FACS
Julius Stoll, MD Professor and Chair
Department of Neurosurgery
The Warren Alpert Medical
   School of Brown University
Providence, Rhode Island, USA

Akua Graf
Fourth Year Medical Student (M4)
Department of Neurosurgery, College of Medicine
University of Illinois at Chicago
Chicago, Illinois, USA

Mari Groves, MD
Department of Neurosurgery
Johns Hopkins University School of Medicine
Baltimore, MD, USA;
Johns Hopkins All Children's Institute for
    Brain Protection Sciences
St. Petersburg, Florida, USA

Jonathan Hobbs, MD
Department of Neurosurgery
The University of Chicago
Chicago, Illinois, USA

Ryan C. Hofler, MD, MS
Assistant Professor
Department of Neurological Surgery
University of Kentucky
Lexington, Kentucky, USA

George I. Jallo, MD
Director, Institute for Brain Protection Sciences
Johns Hopkins All Children's Hospital
Professor, Neurosurgery, Pediatrics and Oncology
Johns Hopkins University School of Medicine
Baltimore, Maryland, USA

G. Alexander Jones, MD
Health System Clinician
Department of Neurological Surgery
Northwestern University Feinberg School of Medicine
Lake Forest, Illinois, USA

Young Jun Lee, MD
Department of Neurosurgery
College of Medicine, University of Illinois at Chicago
Chicago, Illinois, USA

Mark A. Mahan, MD
Assistant Professor of Neurosurgery
Department of Neurosurgery
Clinical Neurosciences Center
University of Utah
Salt Lake City, USA

Hani Malone, MD
Assistant Professor
Department of Neurological Surgery
Scripps Clinic Torrey Pines, La Jolla
California, USA

Luis Manon, MD
Pathology Resident (PGY-4)
Department of Pathology College of Medicine,
    University of Illinois at Chicago
Chicago, Illinois, USA

Ankit I. Mehta, MD, FAANS, FACS
Neurosurgeon
Associate Professor
Director of Spinal Oncology
Associate Program Director
Neurosurgical Residency Program
Department of Neurosurgery;
Adjunct Professor of Chemical Engineering and
    Orthopedic Surgery
University of Illinois at Chicago
Chicago, Illinois, USA

David Nai, MD
Department of Pathology, College of Medicine
University of Illinois at Chicago
Chicago, Illinois, USA

Mohammad Hassan A. Noureldine, MD, MSc
Department of Neurosurgery
University of South Florida
Tampa, Florida, USA

John O'Toole, MD, MS
Professor of Neurosurgery
Co-Director
Coleman Foundation Comprehensive Spine Tumor Clinic
Rush University Medical Center
Chicago, Illinois, USA

Rown Parola, MS
Medical Student
University of Illinois at Chicago
Chicago, Illinois, USA

Alfredo Quinones-Hinojosa, MD
Department of Neurosurgery
Mayo Clinic
Jacksonville, Florida, USA

Abhinav K. Reddy, MS
Department of Neurosurgery
University of Illinois at Chicago
Chicago, Illinois, USA

Karim ReFaey, MB, BCh
Department of Neurosurgery
Mayo Clinic
Jacksonville, Florida, USA

Luca Ricciardi, MD, MSc, PhD
Department of Neurosurgery
Mayo Clinic
Jacksonville, Florida, USA;
A. Gemelli University Hospital;
Department of Neurosurgery
Catholic University of Sacred Heart
Rome, Italy

Jeffrey M. Rogg, MD
Department of Diagnostic Imaging
The Warren Alpert Medical School of Brown University
Providence, Rhode Island, USA

Clayton Rosinski, MD
Department of Neurosurgery
University of Iowa Hospitals and Clinics
Iowa City, Iowa, USA

James S. Ryoo, BS
Department of Neurosurgery
University of Illinois at Chicago
Chicago, Illinois, USA

Nir Shimony, MD
Department of Neurosurgery, Geisinger
  Neuroscience Institute
Danville, Pennsylvania, USA;
Department of Neurosurgery, Johns Hopkins
University School of Medicine
Baltimore, Maryland, USA

Srjan Sreepathy, BS
Department of Neurosurgery
University of Illinois at Chicago
Chicago, Illinois, USA

Nicholas J. Szerlip, MD
Clinical Associate Professor
Department of Neurological Surgery
University of Michigan Medical School
Ann Arbor, Michigan, USA

Matthew K. Tobin, MD, PhD
Resident Physician
Department of Neurological Surgery
Indiana University School of Medicine
Indianapolis, Indiana, USA

Tibor Valyi-Nagy, MD, PhD
Department of Pathology
College of Medicine, University of Illinois at Chicago
Chicago, Illinois, USA

Tito Vivas-Buitrago, MD
Department of Neurosurgery
Mayo Clinic
Jacksonville, Florida, USA;
Universidad de Santander UDES, School of Medicine
Bucaramanga, Colombia, USA

Jack Zakrzewski, MD
Department of Surgery
University of Colorado School of Medicine
Aurora, Colorado, USA

1 Overview of Spinal Canal Tumors

Ankit I. Mehta

Summary

Tumors of the spinal canal provide unique challenges both in the operative realm and in the oncological treatment of disease. Over the past few decades there have been great strides to make operative intervention safer, more precise, and less invasive in a functional and structural manner. Despite these advances, the inherent challenges of tumors in the spinal canal remain due to the specific location of the pathology and the intricate functional tissue surrounding these disease processes. Sometimes to understand the current state of technical surgery, treatment algorithms, and innovative research; we must first understand the early guiding principles of treatment of these tumors of the spinal canal. Through this textbook, a comprehensive yet relevant discussion of spinal pathology, anatomy, management, and future developments will be carried out in a systematic manner.

Keywords: intramedullary spinal tumors, extramedullary spinal tumors, spinal oncology, spinal tumor differential diagnosis

Table 1.1 Spinal tumors

Intramedullary	Intradural extramedullary	Peripheral nerve—paraspinal
Astrocytoma	Meningioma	Schwannoma
Ependymoma	Neurofibroma	Neurofibroma
Dermoid/epidermoid	Schwannoma	Neuroma
Lipoma	Metastatic tumor	Malignant peripheral nerve sheath tumor
Hemangioblastoma		Plasmacytoma
Teratoma		Superior sulcus tumor
Ganglioglioma		Metastatic tumor
Oligodendroglioma		Tuberculous spondylitis
Metastatic tumor		Pseudomeningocele
		Intraforaminal synovial cyst
		Aneurysmal bone cyst
		Extradural arachnoid cyst

1.1 Introduction

The spinal cord provides a necessary conduit for our interaction with the environment both through sensory inputs and motor outputs to our musculoskeletal system. Therefore, when spinal tumors disrupt these pathways in the spinal cord, it can be devastating for the patients and their families. The intricate anatomical relationships between the tumors and normal spinal pathways, the restricted corridors of entry, and the limitations of drug penetration are some of the many challenges in managing spinal tumors.

From an organizational standpoint, tumors of the spinal canal can be divided into three categories based on anatomical location: intradural intramedullary, intradural extramedullary, and peripheral nerve and paraspinal. The pathologies associated with oncological processes are typically from aberrancy in the cells in those regions (primary) or tumors coming from other organ system associated cancers (metastases) (▶ Table 1.1).

This textbook is organized as per these categories, since each of these tumor locations are unique in pathology, presentation, surgical management, treatment algorithms, and research studies.

1.2 Differentiating Tumor Pathology and Neurological Mimickers

It is critical when presented with a patient that a wide differential diagnosis should be entertained and that both imaging and laboratory studies be undertaken to refine the diagnosis. Rigorous workup in this manner has been very useful personally for my practice and can provide a more guided treatment for these patients. Patients who present with a neurological deficit should have an exhaustive differential diagnosis that includes: neoplastic, degenerative, vascular, demyelinating, traumatic, and other etiologies (metabolic, infectious, radiation) (▶ Table 1.2). Obtaining a thorough patient history may refine the differential diagnosis and guide us towards the imaging modality or electrodiagnostic tests to be used. Primarily in neurosurgical practices, the imaging studies are already performed. However, the contrasted studies and other imaging modalities might not be ascertained during the initial consultation. Therefore, it is important that a wide differential is made before looking at the imaging and making a management decision. Once the imaging is obtained, other laboratory studies could guide management including lumbar puncture, inflammatory markers, and infectious disease labs. Ultimately only when a comprehensive analysis is completed should a clinician entertain intervention. There should be an utmost amount of caution in considering surgical treatment as observation can provide a means of determining possible origins of the disease process and the nature of a neoplastic process (slow vs aggressive growth patterns). Through each specific pathology and disease origin we will provide a more granular analysis on the workup of these patients. However, it is important to consider various sources of neurological pathology before considering intervention.

1.3 Research Areas and Future Therapies

It is an exciting time in the treatment of spinal tumors since cutting-edge technology can provide more accurate diagnosis,

Table 1.2 Differential diagnosis

Neoplastic	Degenerative	Vascular	Demyelinating	Traumatic	Other

• Intramedullary
  ○ Astrocytoma
  ○ Ependymoma
  ○ Hemangioblastoma
• Intradural extramedullary
  ○ Meningioma
  ○ Schwannoma
  ○ Neurofibroma
• Extradural
  ○ Metastasis
  ○ Primary bone tumor
	• Disk herniation
	  ○ Cervical stenosis
	    (acquired or
	    congenital)
	• Synovial cyst
		• Arteriovenous
		  malformation
		• Cavernoma
		• Spinal cord infarct
			• Multiple sclerosis
			• Transverse myelitis
			• Neurosarcoidosis
				• Post traumatic
				• Traumatic
				  neuroma
				• Unstable spine
					• Vitamin B12 deficiency
					• Alcoholism
					• Radiation myelopathy
					• Syringomyelia
					• Arachnoid cyst
					• Tethered cord
					• Chiari malformation
					• AIDS
					• Epidural abscess

more effective treatments, and refined drug delivery platforms for these difficult disease pathologies. Throughout this textbook after discussing the pathologies, workup, and standard of care management, we will be discussing new innovations that will transform our management of these pathologies. The world experts on spinal cord tumors will present their unique insight in these chapters and will foster a new means of improving our care for these patients.

1.4 Conclusion

Tumors of the spinal canal provides unique challenges from a diagnostic, therapeutic, surgical, and research standpoint. The following chapters will help clarify the most up-to-date management and research from leaders in the field of spinal oncology. We hope this text will provide you with a more thorough understanding of the field through a systematic approach.

2 Anatomy of the Spinal Cord and Nerve Roots

Jack Zakrzewski and Douglas A. Cotanche

Summary

This chapter offers an extensive overview of the anatomy of the spinal column and spinal cord, the development of the spinal cord, the internal anatomy of the gray matter and the ascending and descending columns in the white matter, the anatomy of the meninges, and the anatomy of the arterial and vascular supply of the spinal cord.

Keywords: vertebral column, spinal cord, spinal nerve, spinal vasculature, development of the spine, meninges, ascending and descending spinal pathways

2.1 Introduction

The spinal cord is one of the two components of the central nervous system (CNS), with the other being the brain. The spinal cord's major function is to provide access to the CNS for the nerves controlling the structures of the neck, body, and limbs of a human being. The spinal cord is composed of a central core of gray matter that contains the neurons and interneurons that communicate with the body. On the periphery of the central gray matter is the white matter, a series of myelinated neuronal processes that communicate with regions up and down the spinal cord and with major tracts to and from the brain. In this chapter we will describe in detail the anatomy of the spinal column and spinal cord, its embryonic development, the organization of the gray matter, and the ascending and descending columns in the spinal cord. We will also describe the meninges in the spinal cord, the arterial and venous supply to the spinal cord, and the anatomy of the spinal nerves. This chapter is intended to serve as an anatomical overview of the vertebral column and spinal cord and will serve as a foundation for the remaining chapters on tumors of the spinal cord.

2.2 Anatomy of the Vertebral Column and Vertebrae

The vertebral column consists of the curved assemblage of the individual vertebrae that make up the spine (▶ Fig. 2.1). The individual vertebrae are connected by synovial facet joints (sometimes referred to as zygapophysial joints), ligaments, muscles, and fascia. There are three main functions of the spine: support the trunk and posture, protect the enclosed spinal cord and nerves, and provide attachment sites for various muscles.[1] The vertebrae also serve as sites of hematopoiesis. The vertebrae of the column receive blood via branches of the intersegmental somatic arteries. Each of these arteries is named based on the level of the column it is found in.

Between each of the vertebrae is an intervertebral disk (▶ Fig. 2.2). Each disk is made of an outer fibrous ring called the anulus fibrosus and an inner gel-like center called the nucleus pulposus. The outer ring is made mostly of type I cartilage, while

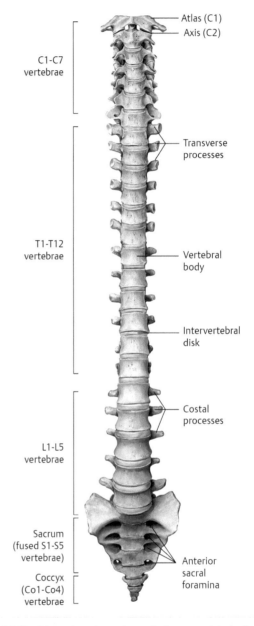

Fig. 2.1 The 31 vertebrae that make up the human vertebral column, anterior view. (Reproduced with permission from Schuenke M, Schulte E, Schumacher U. THIEME Atlas of Anatomy. General Anatomy and Musculoskeletal System. Illustrations by Voll M and Wesker K. Third Edition. © Thieme 2020.)

the nucleus pulposus consists mainly of type II cartilage and water.[2] The intervertebral disks allow for limited amount of vertebral movement, while also acting as quasi-ligaments that hold the column together. Most importantly, they act as shock absorbers that distribute forces along the column.

The anterior aspect of the vertebral column is mostly made up of the vertebral bodies and the intervertebral disks, which are then covered by the anterior longitudinal ligament. This ligament forms a plane with the prevertebral and endothoracic fascia, as well as with the subperitoneal areolar tissue of the posterior abdominal wall, which can act as a route for the spread of pathogens and cancer. The lateral aspect of the column consists of the articular processes in the cervical and lumbar regions and the transverse processes in the thoracic region. The oval intervertebral foramina are found here, behind the bodies themselves and between the pedicles. These foramina allow for interaction between the lumen of the vertebral canal and the paravertebral soft tissues. It is the route of exit of the individual spinal nerves. In addition, it can also act as a route of tumor spread. The posterior aspect of the vertebral column is made of the posterior aspect of the laminae and the spinous processes, as well as the facet joints. It is covered by ligaments and the deep muscles of the back.

2.2.1 The Vertebrae: General Features

Each vertebra consists of three main parts: the vertebral body, the dorsal vertebral arch (sometimes called the neural arch), and the vertebral foramen (▶ Fig. 2.3). The foramen contains the spinal cord, the meninges, and the various vessels that feed and drain the vertebral canal. The vertebrae vary in size and shape depending on the level of the spine they are located in. This section will give a broad overview of vertebral characteristics, as the details are beyond the scope of this text.

The pedicles are located on each side of the posterior surface of the vertebrae and form the lateral walls of the vertebral arch. They are short, thick, and narrower than the rest of the arch, and are continuous with the laminae. The spinous process projects dorsally and caudally from the laminal junction. Its main purpose is to serve as a lever for the antigravity muscles that control posture and movement. The articular processes are paired structures: one superior and one inferior. They originate from the vertebral arch and contribute to the facet joint, allowing for some movement between the vertebrae. The transverse processes project laterally from the laminae, although their exact location varies between spinal levels. Like the spinous process, these projections act as levers for the various back muscles and ligaments.

2.2.2 The Vertebral Canal

The vertebral canal is a continuous series of foramina that is located posterior to the vertebral bodies. It begins at the foramen magnum and terminates in the sacral hiatus. Although it is quite stationary in the thoracic region, it does move slightly in the cervical and lumbar regions. The canal is larger and

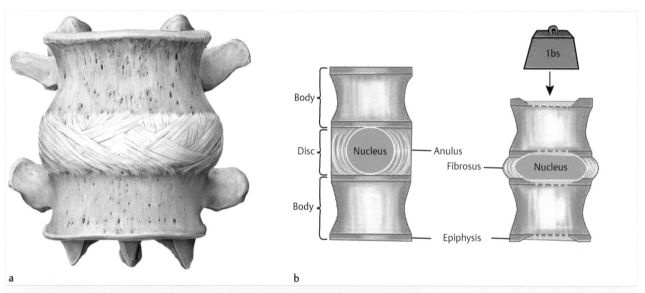

Fig. 2.2 **(a,b)** The intervertebral disks between bony vertebrae and how they adjust to bear weight. (Subpart (a): Reproduced with permission from Schuenke M, Schulte E, Schumacher U. THIEME Atlas of Anatomy. General Anatomy and Musculoskeletal System. Illustrations by Voll M and Wesker K. Third Edition. © Thieme 2020.)

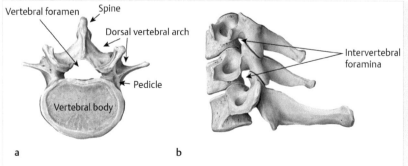

Fig. 2.3 **(a)** Anatomy of a typical vertebra, superior view. (Reproduced with permission from Schuenke M, Schulte E, Schumacher U. THIEME Atlas of Anatomy. General Anatomy and Musculoskeletal System. Illustrations by Voll M and Wesker K. Third Edition. © Thieme 2020.) **(b)** Lateral view of the cervical vertebrae indicating the location of the intervertebral foramina. (Reproduced with permission from Schuenke M, Schulte E, Schumacher U. THIEME Atlas of Anatomy. General Anatomy and Musculoskeletal System. Illustrations by Voll M and Wesker K. Third Edition. © Thieme 2020.)

triangular in shape in the cervical and lumbar regions and smaller and more circular in the thoracic region.

2.2.3 The Intervertebral Foramina

The intervertebral foramina serve as the main route into and out of the vertebral canal. They are found between the posterolateral aspect of the superior vertebral pedicle, the compact bone of the inferior vertebral pedicle, and the ventral aspect of the fibrous capsule of the facet joint. Each foramen is covered by a protective fibrous tissue. The region in which the spinal nerve canal is found is called the true foramina. It also contains the spinal nerves and sheaths, the meningeal nerves, the spinal arteries, and the venous plexus. It is the main site of nerve compression.

2.3 Development of the Spinal Cord

2.3.1 Early Development

The tissues that will become the brain and spinal cord arise early in human embryonic development, shortly after the formation of the trilaminar embryo. Gastrulation is completed by day 18. On day 19, the central region of the ectodermal epithelium begins to thicken and form the pear-shaped neural plate (▶ Fig. 2.4). One day later, the lateral edges of the neural plate begin to elevate and become the neural folds. The neural groove lies centrally between the two neural folds. The neural folds continue to elevate and curl inward toward one another. As they do, the neural groove deepens to become a trench. By day 22, the two neural folds contact one another and begin to fuse into a neural tube, first in the cervical regions and then continuing to zipper up and down the neural plate (▶ Fig. 2.5). The epithelial tissues at the very tip of the neural folds do not become incorporated into the neural tube, but instead separate away from where the folds are merging and migrate out into the mesoderm region between the neural tube and the overlying ectoderm. These tissues are the neural crest cells and they will be discussed below in the development of the sensory components of the spinal nerve and in the development of the meninges.

2.3.2 Neurodifferentiation in the Spinal Cord

Between embryonic days 23 and 25, the neural tube continues to zipper up to enclose the entire neural tube. Closure of the anterior neuropore occurs first and happens on day 25. The posterior neuropore follows by closing up on day 28. During the formation of the neural tube, the tissue is composed of a pseudostratified epithelium, with the basal surface at the outer surface of the neural tube where it rests on a basement membrane. The apical surface of the neuroepithelium faces the lumen of the neural tube. Beginning around day 26, the cells in the lateral walls of the neural tube located closest to the lumen begin to divide rapidly. Some of the progenies of these dividing cells migrate away from the lumen, lose their apical connections to the luminal surface of the neuroepithelium, and begin to differentiate as neuroblasts. The area where these newly formed neuroblasts congregate is known as the mantle layer and it begins to appear by days 31 to 32[3] (▶ Fig. 2.6). As more neuroblasts are generated, they form two distinct clusters of cell bodies in the lateral walls of the neural tube. Those in the upper or more dorsal half of the neural tube are known as the dorsal lamina or the alar plate: They will go on to become the neurons in the dorsal (sensory) horn of the spinal cord. The neuroblasts in the lower or more ventral half of the neural tube form the ventral lamina or basal plate: They will become the motor neurons of the ventral horn of the spinal cord[3] (▶ Fig. 2.7). The shallow, longitudinal groove separating the alar and basal plates is termed the sulcus limitans.

The neuroblasts in the ventral horn begin to mature into neurons beginning on day 28. They form axonal processes that bundle together and begin to exit the ventral spinal cord to form the ventral root. By gestational week 5.5 (GW5.5), the cell bodies of the lower motor neurons are well differentiated in the ventral horn and extend their axons out to form the ventral root of the spinal nerve. As the ventral motor neurons are differentiating, the neuroepithelium begins to create interneurons during GW6.5 that will form communicating links between the primary motor neurons and the primary sensory neurons. Once the neuroepithelium is finished generating neuroblasts, it then switches to produce the glioblasts that will form the glial cells in the dorsal and ventral horns.

The sensory component of the spinal nerves originates not in the spinal cord gray matter, but from the neural crest cells in the mesoderm layer just outside the dorsal half of the neural tube. A group of neural crest cells will differentiate into neurons and congregate just outside the dorsal neural tube to form the dorsal root ganglia. The neurons of the dorsal root ganglia send a bundle of their central neuronal processes into the dorsal horn as the dorsal root of the spinal cord. As they enter the developing spinal cord, these fibers either synapse with sensory neurons in the dorsal horn or they turn and migrate up the spinal cord as the dorsal columns to reach higher centers in the medulla of the brainstem.

The motor axons in the ventral root grow out laterally and eventually come into contact with the peripheral processes of the neurons in the dorsal root ganglion. These two bundles meet to form the true spinal nerve just lateral to the dorsal root ganglion. This is usually located where the dorsal and ventral roots exit through the intervertebral foramina between adjacent vertebrae.

2.3.3 Development of the Spinal Cord White Matter

The developing neurons in the dorsal root ganglia send their proximal processes into the spinal cord beginning in GW5 where they immediately bifurcate into ascending and descending branches. The first synapses form during GW6.5 between the proximal processes and the neurons in the dorsal horn of the cervical spinal cord. Around GW7.5, the ascending proximal processes of the dorsal root ganglion cells begin to form the dorsal funiculi. A distinct fasciculus cuneatus appears in the cervical spinal cord around GW8.5[4] and the fasciculus gracilis appears in a location medial to the fasciculus cuneatus in the cervical region around GW10.[5] The fibers in the fasciculus gracilis formed earlier in the lumbar region of the spinal cord penetrate into the lumbar spinal cord before turning cranially to migrate up the developing spinal cord. Unfortunately, an accurate description of the timing of these events has not been reported in human embryos. Between GW8.5 and GW10.5, there is an overall rostral to caudal gradient in the development

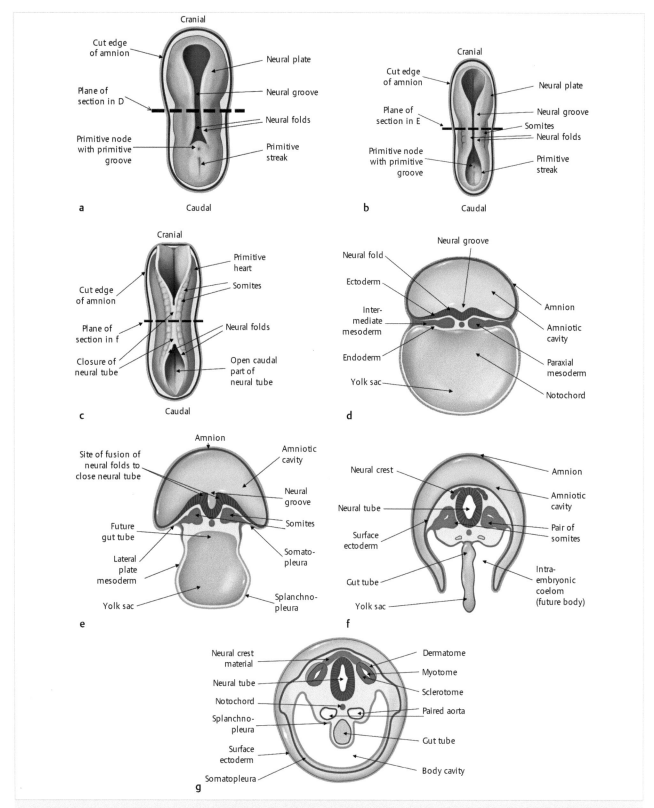

Fig. 2.4 **(a)** Dorsal view of the neural groove. **(b)** Dorsal view of the formation of somites. **(c)** Dorsal view of the closure of the neural groove. **(d)** Transverse view of the beginning of neural crest cell migration. **(e)** Transverse view of the neural groove. **(f)** Transverse view of the neural tube, neural crest, and forming somites. **(g)** Transverse view of the neural tube, notochord, paired aortae, and somites consisting of myotome and sclerotome. (Reproduced with permission from Embryology of the Spine. In: Vaccaro A, Fehlings M, Dvorak M, eds. Spine and Spinal Cord Trauma: Evidence-Based Management. 1st Edition. New York: Thieme; 2010.)

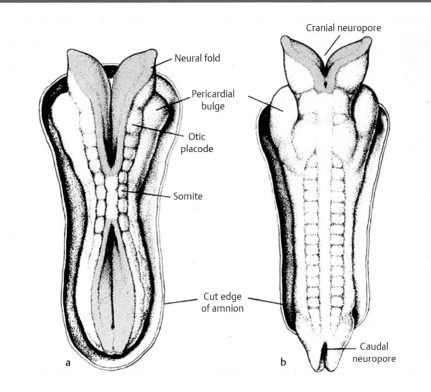

Fig. 2.5 Closure of the anterior and posterior neuropores. **(a)** Closure in the central neural tube with both the rostral and caudal neuropores still widely open throughout most of the neural tube (22 days). **(b)** Closure of almost the entire neural tube with only minimal openings of the rostral and caudal neuropores still present. (Reproduced with permission from Thomas W. Sadler. ed. Langman's Medical Embryology. 12th Edition. Fig. 18.3. Wolters Kluwer Health. 2012.)

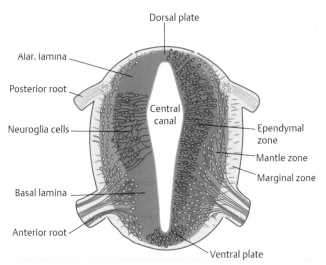

Fig. 2.6 Formation of the mantle layer in the developing neural tube around embryonic days 31 to 32.

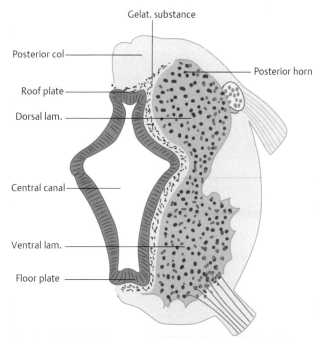

Fig. 2.7 Formation of the basal (motor) and alar (sensory) plates in the developing spinal cord around the end of the third month.

of the spinal cord, with the more caudal regions lagging behind in maturation compared to the cervical region.

The descending corticospinal tract begins to develop first in the cortical white matter of the brain during GW7.5 and descends through the brain during GW19. At this time, the corticospinal tract decussates in the posterior medulla and the crossed fibers begin to descend through the contralateral cervical spinal cord as the lateral funiculus. The tract reaches the cervical spinal cord regions by GW19 (▶ Fig. 2.8), but synaptogenesis with neurons in the ventral horn does not begin for several weeks.[6] The reason for the delay between the arrival of the descending tracts and the onset of synaptogenesis is not currently known.[6]

The descending corticospinal tract enters the thoracic segments of the spinal cord by GW26 and extends throughout the lumbar region by GW29. It reaches the sacral spinal regions by GW31 and is finally present throughout the sacral and coccygeal spinal cord regions by GW37.[7] Once the growth of the corticospinal tract throughout the spinal cord is complete, the myelination of these fibers is much delayed compared with

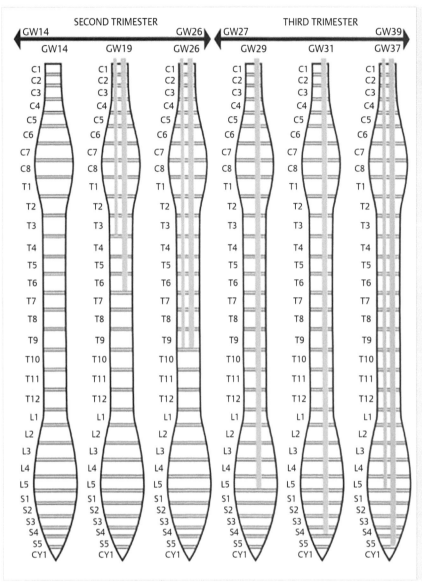

Fig. 2.8 Progression of the growth of the cerebrospinal tract (CST) from the cortex down through the spinal cord. The CST enters the cervical spinal cord just before gestational week 19 (GW19) and moves down the spinal cord to reach the sacral region by GW29 to GW31. (Reproduced with permission from Altman and Bayer, Fig. 7.35.[7])

myelination of the dorsal columns. Myelination in the cervical lateral funiculus begins around the second postnatal month and is complete throughout the cervical region by 4 months.[7] Myelination of the corticospinal tract reaches the lumbar region by 11 months of age and culminates in the sacral spinal cord region by 2 years of age. The behavioral development of motor function seems to correlate well with the time of myelination of the descending lateral funiculus.[6,7]

2.3.4 Development of the Meninges

The classical literature on the development of the meninges states that they develop from the mesodermal tissues surrounding the neural tube; however, more recent studies in developing chicks and mice have identified neural crest cells as the cells of origin of the meninges.[8] These studies also showed that the blood vessels outside and within the meninges are derived from mesodermal cells from the adjacent sclerotomes.[8]

The literature on the development of the human meninges still lists the mesoderm as the source of the meninges, because due to ethical reasons the modern techniques that identified the neural crest origin of the meninges in chicks and mice have not been performed on human embryonic materials. Older human embryonic studies confirmed that the pia on the spinal cord can be first identified at GW6 and forms a layer fully surrounding the spinal cord by GW9.[9] By GW8, a primary meninx can be identified around the spinal cord and a defined dura mater is present under the ventral surface of the spinal cord. By GW9, a distinct dura mater can be seen surrounding the entire spinal cord.[9] The development of a separate arachnoid layer has been clearly seen by GW10 as it begins to differentiate from the developing dura mater. A defined, cell-free subarachnoid space begins to form around GW9. By GW14, the three distinct layers of meninges can be identified surrounding the entire spinal cord[9] (▶ Fig. 2.9).

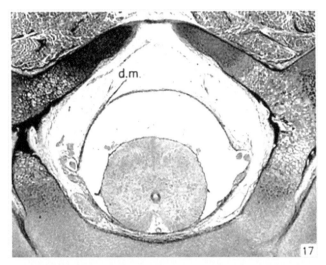

Fig. 2.9 Development of the meninges surrounding the human spinal cord at gestational week 12 (GW12). d.m., dura mater. (Reproduced with permission from Sensenig, Plate 4, Fig. 17.[9])

2.3.5 Length of the Spinal Cord in Relation to the Vertebral Column

The spinal cord fills the entire vertebral canal by 3 months of gestation. This means that the sacral region of the spinal cord is located within the sacral vertebral canal and the dorsal and ventral roots of the sacral nerves exit immediately out of the sacral intervertebral foramina. By the time of birth, the growth of the vertebral canal has exceeded that of the spinal cord and the distal tip of the spinal cord (the sacral and coccygeal parts) is at the level of the third lumbar vertebrae. However, the dorsal root ganglia and the joining of the dorsal and ventral roots to form the spinal nerve still occur near the intervertebral foramina at their appropriate vertebral layers. This means that from vertebral level L3 and below, there is no spinal cord in the vertebral canal. Instead, it is filled with the elongated dorsal and ventral roots of the lower lumbar, sacral, and coccygeal nerves. This bundle of dorsal and ventral roots with no spinal cord resembles a horse's tail and is thus named the cauda equina. By the third year of life, the distal end of the spinal cord has risen up to the level of the first or second lumbar vertebrae. The beneficial clinical result of this uneven growth of the spinal cord versus the vertebral canal is that needles can be inserted epidurally for anesthesia during childbirth or cortisone treatments for spinal nerve pain without risking accidental damage to the spinal cord. Moreover, needles can be inserted directly into the subarachnoid space below the L2 vertebral level to extract cerebrospinal fluid (CSF) for analysis in case of suspected infection or bleeding, again, without risking damage to the spinal cord.

2.4 General Anatomy of the Spinal Cord

The spinal cord emerges from the foramen magnum of the skull. It is continuous with the medulla oblongata and normally

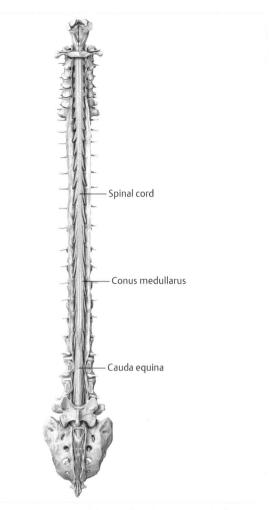

- Spinal cord

- Conus medullarus

- Cauda equina

Fig. 2.10 A posterior view of the spinal cord in situ with the laminae of the vertebrae removed showing the spinal cord, conus medullaris, and cauda equina. (Reproduced with permission from Schuenke M, Schulte E, Schumacher U. THIEME Atlas of Anatomy. Head, Neck and Neuroanatomy. Illustrations by Voll M and Wesker K. Third Edition. © Thieme 2020.)

terminates near the first or second lumbar vertebrae, although this can range from T12 to L3 (▸ Fig. 2.10). At about L1 or L2, the spinal cord tapers and forms a cone-like shape called the conus medullaris. As this happens, the spinal nerves branch out diagonally, forming the cauda equina, which occupies the lumbar cistern in the subarachnoid space inferior to the conus medullaris. The cauda equina provides innervation to the pelvic organs and the lower limbs. In adults, the cord is on average 45 cm in males and 43 cm in females.[10] As the spinal cord ends, a fibrous strand of pia mater, the filum terminale, continues through the spinal canal and attaches to the coccyx, stabilizing the cord within the spinal canal.

The cord varies in diameter not only from one spinal level to another, but also from person to person. Overall, it is largest in the cervical (C5 to T1) and lumbar (L1 to S3) areas, where the sensory input and motor output branch to the extremities. These regions are called the cervical and lumbar enlargements, respectively.[11]

2.4.1 The Anterior Median Fissure and Posterior Median Sulcus

The spinal cord is divided into left and right halves by the anterior median fissure and the posterior median sulcus, which almost completely separate the cord into left and right parts joined together by a commissural band of nervous tissue within a central canal (▶ Fig. 2.11). The anterior (also referred to as ventral) median fissure is about 3 mm deep on average, although its depth increases in the inferior portion of the cord. It contains a double fold, also known as the reticulum, of pia mater. The floor of the fissure is made by a band of white substance called the anterior white commissure, which the spinal vessels pass through as part of their tract into the medulla spinalis. The spinal vessels branch off the anterior spinal artery, which sits within the groove created by the anterior median fissure.[11] This artery, along with the other vessels that provide blood supply to the spinal cord, will be discussed later in this chapter.

The posterior median sulcus is shallower than the anterior fissure, but it gives rise to the posterior median septum, which penetrates almost halfway into the cord. The depth of the septum varies from 4 to 6 mm, but unlike the anterior median fissure, its depth diminishes in the inferior parts of the cord. This central canal also tends to diminish and gets shallower with age.

2.4.2 Regions of the Spinal Cord

The spinal cord can be divided into five regions based on the level of the vertebrae and the spinal nerves that branch off it (the spinal nerves and their numbering will be discussed later in this chapter). The first seven vertebrae, C1–C7, define the cervical region. The next 12 vertebrae, T1–T12, compose the thoracic region. The lumbar region consists of the next five vertebrae, L1–L5. The sacrum is one bone consisting of five fused vertebrae and it gives off five spinal nerves. Finally, the coccyx, known

more colloquially as the tailbone, also consists of one to four fused bones and one spinal nerve.[12]

2.5 Internal Anatomy of the Spinal Cord

When cut into transverse sections, the spinal cord appears almost completely divided into two symmetrical halves by the anterior median fissure and the posterior median septum. There is an inner core of gray matter surrounded completely by the outer white matter, although the ratio between the two and their exact configuration varies by level. The spinal cord in the cervical region has the most white matter, which decreases moving inferiorly down the cord, as the descending nerve tracts shed fibers and the ascending tracts accumulate them. There is a small canal in the center of the gray matter that is lined by columnar ciliated epithelium called the ependyma. It contains the CSF and runs the entire length of the cord, extending superiorly into the medulla oblongata and opening into the fourth ventricle.

2.5.1 The Spinal Gray Matter

On gross inspection, the gray matter of the spinal cord has a "butterfly" or "H" shape and consists of groups of neuronal cell bodies (▶ Fig. 2.12a). It is divided into the dorsal and ventral horns, both of which are then divided into left and right parts. The right and left dorsal horns are the site of termination of the primary afferent fibers that enter the spinal cord through the dorsal roots. The tip of the dorsal horn is connected to the surface of the cord by a thin fasciculus called the tract of Lissauer. The afferent fibers of this tract ascend or descend short distances before terminating within the gray matter inferior to their origin or progressing cranially in the dorsal columns to terminate in the dorsal column nuclei in the medulla. The right and left ventral horns contain efferent neurons with axons leaving the spinal cord via the ventral roots. In the thoracic and upper

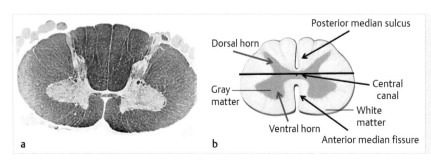

Fig. 2.11 (a) Myelin-stained cross section of the cervical spinal cord (Image from UIC brainstem collection). **(b)** Illustration of the components of the spinal cord. (Reproduced with permission from Schuenke M, Schulte E, Schumacher U. THIEME Atlas of Anatomy. Head, Neck and Neuroanatomy. Illustrations by Voll M and Wesker K. Third Edition. © Thieme 2020.)

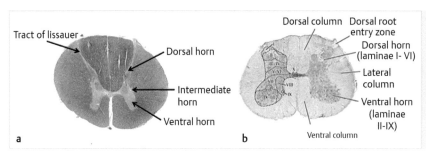

Fig. 2.12 (a) Myelin-stained cross section of the thoracic spinal cord (Image from UIC brainstem collection). **(b)** Illustrations of Rexed's spinal cord laminae stained for Nissl substance. (Reproduced with permission from Purves et al, Fig A7.[25])

lumbar portions of the spinal cord (T1–L2), there is also an intermediate horn, sometimes referred to as the lateral horn. It contains cell bodies of preganglionic sympathetic nerve fibers. The axons of these sympathetic nerves leave the spinal cord through the ventral roots. The dorsal and ventral commissures unite the two sides of the cord on either side of the central canal.

The gray matter is composed of neuronal cell bodies and their processes and synaptic connections, as well as supporting tissue, such as neuroglia and blood vessels. Neurons in this part of the cord are multipolar, varying in size, length, and arrangement. The white matter is mainly composed of longitudinal, myelinated axons collected into large tracts that ascend or descend throughout the length of the spinal cord.[13]

2.5.2 Neuronal Cell Groups: Rexed's Laminae

The gray matter can be divided into 10 different zones based on observed cytoarchitecture and neuron size, shape, and density. These zones are known as Rexed's laminae.[14] Each zone is numbered from dorsal to ventral (▶ Fig. 2.12b). Laminae I to IV are found in the dorsal part of the dorsal horn and are the site of termination for many cutaneous primary afferent nerves. Lamina I is sometimes referred to as lamina marginalis and lamina II is more commonly referred to as the substantia gelatinosa.

Laminae V and VI are in the base of the dorsal horn. They receive the terminal fibers of the proprioceptive primary afferent nerves, profuse corticospinal projections from the motor and sensory cortex, as well as inputs from subcortical levels.

Lamina VII, sometimes referred to as the intermediate zone, lies just ventral to lamina VI and extends across the spinal gray matter. It includes the lateral horn (when present) and varies in size across the regions of the spinal cord. Mechanistically, it contains three nuclear groups: the posterior thoracic nucleus (also known as Clarke's column) in the thoracic and upper lumbar, which gives off the dorsal spinocerebellar tract and the intermediolateral nucleus; the intermediate tract in T1 through L2, which gives rise to the preganglionic sympathetic fibers; and the intermediomedial nucleus, which runs the length of the cord and is possibly involved in control of visceral motor neurons.

Lamina VIII is located at the base of the ventral horn in the thoracic region, but it can be found on the medial aspect of the ventral horn in the cervical and lumbar enlargements. It is mostly made up of propriospinal interneurons receiving terminals from adjacent laminae, commissural fibers from the contralateral lamina VIII, and descending connections from the interstitiospinal, reticulospinal, and vestibulospinal tracts, as well as the medial longitudinal fasciculus. It affects the alpha motor neurons bilaterally, either directly or by excitation of the gamma motor neurons.

Lamina IX is embedded in lamina VIII in the thoracic region and within laminae VII and VIII in the cervical and lumbar regions. It consists of a complex array of alpha, gamma, and interneurons. Alpha neurons supply the motor end plates of striated muscle, while the smaller gamma neurons innervate muscle fibers in muscle spindles. Lamina X surrounds the central canal and is primarily made up of dorsal and ventral gray commissures.

2.5.3 The Dorsal Horn

The dorsal horn is the major site of termination of the incoming primary afferent fibers, which enter the spinal cord through the dorsal roots. These root fibers use many different neurotransmitters, such as glutamic acid, substance P, vasoactive intestinal peptide, somatostatin, and angiotensin II, to name a few. They carry exteroceptive, proprioceptive, and interoceptive information from the peripheral tissue into the spinal cord. Cutaneous fibers tend to terminate in laminae I to IV; fine afferents from the skin, muscle, and viscera end in lamina V; and proprioceptive and cutaneous afferents end in lamina VI. Most (if not all) primary afferent fibers divide into ascending and descending branches after entering the spinal cord. They travel through the tract of Lissauer and send collateral fibers into the gray matter above and below their site of entry. The nerves then run through lamina I at the dorsolateral tip of the dorsal horn, just posterior to the tract of Lissauer, before proceeding through lamina II. Upon receiving these afferent fibers from the dorsal roots, new fibers form within lamina II and create the contralateral spinothalamic tract. This is made possible by the propriospinal neurons of the nucleus proprius, which are ventral to lamina II in laminae III and IV. These neurons link segments of the spinal cord and allow for intraspinal coordination. Propriospinal neurons will be discussed in more detail later in this section.

2.5.4 The Lateral and Ventral Horns

The lateral horn is a small projection of gray matter located between the dorsal and ventral horns in lamina VII. It is only present in C7 or T1 through L2 or L3 and contains cell bodies of preganglionic sympathetic neurons. The axons of these nerves travel through the ventral spinal roots and white rami communicants to the sympathetic trunk. A similar group of cells can sometimes be seen in the lower sacral region, but they do not form a projection like they do in the thoracic region. This group acts as the source of the sacral parasympathetic preganglionic fibers.

The ventral horn consists mainly of the lamina IX neurons, which continue through the ventral roots to innervate the extrafusal fibers of striated muscle. The neurons in lamina IX can be divided into two longitudinal columns: medial and lateral. The medial neurons will innervate the muscles of the axial skeleton, while the lateral neurons will innervate the limb muscles. In the cervical enlargement, it is the lateral neurons that innervate the muscles of the upper limb, whereas in the lumbar enlargement these lateral neurons innervate the muscles of the lower limb. The proximal muscles are innervated by groups of motor cells that are located more rostrally in the enlargement so that, for example, neurons from spinal nerves C8 and T1 innervate the hand, while neurons from C5 and C6 innervate the shoulder.

2.5.5 The Spinal White Matter

The white matter of the spinal cord surrounds the gray matter. It consists mostly of longitudinal nerve fibers. Fibers that travel to or from the same place can be grouped into tracts (sometimes referred to as fasciculi). These tracts can then be classified

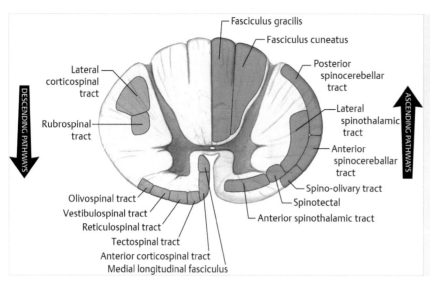

Fig. 2.13 Drawing of the ascending and descending tracts in the spinal cord. (Illustration by Christa Wellman, Biomedical Visualization faculty at University of Illinois Chicago).

as ascending, descending, or propriospinal. The ascending tracts are normally made up of afferent fibers that enter the spinal cord through the dorsal roots, while the descending tracts are fibers that are coming down the cord originating from the cerebral cortex or brainstem and control the activity of the spinal nerves. Propriospinal tracts are located completely within the spinal cord and can ascend, descend, or even run transversely. They help coordinate intersegmental and intrasegmental communication.

The white matter is typically described as three large, bilateral paired regions: dorsal, lateral, and ventral funiculi. Each one contains a certain number of tracts (▶ Fig. 2.13). The dorsal funiculus is located between the dorsal horn and the posterior median septum. The lateral is between the dorsal root entry and the ventral root exit. The ventral (sometimes referred to as anterior) funiculus is found between the anterior median fissure and the emergence of the ventral roots.

2.5.6 The Ascending White Matter Tracts

- **The dorsal columns**: The dorsal funiculus contains two large ascending tracts, the fasciculus gracilis and the fasciculus cuneatus, separated by the posterior intermediate septum (▶ Fig. 2.13). These two tracts are commonly referred to as the dorsal columns. Both tracts contain numerous myelinated fibers that carry proprioceptive, exteroceptive, and vibratory sensations further up the CNS. Nerves feeding into these tracts enter the spinal cord through the dorsal roots and ascend to the dorsal column nuclei in the medulla oblongata. The fasciculus gracilis originates at the caudal end of the cord and carries ascending nerves that enter the cord through the ipsilateral dorsal roots. Most of its fibers are from the deep and cutaneous receptors in the lower limb. As more fibers enter the cord and join the tract, it is shifted more medially into the spinal cord. The fasciculus cuneatus begins in the midthoracic portion of the cord and lies lateral to the gracilis. Most of its nerves are from the deep and cutaneous receptors of the upper limbs. The majority of the nerves terminate in the medulla oblongata and synapse with neurons in the

dorsal column nuclei. These nerves then decussate to form the medial lemniscus and traverse rostrally through the brainstem to reach the thalamus.

- **The spinocerebellar tract**: This tract is located in the periphery of the lateral aspect of the white matter. It can be divided into dorsal (posterior) and ventral (anterior) tracts (▶ Fig. 2.13). The dorsal spinocerebellar tract begins in the lumbar region and increases in size as it ascends the spinal cord. The dorsal tract draws axons from the ipsilateral neurons in lamina VII. It mainly carries information from the upper limbs. The ventral tract is located just anterior to the dorsal tract and receives axons from neurons in laminae V, VI, and VII, and carries information from the lower limbs. Both the dorsal and ventral tracts propagate proprioceptive and cutaneous information into the cerebellum that ultimately helps with coordination and movement.

- **The spinothalamic tract**: The spinothalamic tract primarily contains second order neurons that carry information mostly regarding pain and temperature, but also coarse touch, and pressure from the skin to the thalamus. It receives axons from neurons in multiple laminae originating in the contralateral gray matter. The axons from these neurons immediately cross through the anterior white commissure to reach the tract which is located ventrolateral to the ventral horn on the opposite side of the spinal cord (▶ Fig. 2.13). This tract is less well defined than others, as it is intermingled with the ascending spinoreticular and descending reticulospinal tracts. There is some debate about whether to divide this tract into lateral and ventral spinothalamic tracts, but research seems to indicate that they are structurally and functionally the same. Still, some evidence suggests that the lateral tract, located in the lateral funiculus medial to the ventral (anterior) spinocerebellar tract, transmits pain and temperature, while the ventral tract, located in the ventral funiculus medial to the exit point of the ventral spinal roots and dorsal to the vestibulospinal tract, transmits coarse touch and pressure.[15] Unlike many other tracts, the spinothalamic fibers decussate at the level of the spinal cord close to where the processes enter the cord and ascend contralaterally to reach the brainstem.

- **The spinoreticular tract**: The spinoreticular tract can be found intermingled with the spinothalamic tract in the ventrolateral quadrant of the spinal cord with neurons originating from laminae V, VII, and VIII. (▶ Fig. 2.13). Fibers in the lumbar enlargement and some of the fibers in the cervical enlargement cross the midline. This tract is responsible for carrying sensory inputs from the skin and deep tissues to the brain.
- **The spinomesencephalic pathway**: The spinomesencephalic pathway is made up of a series of ascending tracts that connect the spinal cord to various parts of the midbrain. It is located in the ventrolateral quadrant of the cord, along with neurons in the spinothalamic and spinoreticular tracts (▶ Fig. 2.13). Most of the fibers in this pathway receive inputs from the lumbosacral and cervical enlargements, mainly from neurons in lamina I and laminae IV to VIII (although mostly concentrated in lamina V). The majority of fibers are contralateral, but there are many ipsilateral groups in the upper cervical region. The nerves in this pathway carry various inputs from large portions of body surface areas.

2.5.7 The Descending White Matter Tracts

The descending tracts originate from the cerebral cortex or from the brainstem. They carry the signals that control movement, muscle tone, and posture, as well as signals that modulate the spinal reflexes. Certain tracts also have control over the spinal autonomic nerves.

- **The corticospinal tract**: This tract begins in the cerebral cortex and enters the spinal cord through the medulla oblongata. Upon reaching the spinomedullary junction, 75 to 90% of the corticospinal nerves cross the median plane in the region known as the motor decussation (also called the decussation of the pyramids) and continue inferiorly as the lateral corticospinal tract (▶ Fig. 2.13). The remaining 10 to 25% of the nerves do not cross the median and continue as the ventral (anterior) corticospinal tract. The lateral tract descends within the lateral funiculus, in the area ventrolateral to the dorsal horn and medial to the dorsal spinocerebellar tract, before terminating in the region of the fourth sacral cord segment (the spinal cord itself ends at the level of the L2 vertebra). The nerves that exit the cord into the upper limbs are located more laterally, and the tract becomes smaller and more superficial as it descends the spinal cord below the cervical region. The ventral (anterior) corticospinal tract descends within the ventral funiculus close to the ventral median fissure. The small amount of tissue that separates the tract from the fissure is called the sulcomarginal fasciculus. This tract also decreases in size as it descends the spinal cord before disappearing in the midthoracic region. These nerves affect the activity of various motor neurons throughout the body.
- **The rubrospinal tract**: The rubrospinal tract starts in the midbrain, although its exact origin and functions are yet to be well described in humans. It crosses within the ventral tegmental decussation and descends within the lateral funiculus, intermingled with fibers from the lateral corticospinal tract, although a cluster of the tract appears to be concentrated ventrally to the corticospinal tract as well (▶ Fig. 2.13). The rubrospinal tract is short and most likely ends within the upper three cervical segments. These neurons are thought to have similar roles as those of the corticospinal tracts.
- **The tectospinal tract**: This tract also originates from the midbrain. It crosses over the midline in the dorsal tegmental decussation and descends in the medial part of the ventral funiculus (▶ Fig. 2.13). Like the rubrospinal tract, the tectospinal tract is quite short and terminates in the upper portion of the cervical region. It provides efferent signals to the muscles of the neck, innervating the contralateral side and inhibiting the ipsilateral side.
- **Vestibulospinal tracts**: These tracts are formed in the vestibular nuclear complex, which is located in the lateral part of the floor of the fourth ventricle. It gives rise to two distinct tracts: the lateral and medial vestibulospinal tracts. Both tracts are responsible for stimulating the antigravity muscles, which are the epaxial muscles of the vertebral column and the extensor muscles of the lower limbs. The lateral vestibulospinal tract arises from the lateral aspect of the vestibular nucleus and descends on the ipsilateral side, along the edge of the ventrolateral spinal white matter (▶ Fig. 2.13). As the tract descends, it projects into and ends in the medial parts of laminae VII and VIII. All the nerve fibers end ipsilaterally. The medial vestibulospinal tract arises in the medial aspect of the vestibular nucleus as well as from the inferior and lateral nuclei. It descends along the medial longitudinal fasciculus near the midline of the sulcomarginal fasciculus (▶ Fig. 2.13). Unlike the lateral tract, the medial tract has both crossed and uncrossed fibers. It ends in the midthoracic region.
- **The reticulospinal tract**: This tract originates in the reticular formation of the brainstem and descends into the spinal cord in the ventral funiculus (▶ Fig. 2.13). Its exact location and course through the spinal cord are poorly described in humans, but it is believed to activate the antigravity muscles. Unlike the vestibulospinal tract, it is thought that the reticulospinal tract also contains some inhibitory fibers.

2.5.8 The Propriospinal White Matter Pathways

The propriospinal pathways are a series of ascending and descending fibers that are intrinsic to the spinal cord. They communicate with neurons in the same segment, as well as in more distant segments, and allow for neuronal integration and coordination. Most of the nerves that make up the spinal cord are propriospinal nerves. They reside primarily in laminae V to VIII around the margins of the gray matter. They are characterized by the length of their axons as either long, intermediate, or short neurons. The long nerves can be found throughout the spinal cord, mostly in the ventral and lateral funiculi, but their cell bodies are generally in lamina VIII. Most of the long neurons are bilateral in the cervical region and descend. In the lumbar region, they generally ascend contralaterally. The intermediate nerves are located in the central and medial parts of lamina VII and are mostly ipsilateral. The short neurons are normally found in the lateral funiculus, specifically in the lateral parts of laminae V to VIII, and are also ipsilateral.

The propriospinal nerves are distributed in specific regions of the spinal gray matter. In the cervical and lumbar enlargements, the propriospinal fibers in the dorsolateral funiculus project their axons onto neurons in the dorsal and lateral parts of the intermediate zone, as well as to the spinal motor neurons that innervate the muscles of the proximal limbs. Other propriospinal nerves, such as those in the ventral funiculus, communicate with the long propriospinal nerves and with the motor nerves of the axial and girdle muscles.

2.5.9 The Track of Lissauer

The track of Lissauer, sometimes referred to as the dorsolateral tract, is located between the dorsal horn and the spinal cord and surrounds the entering dorsal root fibers (▶ Fig. 2.12). It is found throughout the spinal cord but is best seen in the upper cervical region. Most of this tract is made of the branches of axons from the lateral bundles of the dorsal roots, which divide and become either ascending or descending branches upon entering the spinal cord. From there, they travel in the respective direction for one or two spinal segments before branching off collaterals to the nearby dorsal horns. The tract also contains some propriospinal fibers, mostly short, which re-enter the dorsal horns.

2.6 The Meninges

The three meninges form a protective covering over the brain and continue onto the spinal cord.[16] The three layers from most external to most internal are the dura mater, the arachnoid mater, and the pia mater (▶ Fig. 2.14).

2.6.1 The Dura Mater

The dura mater is made of dense, irregular, fibrous connective tissue that forms a thick membrane. It is tightly adherent to the inner surface of the bone throughout the cranium and fuses with the endosteum at the base of the skull. The dura remains attached to the bone of the foramen magnum and to the posterior periosteum of three superior cervical vertebrae, as well as to the posterior longitudinal ligament by fibrous bands.[16] It then separates from the tissues that line the vertebral canal, creating the epidural space. The dura mater creates a tube that surrounds the spinal cord and continues down the length of the vertebral canal. This tube begins to narrow at about S2 before it invests in the thin spinal filum terminale and merges back with the periosteum and the end of the coccygeal vertebrae.

2.6.2 The Epidural Space

The epidural space is formed between the spinal dura and the tissues that line the vertebral canal. It is enclosed superiorly by the foramen magnum and inferiorly by the sacrococcygeal ligament. Inside the space, there are loose connective tissue, fat, the vertebral venous plexus, small arterial branches, and fine bands of fibrous tissue that connect the theca to the tissue lining the vertebral canal. These fibrous bands are called the meningovertebral ligaments and they can be appreciated best anteriorly and laterally. The venous plexus is a series of longitudinally arranged chains of vessels that are interconnected by venous rings. The anterior-most vessels receive the basivertebral veins before they drain into the vertebral vein.[17]

The epidural space is not of uniform size throughout its length; rather, it follows a segmental pattern that repeats itself several times. In the lumbar region of the spine, the dura is attached to the walls of the vertebral canal anteriorly by connective tissue, which allows for movement of the dural sac during body motion or venous filling. Adipose tissue located posteriorly between the ligamentum flavum and the dura acts as a cushion during flexion or extension.

The epidural space has many clinical correlations. Due to of its hollow nature, it can be the site of tumors and hematomas. The dense connective tissue can be host to various infectious

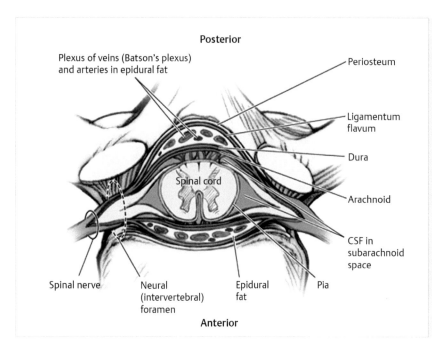

Fig. 2.14 Cross section of the meninges surrounding the spinal cord. (Reproduced with permission from Blumenfeld, Fig. 8.2d.[13])

Posterior

Plexus of veins (Batson's plexus) and arteries in epidural fat

Periosteum

Ligamentum flavum

Dura

Spinal cord

Arachnoid

CSF in subarachnoid space

Spinal nerve

Neural (intervertebral) foramen

Epidural fat

Pia

Anterior

agents. Drugs and other agents such as contrast media can be injected into the epidural space in the sacral level and spread anteriorly to the base of the skull.

2.6.3 The Subdural Space

The subdural space is a potential (also called artificial) space that is only open when the arachnoid mater and dura mater, which are normally closely apposed, are separated. This can occur with accidental subdural catheterization during epidural injections, as a result of hemorrhage or trauma, or from the absence of CSF.[18] The subdural space is not connected with the subarachnoid space. It does, however, continue along the cranial and spinal nerves for a short distance after they emerge from the spinal cord.

2.6.4 The Arachnoid Mater

The arachnoid mater surrounds the entirety of the spinal cord and is continuous with the arachnoid that surrounds the brain. Normally, it is closely attached to the dura mater. The arachnoid mater follows the spinal nerves and vessels out of the spinal cord and into the intervertebral foramina, forming a thin membrane around them. In doing so, the subarachnoid angle is made. At the angle, the arachnoid mater and the pia mater fuse, forming the leptomeninges which then fuse with the perineurium that surrounds the nerves and is continuous with the dura mater. The perineurium is important for sealing the subarachnoid space and preventing any particulate matter from passing into the nerves directly.

2.6.5 Cerebrospinal Fluid

CSF is a clear, colorless liquid that contains small amounts of protein and electrolytes. It is an ultrafiltrate of blood that is made and secreted in the choroid plexuses of the lateral, third, and fourth ventricles of the brain at a rate of about 600 to 700 mL per day. The total amount of CSF in adult humans can be between 140 and 270 mL, meaning that the entire volume of CSF is replaced about four times a day. It is believed that most of the CSF is reabsorbed in the superior sagittal sinus, but absorption here alone would not allow for the high rate of CSF turnover that is observed. It is therefore thought that there are several other sites of absorption that are yet to be described.[19] Some CSF is thought to be absorbed into the pial and subarachnoid vessels, via the ependymal ventricular and pial surfaces, and through extracranial lymphatics.[20]

CSF flow is described as pulsating and bidirectional in the ventricular system with a net forward flow toward the fourth ventricle.[21] The CSF flows into the subarachnoid space from the fourth ventricle, as the two are continuous with one another. Once the CSF enters the subarachnoid space of the spinal cord, its flow mechanics are poorly understood and described.

The CSF has several main functions. The first is to suspend the brain within the skull and provide it natural buoyancy. This allows the brain to maintain adequate density and blood flow to perform all its functions.[22] The CSF also provides protection to the brain and the spinal cord by acting as a shock absorber from certain kinds of mechanical injury.[22] Lastly, CSF controls homeostasis in the CNS by maintaining the concentrations of certain neuroendocrine factors, pH, and cleaning waste.[23]

2.6.6 The Pia Mater

The pia mater sits on top of and invests into the spinal cord, eventually passing into the ventral median fissure. It also creates a sheath around the anterior spinal artery.[16] The layer of collagen underneath the pia in the subpial space becomes continuous with the collagen core of the medial ligamentum denticulatum, also known as the denticulate ligament.

The denticulate ligament is a flat, fibrous sheet of tissue that lies on either side of the spinal cord, between the ventral and dorsal spinal roots. It is continuous with the subpial collagen medially. Its lateral border forms a series of triangular processes that attach at fixed intervals to the dura mater. The first of these processes is located behind the vertebral artery attached to the dura mater above the rim of the foramen magnum, behind the hypoglossal nerve with the accessory nerve on its posterior aspect. It separates from the artery when they reach the first cervical ventral root. The last denticulate ligament process is attached between the twelfth thoracic and first lumbar vertebrae, descending laterally from the conus medullaris. Past the conus, the pia mater continues as a thin membrane over the filum terminale.

2.6.7 The Intermediate Layer

The intermediate layer is a loosely defined protective coating over the spinal cord made up of the leptomeninges, which are the product of the fusion of the arachnoid and pia maters. It is a highly perforated, lace-like structure that is compacted in certain regions of the cord to make the dorsal, dorsolateral, and ventral ligaments of the spinal cord. It is believed to function as a wave dampener for rapid shifts of CSF.

The layer is most evident in the dorsal and ventral regions of the cord. Dorsally, the intermediate layer adheres to the arachnoid mater and forms ligaments that attach the cord to the arachnoid. Dorsolaterally, the ligaments run from the dorsal roots to the parietal arachnoid. As the intermediate layer continues down the dorsal aspect of the dorsal roots, it becomes more fenestrated and eventually disappears. There is a similar layout on the ventral side, but the intermediate layer is even less obvious.

2.7 The Vasculature of the Spinal Cord

The spinal cord and spinal roots and nerves are supplied with oxygenated blood by longitudinal and segmental vessels. Due to the importance and high metabolic activity of the CNS, there are extensive networks of collateral supplies and anastomoses throughout the spinal cord.

2.7.1 The Longitudinal Arteries

One anterior and two posterior longitudinal arteries run along the length of the spinal cord (▶ Fig. 2.15). At times, each of the arteries can form a doublet in order to pass on either side of a

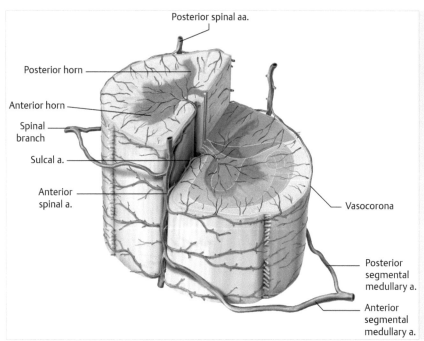

Posterior spinal aa.

Posterior horn

Anterior horn

Spinal branch

Sulcal a.

Anterior spinal a.

Vasocorona

Posterior segmental medullary a.

Anterior segmental medullary a.

Fig. 2.15 Arteries that surround and supply the spinal cord. (Reproduced with permission from Schuenke M, Schulte E, Schumacher U. THIEME Atlas of Anatomy. Head, Neck and Neuroanatomy. Illustrations by Voll M and Wesker K. Third Edition. © Thieme 2020.)

rootlet emerging from the cord. All three of these arteries originate from the vertebral artery intracranially and terminate as a plexus formed around the conus medullaris.

The anterior spinal artery forms from the fused anterior spinal branches of the vertebral artery and descends the spinal cord within the ventral median fissure (▶ Fig. 2.16). As the artery proceeds inferiorly, it gives off central branches that pierce through the ventral median fissure and supply the ventral gray matter, as well as the base of the dorsal gray column. This includes the dorsal nucleus and the adjacent white matter.

The posterior spinal arteries can originate either from the ipsilateral vertebral artery or from its posterior inferior cerebellar branch and descend within their own posterolateral sulcus of the spinal cord (▶ Fig. 2.16). Along the way, each posterior artery contributes to two longitudinal anastomotic channels that form anterior and posterior to the dorsal roots. They are then reinforced by posterior medullary feeders and posterior radicular arteries, which are variable in number and tend to be quite small but are more evenly distributed than other collateral vessels. The anterior anastomose channel joins with the ramus of the descending branch of the artery of Adamkiewicz, completing the pathway.

All three longitudinal arteries vary in width along their path and can have complete interruptions. They form anastomotic loops in the conus medullaris.

2.7.2 The Segmental Spinal Arteries

The segmental spinal arteries branch off the spinal branches of the vertebral, deep cervical, intercostal, and lumbar arteries in a craniocaudal sequence. Generally, there is one large segmental branch every four to six vertebrae, with smaller branches present in between them. Each branch then enters the vertebral canal via the intervertebral foramina and forms an anastomose

with branches of the longitudinal arteries. As these vessels anastomose, they form a plexus in the pia mater on the surface of the spinal cord. The segmental arteries are also responsible for sending anterior and posterior radicular branches along the surface of the ventral and dorsal roots. The anterior radicular arteries are smaller and end within the ventral nerve root or in a pial plexus, as described above. The posterior radicular arteries are the primary arterial supply to the dorsal root ganglia. Branches of these arteries enter through both ganglionic poles and distribute themselves around the ganglionic cells and nerves.

2.7.3 The Segmental Radiculomedullary Feeder Arteries

Some of the larger radicular arteries, mostly the ones found in the lower cervical, lower thoracic, and the upper lumbar, can reach the ventral median fissure, at which point they divide into ascending and descending branches, making what are called the anterior radiculomedullary feeder arteries. These arteries form anastomoses with the anterior spinal arteries and form a single longitudinal vessel that runs along the ventral median fissure. This vessel is very irregular and uneven in diameter; in fact, the arteries can sometimes come together in such a way that it becomes a partly double longitudinal vessel.

The largest of the anterior medullary feeder arteries is called the greater anterior radiculomedullary artery of Adamkiewicz, or more simply, the artery of Adamkiewicz.[24] It comes off the spinal branch of either one of the lower posterior intercostal arteries (between T9 and T11), the subcostal artery (T12), or, less frequently, the upper lumbar arteries (L1 or L2). The artery normally arises on the left side of the spinal column. Upon reaching the spinal cord, the artery splits into branches: one proceeds to the anterior longitudinal spinal artery inferiorly and another branch anastomoses with the ramus of the posterior spinal artery anteriorly to the dorsal roots. The artery of

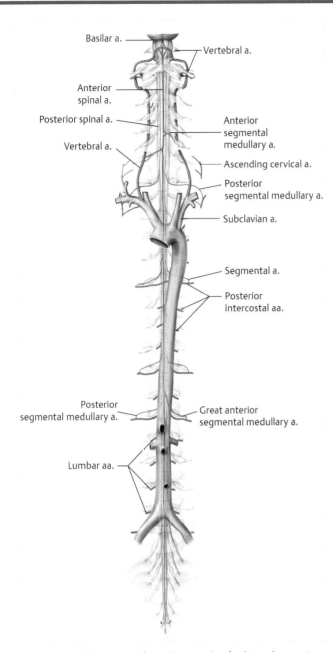

Fig. 2.16 Radicular arteries from the aorta that feed into the anterior and posterior spinal arteries along the length of spinal cord. Note in particular the great anterior segmental artery, also known as the artery of Adamkiewicz. (Reproduced with permission from Schuenke M, Schulte E, Schumacher U. THIEME Atlas of Anatomy. Head, Neck and Neuroanatomy. Illustrations by Voll M and Wesker K. Third Edition. © Thieme 2020.)

Adamkiewicz is sometimes the main source of oxygenated blood for the lower two-thirds of the spinal cord.

2.7.4 The Intramedullary and Small Radial Arteries

The intramedullary arteries are central branches of the anterior spinal artery that infiltrate the cord and supply two-thirds of its cross-sectional area. The remaining gray and white columns, along with the peripheral parts of the lateral and ventral white columns, receive most of their blood from small radial vessels that branch off the posterior spinal arteries, as well as from the pial plexus. Their numbers can vary between sections of the spinal cord, as well as between individuals.

2.7.5 Proper Oxygenation and Watershed Areas of the Spinal Cord

The spinal cord requires both transverse and longitudinal blood supply to survive and function properly. Like all other nervous tissue, the spinal cord is particularly sensitive to oxygen deprivation because of its high metabolic demand.[25]

Damages to the anterior longitudinal artery can lead to a loss of function of the anterior two-thirds of the cord, as this artery and the intermedullary arteries are functional end arteries. This will normally manifest as motor deficits, whereas loss of the posterior longitudinal arteries is more likely to manifest as sensory loss.[25]

The longitudinal arteries do not supply the whole length of the spinal cord, which is why the segmental medullary feeders are necessary for proper blood delivery. The artery of Adamkiewicz is especially important, as it is the major supplier of oxygenated blood to the inferior aspects of the spinal cord. Damage to or occlusion of this artery can lead to paraplegia and is the suspected cause of postaortic bypass surgery paraplegia.[26]

A watershed zone exists in the midthoracic cord and the medullary feeder arteries that branch off there; this area is particularly susceptible to ischemia in hypotension. T4–T9 is described as the "critical zone" of vasculature for the spinal cord, as issues with circulation here are likely to result in paraplegia.

2.7.6 Venous Drainage of the Spinal Cord

A series of intramedullary veins form a circumferential plexus of surface veins known as the coronal plexus, sometimes called the venous plexus of the pia mater. This plexus is composed of six tortuous longitudinal channels: the anterior and posterior spinal veins, as well as four smaller veins that run along either side of the ventral and dorsal nerve roots (▶ Fig. 2.17). The anterior vein drains most of the central gray matter and sulcal and small pial veins (also a part of the coronal plexus). It is the only vein in the plexus that is present throughout the length of the spinal cord, and peaks in caliber in the lumbosacral region. The posterior vein has a variable tract, being plexiform in some regions of the spinal cord and a channel in others.

All the vessels of the coronal plexus converge together and drain superiorly into the cerebellar veins, as well as the cranial sinuses (▶ Fig. 2.18). Some drainage also occurs segmentally into the medullary veins. These veins then connect with the intervertebral veins, through which the blood goes into the external vertebral venous plexus, before finally reaching the caval and azygous systems.

The Batson's venous plexus is made up of valveless veins that connect the deep pelvic and thoracic veins to the vertebral venous plexuses.[27] The lack of valves in these veins is believed to allow for the spread of cancer metastasis, and the Batson's plexus is commonly used to explain the high rate of pelvic cancers (rectal, prostate) metastasizing to the vertebral column and brain.[28] Other pathologies, such as infectious pathogens, also likely use this plexus to spread from the pelvic region to the vertebrae.

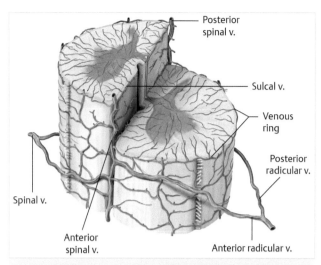

Fig. 2.17 Veins that surround and drain the spinal cord. (Reproduced with permission from Schuenke M, Schulte E, Schumacher U. THIEME Atlas of Anatomy. Head, Neck and Neuroanatomy. Illustrations by Voll M and Wesker K. Third Edition. © Thieme 2020.)

2.7.7 The Anterior and Posterior Radiculomedullary Veins

The anterior and posterior radiculomedullary veins act as segmental veins that run along some of the ventral and dorsal roots. These veins are the largest in the cervical and lumbar parts of the spinal cord, but they are not located in the same areas as the medullary feeders. Although they are in proximity to the roots, they only drain the spinal cord. The roots are drained by very small anterior and posterior radicular veins that are in most segments of the cord along the entry and exits of the rootlets. They eventually drain into the intervertebral veins.

2.8 Anatomy of the Spinal Nerves

The dorsal and ventral root filaments are attached immediately lateral to the cord via root filaments (▶ Fig. 2.19). Each dorsal nerve root begins from either within or near the intervertebral foramen as a swelling, which forms the dorsal root ganglion. The ganglion then merges with the corresponding ventral root and forms a spinal nerve. The spinal nerves are quite short, as they are the intermediate chute that forms after the union of the roots, but before the branching of the nerve into dorsal and ventral rami. There are a total of 31 pairs of spinal nerves: 8 cervical (C), 12 thoracic (T), 5 lumbar (L), 5 sacral (S), and 1 coccygeal (Co). Each spinal nerve is labeled by the vertebra immediately above it: for example, the L2 nerve is found between the L1 and L2 vertebrae. The exceptions to this rule are the cervical spinal nerves, which are named by the vertebra immediately below: for example, the C1 spinal nerve comes out from between the skull base and the C1 vertebra. However, the C8 spinal nerve exits between vertebrae C7 and T1. The nerve directly below T1 is now named the T1 spinal nerve and this pattern continues down through the rest of the spinal cord and vertebrae.

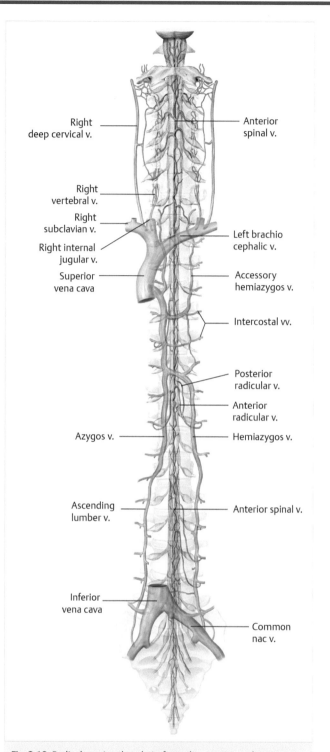

Fig. 2.18 Radicular veins that drain from the anterior and posterior spinal veins along the length of the spinal cord. (Reproduced with permission from Schuenke M, Schulte E, Schumacher U. THIEME Atlas of Anatomy. Head, Neck and Neuroanatomy. Illustrations by Voll M and Wesker K. Third Edition. © Thieme 2020.)

2.8.1 Basic Anatomy of the Spinal Nerves

Although the spinal nerves are named based on the level of the spine they emerge from, anatomically, they are quite similar. The dorsal rami, also known as the epaxial rami, pass posteriorly and

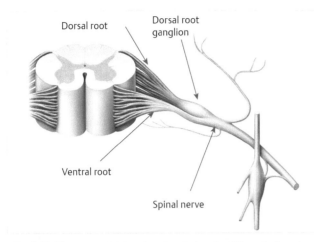

Fig. 2.19 The segmental dorsal and ventral roots of the spinal cord that meet to form the segmental spinal nerve. (Reproduced with permission from Schuenke M, Schulte E, Schumacher U. THIEME Atlas of Anatomy. Head, Neck and Neuroanatomy. Illustrations by Voll M and Wesker K. Third Edition. © Thieme 2020.)

laterally to the articular process of the vertebrae and divide into medial and lateral branches. These branches normally penetrate and innervate the deep muscles of the back, as well as the skin on the posterior of the body. The ventral rami, also known as the hypaxial rami, connect to the corresponding sympathetic ganglion via the white rami (T1–L2) and gray rami (superior cervical ganglion to S5). They innervate the prevertebral muscles and continue along their track around the body wall, where they innervate the lateral muscles, the anterior muscles, and the muscles of the upper and lower limbs.

The segment of spinal cord from which a pair of dorsal and ventral roots emerges is called a myelomere. As mentioned above, the spinal cord does not extend throughout the vertebral column, terminating in the superior portion of the lumbar region. This means that the lower myelomeres are not paired with their corresponding numbered vertebrae. Instead, the nerves that make up the cauda equina leave the appropriate myelomere and descend to exit from the vertebral column at the intended vertebral level: for example, the S1 myelomere emerges adjacent to the T12 vertebra but descends to exit through the S1 foramina in the sacrum.[11]

2.8.2 The Spinal Roots

Ventral roots contain axons from the ventral and intermediate horns of the spinal gray matter. They emerge from the spinal cord as a series of smaller roots, normally in a configuration with two to three irregular rows about 3 mm in width. The dorsal roots, on the other hand, emerge from the spinal cord as centripetal processes made up of neurons within the spinal ganglia. These processes begin as medial and lateral fascicles which come together to form rootlets. The rootlets extend into the spinal cord along the posterolateral sulcus and are often connected to each other and the cord via oblique filaments, especially in the cervical and lumbosacral parts of the cord.

Each part of the spinal cord has a unique appearance, orientation, size, and direction to its roots. The first four cervical roots are small, while the bottom four tend to be larger. The dorsal roots are, on average, three times thicker than the ventral roots (the first cervical root is the exception to this rule, in that its dorsal root is smaller than its ventral root and is sometimes completely absent). The orientation and direction of the cervical roots can be described in two ways. Conventionally, the first and second roots are short and run almost horizontally after they emerge from the spinal cord, while the remaining roots (C3–C8) exit the cord and run inferiorly at an oblique angle. The slope and length of each root increase for each progressive vertebra, but the root is never longer than the height of its respective vertebra. The alternative view was presented by Kubik and Müntener: they described the roots as descending in C1–C4, horizontal at C5, and ascending in C6–C8.[29] This is based on their observation that the cervicothoracic cord grows more in length during development than the other parts.

The thoracic roots are all relatively small, except for T1. The dorsal and ventral roots are comparable in thickness, but the dorsal root is slightly thicker. Each root is progressively longer than the previous one. In the lower thoracic spine, the roots descend with the spinal cord for at least two vertebrae before they emerge from the vertebral canal. Kubik and Müntener described the thoracic roots as horizontal in T1 and T2, ascending in T3–T5, horizontal again in T6, and descending in T7–T12.[29]

The lower lumbar and the upper sacral spinal roots are the largest and are composed of the most rootlets, while the coccygeal roots are the smallest. As the spinal cord ends near the lower part of L1, each successive root gets longer, creating a collection of roots called the cauda equina. The nerves that compose the cauda equina will innervate the pelvic organs and the lower limbs with both sensory and motor innervation.

The spinal roots and nerves are protected by the meninges. The spinal dura mater and arachnoid mater surround them as they pass through the lateral zone of the vertebral canal and through the intervertebral foramina. Each dorsal and ventral root is covered with pia mater as it runs within the subarachnoid space. As each root passes through the dura, it takes its arachnoid lining with it until it reaches the ganglion.

2.8.3 The Spinal Ganglia

The spinal ganglia, also known as the dorsal root ganglia, are large groups of neurons that can be found on the dorsal spinal roots. These neurons are first-order neurons and are responsible for relaying sensory information to the cord.[25] The ganglia normally have an oval shape and are reddish in color. Their size is related to the size of their respective roots. Each ganglion is divided into two parts where the two fascicles of the dorsal root emerge to then enter the spinal cord. Most of the ganglia can be found in the intervertebral foramina, lateral to the perforation of the dura mater, but near the roots. There are a few exceptions to this rule: The first cervical ganglia, if present at all, is normally found on the vertebral arch of the atlas; the C2 ganglion is normally found behind the lateral atlantoaxial joint; the sacral ganglia are found inside of the vertebral canal; and the coccygeal ganglia are inside of the dura mater.

2.8.4 The Spinal Nerves Proper

The spinal nerves proper are located distal to the spinal ganglia, where the ventral and dorsal roots come together and form the spinal nerves. The spinal nerve is short-lived, however, and quickly divides again into the dorsal and ventral rami. Both rami receive nerve fibers from the dorsal and ventral roots, so these rami are now mixed fibers with both motor and sensory components. The division into the dorsal and ventral rami occurs within the intervertebral foramen throughout the spinal column, except in the sacral portion: There, the spinal nerves split into the rami within the sacral vertebral canal. From there, the dorsal and ventral rami leave separately through the posterior and anterior sacral foraminae, respectively. Most of the spinal nerves bifurcate; however, some nerves in the cervical and thoracic levels can trifurcate. When this happens, the third branch that is formed is called the ramus intermedius. The ventral rami give off recurrent meningeal branches that begin at or just distal to the origin of the ramus. These branches receive gray ramus communicans from their respective sympathetic ganglia. The thoracic and the first and second lumbar ventral rami also contribute to the white ramus communicans of their respective sympathetic ganglia. The S2–S4 nerves supply visceral branches called the pelvic splanchnic nerves (which are not connected to the sympathetic ganglia) and carry the parasympathetic outflow of the spinal cord to the pelvic plexuses.

The spinal nerve size is independent of the size of the related vertebrae and varies tremendously throughout the levels of the spine. Each of the first six cervical spinal nerves gets progressively larger than the last before the size plateaus and remains about the same for C6, C7, C8, and T1. These spinal nerves are larger because they carry the nerve fibers for the upper limb that will form the brachial plexus. After T1, the remaining thoracic spinal nerves decrease in size and are relatively small, as they contribute only to the muscles and skin of the thoracic body wall. The lumbar spinal nerves are once again large and get progressively larger when moving inferiorly. This is due to the large nerve outflow to the lower limb and is continued down into the sacral spinal nerves. The spinal nerve for S1 is the largest spinal nerve in the body. After S1, the rest of the sacral nerves decrease in size. Finally, the coccygeal spinal nerve is the smallest. Just as the size of the nerve is not related to the size of the vertebra, it is also not related to the size of the intervertebral foramen. The best example of this can be seen in the fifth lumbar nerve: L5 has the largest spinal nerve of all the lumbar nerves, but the smallest foramen of the lumbar portion of the spine. This is the reason why the L5 nerve is commonly compressed and results in sciatic pain.

Each of the spinal nerves contains somatic efferent and somatic and visceral afferent nerve fibers. In addition, some of the nerves also contain preganglionic autonomic nerves. The somatic efferent fibers innervate the skeletal muscles using the axons of alpha, beta, and gamma neurons of the ventral gray column. The afferent fibers carry information of the skin, subcutaneous tissues, muscles, tendons, fascia, and joints to the CNS via the peripheral processes of unipolar neurons in the dorsal root ganglia.

The visceral components include the efferent sympathetic fibers, efferent visceral parasympathetic fibers, and visceral afferent fibers. The preganglionic efferent sympathetic fibers are the axons of neurons located in the spinal intermediolateral gray column of the T1–T12 thoracic spinal cord and L1–L2 (and sometimes L3) spinal cord. The sympathetic preganglionic fibers leave their respective spinal nerves and merge

with the sympathetic trunk at their respective white rami communicans. They then synapse with postganglionic neurons in smooth muscle, myocardium, the intestinal organs, and exocrine glands. The preganglionic efferent visceral parasympathetic fibers are the axons of neurons located in the spinal lateral gray column within the S2–S4 region of the spinal cord. These fibers exit the ventral rami of S2–S4 as the pelvic splanchnic nerves and synapse with postganglionic neurons in the pelvic ganglia, which innervate the organs, smooth muscle, and glands in the pelvic viscera. The visceral afferent fibers have their cell bodies within the dorsal root ganglia. Their peripheral processes that follow the sympathetic efferents pass through the white rami and through at least one sympathetic ganglion before terminating in the walls of the viscera. The afferents following the parasympathetic efferents join the spinal nerves directly and return to the dorsal roots of their respective spinal nerves. All of this occurs without a synapse.

The unipolar neurons in the dorsal root ganglion have central processes that enter the spinal cord through the dorsal roots and synapse on the somatic and sympathetic efferent neurons via specialized interneurons. Through this mechanism, the reflex pathways are completed. Alternatively, some unipolar neurons can also synapse with neurons in the spinal or brainstem gray matter to trigger other ascending reflex pathways.

2.8.5 Meningeal Nerves

The meningeal branches of the spinal nerves are known by many names including the recurrent meningeal nerves, the sinuvertebral nerves, and the recurrent nerves of Luschka. These nerves contain mixed sensory and sympathetic nerves: the sensory fibers innervate the intraspinal ligaments, vertebral periosteum, anulus fibrosus, and the zygapophysial joint capsules.[23] Vascular branches can also be found following the arteries and veins of the vertebral canal, as well as the vessels of the vertebral bodies. The meningeal nerves are made up of numerous fine filaments and can sometimes have one to four larger trunks as well. Their connections and orientations vary throughout the levels of the spinal cord.

The cervical meningeal nerves are mostly autonomic roots that come from the gray rami. The C1–C3 meningeal nerves ascend through the foramen magnum and proceed into the posterior cranial fossa, where they innervate the dura mater over the clivus and the median atlantoaxial joint and associated ligaments which they pass through. In the thoracic and lumbar regions of the spine, each meningeal nerve originates from a somatic root as well as from an autonomic root from the gray ramus communicans.

Regardless of their spinal level, each meningeal nerve runs a recurrent course (hence their pseudonyms) through the intervertebral foramen. They pass the spinal nerve ventrally and enter the vertebral canal before dividing into ascending, descending, and transverse branches. Each of these branches then communicates with their respective branches from the other vertebrae, creating a nervous arcade along the floor of the vertebral canal. On the ventral side of the dural sac and nerve root sleeve, the meningeal nerves of this arcade form a nerve plexus before they attenuate laterally and completely disappear before they reach the posterior paramedian dura.

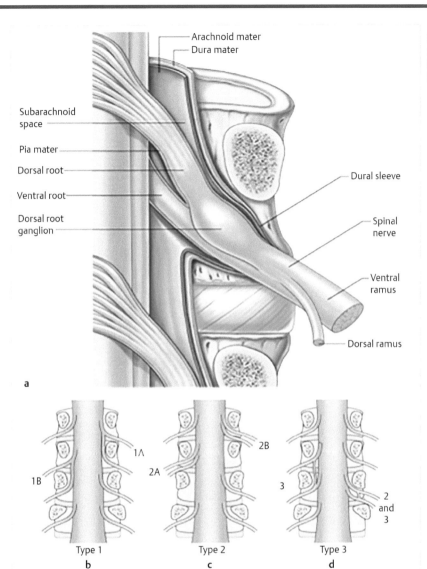

Arachnoid mater
Dura mater
Subarachnoid space
Pia mater
Dorsal root
Ventral root
Dorsal root ganglion
Dural sleeve
Spinal nerve
Ventral ramus
Dorsal ramus

a

1A
1B
2A
2B
3
2 and 3

Type 1
b

Type 2
c

Type 3
d

Fig. 2.20 Anomalies in the branching of spinal nerves. (Reproduced with permission from Standring et al.[1], Fig 45.6; based on Neirde and MacNab.[30])

Variations of the Spinal Roots and Nerves

It can be very difficult to describe the courses that the spinal roots and nerves take in relation to the thecal sac or the vertebral and radicular canals because they tend to vary significantly from vertebrae to vertebrae: one intervertebral foramen can contain a duplicated sheath with the nerve and roots while the foramen directly inferior will contain none of these. The communications between roots within the vertebral canal also do not follow a standard or predictable pattern. Some of the more common patterns of spinal root and nerve distributions described by Neidre and MacNab[30] can be seen in ▶ Fig. 2.20.

Spinal Nerve Rami

The ventral rami are generally larger than the dorsal rami. They supply the limbs and the anterolateral aspects of the trunk. In the thoracic region of the spine, the ventral rami run independently and have a segmental distribution. In the cervical, lumbar, and sacral regions, the ventral rami connect to form a nerve plexus, though the dorsal rami in these areas do not contribute to it.

The dorsal rami are smaller than the ventral rami and project posteriorly. Most of the rami divide into medial and lateral branches, which then innervate the muscles and skin of the posterior neck and trunk. C1, S4, S5, and the coccygeal dorsal rami are exceptions to this rule, as they do not divide into branches.

2.9 Conclusion

The spinal cord is one of the two organs that make up the central nervous system. It begins to form around day 20 of gestation, when the neural plates fold and create neural folds, which eventually becomes the neural tube. From there, the neuroblasts continue to differentiate into various components and support cells that can be found in the central nervous system. In adults, the spinal cord is well protected, first by three layers of meninges the dura mater, the arachnoid mater, and the pia mater, and then by the vertebrae and the various ligaments. The spinal cord itself is made up of neuronal cell bodies, the gray matter, as well as axons that travel up-and-down the cord, the white matter. These tracks allow the brain to communicate with the rest of the body via the ventral roots and the body to communicate with the brain via the dorsal roots. The spinal cord has distinct histological appearances at its various levels before terminating as a loosely organized bundle of nerve tracts, termed the cauda equina. Blood supply is plentiful, but there are several watershed areas that can be compromised during certain physiological states. Tumors can arise in various places throughout the spinal cord and become symptomatic once they begin to impede some of the essential functions that the cord serves.

Acknowledgments

The authors would like to express their thanks to Alexandra Lamacki, University of Illinois College of Medicine (class of 2021), for her editorial comments and for proofreading the chapter, and Christa Wellman, Clinical Assistant Professor in the UIC Department of Biomedical Visualization for the illustration used in ▶ Fig. 2.13.

References

[1] Standring S, ed. Gray's Anatomy: The Anatomical Basis of Clinical Practice. 41st ed. Elsevier Limited; 2016 [This reference was used for a majority of the anatomical descriptions in this chapter.]

[2] Urban JP, Roberts S. Degeneration of the intervertebral disc. Arthritis Res Ther. 2003; 5(3):120–130. doi: 10.1186/ar629 [Open Access]

[3] Keith A. Human Embryology and Morphology. New York: Longman, Greens & Co.; 1921

[4] Ma X, Goto N, Goto J, Ezure H, Nonaka N. Development of the human cuneatus medialis nucleus: a morphometric evaluation. Early Hum Dev. 2005; 81(4):369–377

[5] Ma X, Goto N, Goto J, Ezure H, Lu S. Development of the human gracilis nucleus: a morphometric evaluation. Okajimas Folia Anat Jpn. 2001; 78(4):115–122

[6] Eyre JA. Corticospinal tract development and its plasticity after perinatal injury. Neurosci Biobehav Rev. 2007; 31(8):1136–1149

[7] Altman J, Bayer SA. Development of the Human Spinal Cord. New York: Oxford University Press; 2001. Chapters 5–8

[8] Batarfi M, Valasek P, Krejci E, Huang R, Patel K. The development and origins of vertebrate meninges. Bio Comm. 2017; 62(2):73–81

[9] Sensenig EC. The early development of the meninges of the spinal cord in human embryos. Contrib Embryol. 1951; 228:147–157

[10] Maton A. Human Biology and Health. Englewood Cliffs, NJ: Prentice Hall; 1993:132–144

[11] Swenson RS. "Chapter 5 - Spinal Cord." Review of Clinical and Functional Neuroscience, Dartmouth Medical School. www.dartmouth.edu/~rswenson/NeuroSci/chapter_5.html. 2006

[12] Fletcher TF. Spinal Cord Anatomy Lab, College of Veterinary Medicine, University of Minnesota. 2006. http://vanat.cvm.umn.edu/neurLab2/SpCdGross.html

[13] Blumenfeld H. Neuroanatomy Through Clinical Cases. Sunderland, MA: Sinauer Associates, Inc.; 2010. Chapter 2

[14] Rexed B. The cytoarchitectonic organization of the spinal cord in the cat. J Comp Neurol. 1952; 96(3):414–495

[15] Foreman RD, Blair RW. Neural mechanisms of cardiac pain. In: Max MB, Lynn J, eds. Interactive Textbook on Clinical Symptom Research. NIDR: 2010. http://symptomresearch.nih.gov/chapter_25/index.htm

[16] O'Rahilly, Muller F, Carpenter S, Swenson R. Basic Human Anatomy: A Regional Study of Human Structure. Dartmouth Medical School Online Version: https://www.dartmouth.edu/~humananatomy/ Chapter 7, Section 41: The Back: Spinal Cord and Meninges. 2004

[17] Moore KL. Clinically Oriented Anatomy. Lippincott Williams & Wilkins; 2010:472–473

[18] Haines DE, Harkey HL, al-Mefty O. The "subdural" space: a new look at an outdated concept. Neurosurgery. 1993; 32(1):111–120

[19] Pollay M. The function and structure of the cerebrospinal fluid outflow system. Cerebrospinal Fluid Res. 2010; 7:9

[20] Zakharov A, Papaiconomou C, Koh L, Djenic J, Bozanovic-Sosic R, Johnston M. Integrating the roles of extracranial lymphatics and intracranial veins in cerebrospinal fluid absorption in sheep. Microvasc Res. 2004; 67(1):96–104

[21] Yamada S, Miyazaki M, Kanazawa H, et al. Visualization of cerebrospinal fluid movement with spin labeling at MR imaging: preliminary results in normal and pathophysiologic conditions. Radiology. 2008; 249(2):644–652

[22] Saladin KS. Anatomy & Physiology, The Unity of Form & Function. 6th ed. McGraw-Hill Education; 2012

[23] Ropper AH, Brown RH. Adams and Victor's Principles of Neurology. 8th ed. McGraw-Hill Education Medical; 2005

[24] Adamkiewicz AA. "Die Blutgefässe des menschlichen Rückenmarkes. II. Die Gefässe der Rückenmarksoberfläche". Sitzungsberichte der Kaiserlichen Akademie der Wissenschaften. Mathematisch-Naturwissenschaftliche Classe. 1882; 85:101–130

[25] Purves D, Augustine GJ, Fitzpatrick D, et al. Neuroscience. 6th ed. Sinauer Associates; 2018

[26] Yoshioka K, Niinuma H, Ohira A, et al. MR angiography and CT angiography of the artery of Adamkiewicz: noninvasive preoperative assessment of thoracoabdominal aortic aneurysm. Radiographics. 2003; 23(5):1215–1225

[27] Wiltse LL, Fonseca AS, Amster J, Dimartino P, Ravessoud FA. Relationship of the dura, Hofmann's ligaments, Batson's plexus, and a fibrovascular membrane lying on the posterior surface of the vertebral bodies and attaching to the deep layer of the posterior longitudinal ligament. An anatomical, radiologic, and clinical study. Spine. 1993; 18:1030–1043

[28] Geldof AA. Models for cancer skeletal metastasis: a reappraisal of Batson's plexus. Anticancer Res. 1997; 17 3A:1535–1539

[29] Kubik S, Müntener M. [Topography of the spinal nerve roots. II. The influence of the growth of the dural sac as well as of the curvatures and of the movements of the vertebral column upon the course of spinal nerve roots]. Acta Anat (Basel). 1969; 74(2):149–168

[30] Neidre A, MacNab I. Anomalies of the lumbosacral nerve roots. Review of 16 cases and classification. Spine. 1983; 8(3):294–299

Section I

Intramedullary Spinal Tumors

3 Intramedullary Spinal Tumors: Histopathology and Radiology

Hamidou Drammeh, Matthew K. Tobin, and Jonathan Hobbs

Summary

Intramedullary spinal cord tumors are rare neoplasms, accounting for 4 to 10% of all central nervous system tumors. Pain and neurological dysfunction such as sensory loss, reflex changes, weakness, and bladder and bowel dysfunction are common clinical manifestations. Magnetic resonance imaging (MRI) is the modality of choice to narrow the differential diagnosis, guide surgical resection, and it is used postoperatively as a screening tool for recurrence. MRI with contrast manifests as cord widened in all views and some degree of contrast enhancement. Spinal ependymoma is the most common type in adults and spinal astrocytoma is the most common type in children. Both tumors account for 70% of all intramedullary neoplasms. Spinal ependymoma is commonly located in the cervical cord and on sagittal imaging, the tumor is centrally located with adjacent syrinx extending above and below the tumor. Spinal astrocytoma arises from parenchyma and is usually eccentrically located, has ill-defined borders and patchy enhancement after intravenous contrast administration, which usually means more active tumor and may directly involve biopsy to confirm diagnosis. Spinal astrocytoma and ependymoma are tough to differentiate based on imaging features alone. Cord hemangioblastomas are the third most common type of intramedullary spinal tumor, usually dorsally located and are associated with von Hippel-Lindau syndrome. Ganglioglioma is more common in children and spans more than eight vertebral segments. Paragangliomas are neuroendocrine tumors that arise from sympathetic ganglion and are usually located in filum terminale and cauda equina. Spinal cord metastasis is usually well-circumscribed, solitary lesion with extensive edema out of proportion to tumor size.

Keywords: intramedullary, cord, tumors, ependymoma astrocytoma

3.1 Introduction

Intramedullary spinal cord tumors (IMSCTs) account for about 4 to 10% of all central nervous system (spinal cord) tumors and about 2 to 4% of all spinal cord tumors. The majority of intramedullary tumors are glial tumors; about 90% are ependymomas or astrocytomas. Ependymomas are the most common glial tumors in adults, whereas astrocytomas are the most common intramedullary tumors in children and adolescents. Ependymomas are rare in children outside the setting of neurofibromatosis type 2 (NF2).[1] Nonglial neoplasms, including hemangioblastomas (HBs), gangliogliomas, germinomas, primary CNS lymphomas, and melanomas, are less common. Although IMSCTs can be seen in any location throughout the length of the spinal cord, astrocytomas and ependymomas are more frequent in the thoracic and the cervical regions, respectively, while myxopapillary ependymomas are typically seen in the region of the conus medullaris, filum terminale, and cauda equina.[1,2]

Magnetic resonance imaging (MRI) is the preoperative study of choice for identification and evaluation of IMSCTs. MRI can narrow the differential diagnosis and guide surgical resection. The imaging protocol should include sagittal and axial T1-weighted and T2-weighted sequences, including contrast-enhanced T1-weighted sequences in the sagittal, axial, and coronal planes. Spinal cord neoplasms enhance after the administration of contrast material. Enhanced areas probably represent more active portions of the tumors and could aid in biopsy if resection is not feasible.

The most common presenting symptom in patients with IMSCTs is localized pain, which is either radicular or diffuse. The quality of the pain varies but often worsens in the evening. Other symptoms like sensory and motor disturbances, including bowel and bladder dysfunction, may occur.[2,3] In young patients, IMSCTs are especially difficult to diagnose because they usually remain asymptomatic for a prolonged period of time and often manifest as nonspecific complaints.[1,2,3]

In this chapter, we highlight the imaging features of intramedullary spinal neoplasms with the underlying pathologic findings. We start off with a description and illustrate the prevalence, and clinical, pathologic, and imaging characteristics of ependymoma and its variants, astrocytomas, HBs, gangliogliomas, germinomas, primary CNS lymphomas, amputation neuromas, and melanomas. We then review the use of MRI in the evaluation of spinal cord neoplasms.

3.2 Amputation Neuroma

Amputation or traumatic neuromas are benign nonneoplastic overgrowth that form when a nerve is sectioned or traumatized in some way, and continuity cannot be re-established. Neuromas are regarded as a reactive process that results in an abnormal regeneration of sprouting axons, Schwann cells, and scar tissue deposited by fibroblasts. Neuromas usually originate within the spinal cord and rarely in the CNS.[4,5] Although amputation neuromas are typically associated with a history of traumatic nerve injury, there are reports of amputation neuromas occurring without a subjective history of traumatic events.[4] Most neuromas are asymptomatic. Painful neuroma can develop if the nerves are chronically irritated or constantly stimulated. Patient typically presents with back pain, weakness, or numbness in the arms and legs, loss of bladder or bowel function, and paralysis.[6] Neuromas are well-circumscribed making gross total resection generally achievable, which allows for good results. Some complications reported in the literatures are spinal arachnoiditis and vertebral deformities, but the rate of such complications is not well known.[7] Care must be taken at the time of surgery to prevent formation of a second traumatic neuroma.

3.2.1 Histopathology

Amputation neuromas are composed of an irregular arrangement of nerve fascicles embedded in fibrous scar tissue.[8] Microscopic finding shows a haphazard arrangement of small nerve fascicles, containing axons, Schwann cells, and perineurial cells, surrounded by fibrosis.[8] Concentric condensations of fibrous tissue around individual fascicles, giving the appearance of multiple separate nerves, may be seen.[8] Immunohistochemistry (IHC) showed positivity for S-100 and vimentin, and neurofilament immunostaining highlighted the axons within tumor (▶ Fig. 3.1).[4]

3.2.2 Imaging Characteristic

On MRI, amputation neuromas are intermediate signal on T1-weighted images and intermediate to high signal on T2-weighted imaging, occasionally with a heterogeneous ring (fascicular) pattern (▶ Fig. 3.2).[9]

3.3 Ependymoma

Ependymoma is the most common intramedullary spinal neoplasm in adults (60% of all glial spinal cord neoplasm) with a peak incidence in the fourth or fifth decades.[1] They are the second most common primary spinal cord tumor in the pediatric population.[1] These tumors arise from the ependymal cells lining the spinal cord central canal or from the wall of the ventricle.[1,10] WHO currently classifies ependymomas into three grades: grade I myxopapillary ependymomas and subependymomas, grade II includes classic ependymomas, and grade III includes anaplastic ependymomas.[3,11]

Intramedullary ependymomas are most commonly found in the cervical (44%) or cervicothoracic (23%) locations (cellular ependymomas), with the exception of the myxopapillary subtype, which are located in the conus medullaris or filum terminale and found predominately in young men.[1,4] These tumors are slow growing and tend to compress adjacent spinal cord tissue rather than infiltrate it, resulting in a cleavage plane, which facilitates gross total resection, the treatment of choice, substantially reducing recurrence when achieved.[1,4]

3.3.1 Histopathology

Most ependymomas displace adjacent neural tissue rather than infiltrate. Since ependymomas arise from ependymal cells of the central canal within the spinal cord, symmetric cord expansion is usually seen. There are six histologic ependymoma subtypes: cellular (the most common intramedullary type), papillary, clear cell, tanycytic, melanotic, and myxopapillary (always located along the filum terminale).[1]

Cellular ependymomas consist of cellular sheets of uniform cells with moderately hyperchromatic nuclei which are often interrupted by perivascular anuclear zones or pseudorosettes. Less frequently, true rosettes can be seen.[1] There may also be collagenized tissue and foamy macrophages identified on specimens.[1]

Some specific genetic changes have been identified in ependymomas. Intramedullary ependymomas in NF2 patients commonly harbor a mutation on chromosome 22q that differs from intracranial ependymomas, myxopapillary ependymomas, or tanycytic ependymomas. Intracranial ependymomas also have loss of material on 22q; however, they do not have the NF2 mutations. Patients with multiple endocrine neoplasia type 1 are also associated with IMSC ependymomas, where there is a mutation of a tumor suppressor gene on chromosome 11q13, resulting in 11q loss of heterozygosity (LOH) and is associated with malignant transformation of these tumors (▶ Fig. 3.3).[1]

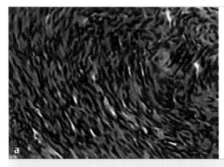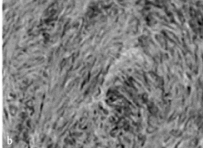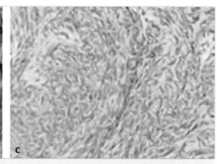

Fig. 3.1 (a) Hematoxylin and eosin, (b) S-100, and (c) neurofilament-stained tissue samples.

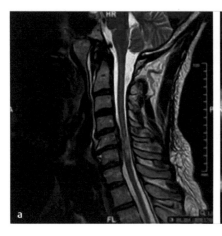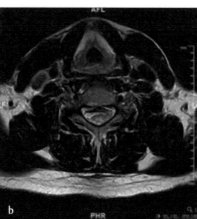

Fig. 3.2 (a, b) Magnetic resonance imaging (MRI) of the lesion. T2 fluid-attenuated inversion recovery (FLAIR) fast relaxation-fast spin echo (FR-FSE) sequence, sagittal and axial orientations.

3.3.2 Imaging Characteristic

Plain radiograph may show features of scoliosis, spinal canal widening, vertebral body scalloping, pedicle erosion, and laminar thinning.[1] Computed tomography (CT) may show nonspecific canal widening, isoattenuating to slightly hyperattenuating compared with normal spinal cord, intense enhancement with iodinated contrast and large lesions may cause scalloping of the posterior vertebral bodies and neural exit foraminal enlargement.[1] MRI is the modality of choice for evaluating suspected spinal cord tumors. Features include widened spinal cord; well-circumscribed tumoral cysts are present in 22% of cases. Non-neoplastic cysts are present in 62%, having an average length of four vertebral body segments.[1,11] Typical signal characteristics for T1-weighted images are mostly isointense to hypointense; mixed signal lesions are seen if cyst formation, tumor necrosis, or hemorrhage has occurred. T2-weighted images are hyperintense. Peritumoral edema is seen in 60% of cases, most commonly with large, multisegment tumors.[1] These tumors demonstrate intense, but heterogenous, enhancement with gadolinium contrast. Associated hemorrhage leads to the "cap sign" (a hypointense hemosiderin rim on T2-weighted images) in 20 to 33% of cases. The cap sign is suggestive of, but not pathognomonic for, ependymoma as it may also be seen in hemangioblastomas and paragangliomas. Syrinx is often seen with tumors located in the cervical spinal cord (▶ Fig. 3.4).[1]

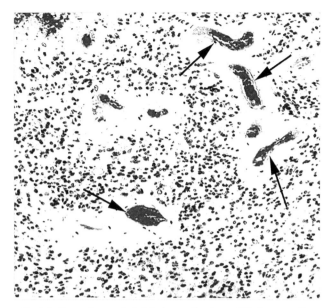

Fig. 3.3 Photomicrograph (original magnification, × 100; hematoxylin-eosin [H-E] stain) of a spinal cord ependymoma shows ependymal cells with uniform hyperchromatic nuclei arranged in perivascular pseudorosettes (*arrows*). (Reproduced with permission from Koeller et al, p. 1727.[1])

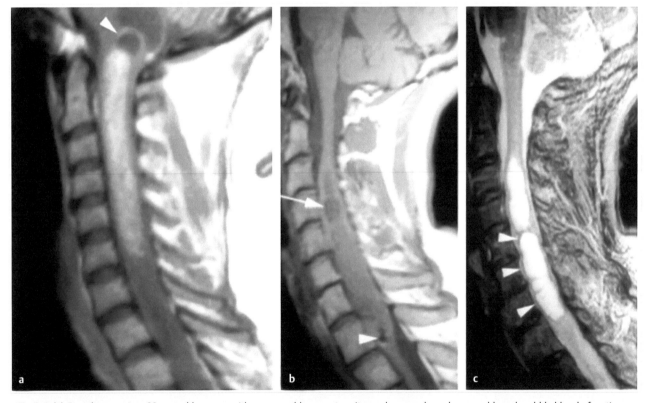

Fig. 3.4 (a) Ependymoma in a 32-year-old woman with upper and lower extremity weakness and numbness and bowel and bladder dysfunction. Contrast-enhanced sagittal T1-weighted magnetic resonance (MR) image demonstrates a heterogeneously enhancing mass expanding the cervical spinal cord. A cyst with faint peripheral enhancement (*arrowhead*) is seen at the superior pole of the mass. **(b)** Intramedullary ependymoma in a 42-year-old man with a 3-month history of neck pain and upper extremity numbness. Sagittal T1-weighted MR image shows an expanded spinal cord from C2 through T2, with associated septated syringohydromyelia (*arrow*). The expanded cord is slightly hyperintense relative to cerebrospinal fluid. There is a focal area of low signal intensity (*arrowhead*) at the caudal pole of the tumor, which is suggestive of calcification or hemosiderin deposition. **(c)** Sagittal T2-weighted MR image reveals a septated syringohydromyelia. The inner surface of the cyst has low signal intensity (*arrowheads*), which is consistent with prior hemorrhage. The mass fragmented into multiple, irregular, nodular, reddish-brown masses at surgical resection. Results of histologic examination revealed ependymoma. (Reproduced with permission from Koeller et al, p. 1728.[1])

3.4 CNS Lymphoma

Intramedullary CNS lymphoma is an uncommon type of extranodal non-Hodgkin's lymphoma (NHL). It is thought to arise from adjacent lymphoid tissue and subsequently invade the spinal cord. It is usually a highly aggressive NHL that resembles diffuse large B-cell lymphocytes. Intramedullary spinal lymphoma accounts for 3.3% of all CNS lymphoma, which constitutes only 1% of all lymphomas in the body.[3,12,13] Clinical presentation typically includes numbness, back pain, paresthesia, and radicular pain followed by extremity weakness, paresis, and paralysis, but can also be asymptomatic.[1] Patients are classified as "primary CNS lymphomas" if there is no evidence of systemic lymphoma detected by screening at the time of diagnosis.[12] Spinal cord lymphomas may be primary and originate in the spinal cord, may accompany tumors in other locations throughout the CNS sequentially or concurrently, or may occur as part of a systemic lymphoma.[12]

Due to lack of localization, high-dose methotrexate-based chemotherapy in combination with radiotherapy is the primary therapy recommended for all spinal cord lymphomas for potential preservation of neurologic function and extension of survival.[3,14] The prognosis for patients with intramedullary spinal lymphoma is poor despite aggressive treatment. Early diagnosis and initiation of treatment is critical because effective treatment in early period of the disease may provide quite long survival. The survival rate at 2.5 years is less than 50%.

Local radiation therapy has been shown to generally increase survival in patients with primary CNS lymphoma. Resistant cases have been reported and are thought to be associated with multifocal disease.

3.4.1 Histopathology

Pathologic specimen is obtained through spinal cord biopsy. Hematoxylin and eosin staining studies showed dense infiltrate of large atypical mononuclear cells surrounding the nerve roots. The cells were large with hyperchromatic nucleus and scant cytoplasm.[15] Many neoplastic cells have prominent central nucleoli with a high mitotic activity. IHC showed intense positivity for cluster differentiation (CD) 20 and the cells were negative for CD 3 and CD 99 (▶ Fig. 3.5 and ▶ Fig. 3.6).[15]

3.4.2 Imaging Characteristic

Spinal cord lymphomas have an ill-defined, yet high intensity, signal on T2-weighted images. T1-weighted images show lesion that is isointense relative to the spinal cord. However, they show solid and homogeneously enhancing enlarged area of the spinal cord with contrast administration.[1,11,13,14] Lymphomas may present as solitary lesions, or may be multifocal in the spinal cord. They do not cause as significant enlargement of spinal cord as seen in other IMSCTs (▶ Fig. 3.7).

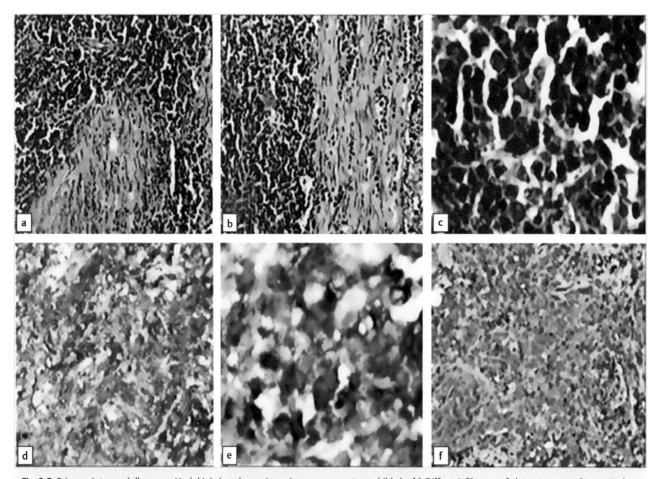

Fig. 3.5 Primary intramedullary non-Hodgkin's lymphoma in an immunocompetent child. (a, b) Diffuse infiltrates of the nerve roots by atypical mononuclear large lymphocytes (small round cells). (c) The cells are large with hyperchromatic nuclei and scant cytoplasm. Hematoxylin and eosin stain, × 400. (d, e) The cells showed diffuse cytoplasmic positivity for CD 20 (horseradish peroxidase [HRP] polymer CD 20) and (f) negativity for CD3 (HRP polymer, CD3). (Reproduced with permission from Bhushanam et al, p. S22.[15])

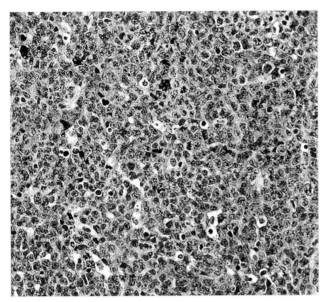

Fig. 3.6 Photomicrograph (original magnification, ×200; hematoxylin-eosin [H-E] stain) of a spinal cord lymphoma dense infiltrate of large atypical mononuclear lymphocytes surrounding small blood vessels. Many neoplastic cells have prominent central nucleoli with a high mitotic activity. (Reproduced with permission from Koeller et al, p. 1743.[1])

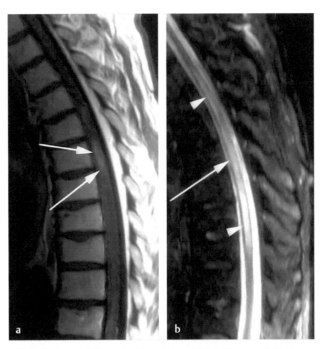

Fig. 3.7 Intramedullary spinal lymphoma. **(a)** Sagittal T1-weighted magnetic resonance (MR) image shows an ill-defined region of slightly high signal intensity (*arrows*) in the midthoracic spinal cord. **(b)** Sagittal T2-weighted MR image reveals abnormal high signal intensity (*arrow*) in the same region. Extensive cord edema (*arrowheads*) is also seen. (Reproduced with permission from Koeller et al, p. 1743.[1])

3.5 Ganglioglioma

Intramedullary gangliogliomas are rare, slow growing (WHO Grade I or II) benign tumors that are typically seen in children and young adults, predominantly localized in the cervical and thoracic spine.[1,3,11] Gangliogliomas are composed of a combination of neoplastic ganglion cells and glial elements. In 5% of cases, gangliogliomas show aggressive behavior and anaplastic changes in the glial component characteristic of WHO grade III.[11] Spinal cord gangliogliomas account for 1.1% of all spinal neoplasms.[1] They most frequently affect children, representing 15% of intramedullary neoplasms in pediatric age group.[16]

The most common clinical presentations are paraparesis (limb weakness), sensory changes, and radicular pain.[1,4] However, scoliosis is an important presentation, as it can be indicative of this lesion. Primary treatment is surgical resection. Studies have noted an 88%, 5-year survival rate after gross surgical resection.[1,3,16] There is a 27% rate of recurrence, which is likely due to increased difficulty of complete surgical excision of the spinal tumor.[1]

3.5.1 Histopathology

Gangliogliomas comprise of a mixture of dysplastic neuronal elements (ganglion cells) and glial elements (primary neoplastic astrocytes) on histological examination (▶ Fig. 3.6).[1] Since tumors vary in composition of cells, various synonyms are used to describe these lesions, including ganglioglioneuroma, ganglionic neuroma, neuroastrocytoma, neuroganglioma, ganglionic glioma, neuroma gangliocellulare, and neuroglioma.[1] Proving the neoplastic nature of neuronal cells requires dysmorphic features, such as abnormalities of localization, irregular clustering, loss of polarity, multinucleation, and presence of bizarre processes.[17] Other features typical of gangliogliomas, such as perivascular lymphocytic infiltrates, Rosenthal fibers, small foci of calcification, and eosinophilic droplets or granular bodies, are frequently

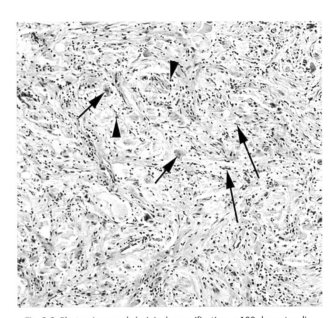

Fig. 3.8 Photomicrograph (original magnification, ×100; hematoxylin-eosin [H-E] stain) of a spinal cord ganglioglioma shows groups of irregular ganglion cells (*short arrows*) and neoplastic glial cells (*long arrows*) with scattered lymphocytes (*arrowheads*). (Reproduced with permission from Koeller et al, p. 1735.[1])

seen with mitotic figures rarely identified.[1,17] Immunophenotypic expression of neuronal markers such as synaptophysin, neurofilament protein, neuron-specific enolase, and chromogranin A also serve to identify neurons (▶ Fig. 3.8).[1,17]

3.5.2 Imaging Characteristic

Gangliogliomas of the spinal cord are typically circumscribed solid or mixed solid and cystic masses that span a long segment of the cord, often greater than eight vertebral body segments and are associated with bony erosion or scalloping.[1,11,16] T1-weighted image shows mixed signal intensity due to the dual cellular population (neuronal and glial elements) and is a unique finding among spinal cord tumors.[1,11,16] T2-weighted image shows high signal intensity with no surrounding edema.[1] In a large series of 27 patients with spinal cord gangliogliomas, Patel et al described several clinical and imaging findings characteristic of gangliogliomas: young patient age, long tumor length, tumoral cysts, absence of edema, mixed signal intensity on T1, patchy tumor enhancement, and cord surface enhancement.[18] Enhancement patterns can be highly variable, ranging from patchy to no enhancement.[11] A gradient echo shows low signal with blooming representing calcification.[1] There is a lack of edema and hemosiderin associated with these tumors (▶ Fig. 3.9).[1]

3.6 Hemangioblastoma

HBs are benign, discrete, highly vascular, and often lipid rich neoplasms (WHO Grade I) occurring primarily in adults in their third to fifth decades with a slight gender predilection for males. They account for 2 to 6% of all intramedullary spinal neoplasm and 60 to 75% of HBs are disseminated due to malignant spread of the original primary tumor with recurrence at the surgically resected site.[1,11] HBs commonly involve the thoracic cord (50%) and the cervical cord (40%) and are most often located posteriorly within the cord. HBs commonly occur as sporadic isolated lesion (80%) or as multiple lesions in association with von Hippel-Lindau disease.[1] Clinical presentation is similar to other IMSCTs with pain, weakness, and sensory changes.[1,4] Complete microsurgical resection with preceding endovascular embolization is curative of sporadic cases.[3,11] The recurrence rate post resection has been reported to be 15 to 27%.[11]

3.6.1 Histopathology

Gross examination reveals well-circumscribed mural nodule (containing tumor) associated with large fluid filled cyst (syrinx).[1] Histologic examination reveals dense network of vascular capillary channels that contain endothelial cells, pericytes, and large neoplastic stromal cells with pink to clear foamy cytoplasm with fine vacuoles containing PAS + lipid.[1] These stromal cells dominate the cellular portions of these benign neoplasms. Many of the cytoplasmic vacuoles contain fat and are visible with fat stains such as oil red O. However, one must be careful when interpreting frozen sections, as HBs can resemble an astrocytoma due to the cellular crowding and occasional nuclear pleomorphism accentuated by the freezing process. A fat stain may be helpful in the differentiation (▶ Fig. 3.10).

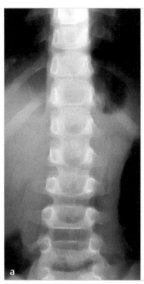
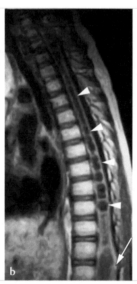
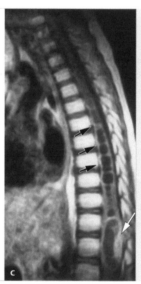

Fig. 3.9 Ganglioglioma in a 7-year-old boy with abdominal pain. **(a)** Frontal radiograph demonstrates a widened interpedicular space, which is suggestive of an intraspinal lesion. **(b)** Sagittal T1-weighted magnetic resonance (MR) image of the spine shows expansion of the lower thoracic cord and conus medullaris region with an associated syringohydromyelia (*arrowheads*) and an irregularly thickened posterior wall (*arrow*). **(c)** Contrast-enhanced sagittal T1-weighted MR image demonstrates enhancement of the posterior thickening in the distal cord (*white arrow*) and along the anterior margin of the midthoracic cord (*black arrows*). (Reproduced with permission from Koeller et al, p. 1736.[1])

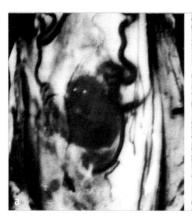
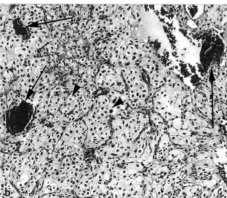

Fig. 3.10 Hemangioblastoma of the conus medullaris. **(a)** Intraoperative photograph demonstrates a vascular mass with enlarged draining veins. **(b)** Photomicrograph (original magnification, ×100; hematoxylin-eosin [H-E] stain) of a spinal cord hemangioblastoma demonstrates a hypervascular neoplasm with prominent zones of hemorrhage (*arrows*) and densely packed large stromal cells with hyperchromatic nuclei (*arrowheads*). (Reproduced with permission from Koeller et al, p. 1737.[1])

3.6.2 Imaging Characteristic

Noncontrast CT reveals soft tissue nodule, often with a prominent hypodense cyst-like component. Contrast administration results in vivid enhancement of the solid component.[1]

On MRI, most HBs present as a focal mass within the spinal cord. Smaller lesions tend to be isointense on T1-weighted images with concordant hyperintensity on T2 lesions with homogeneous enhancement.[1,11] Large lesions tend to be more variable in signal intensity, appearing iso- to hypointense on T1-weighted images and a heterogenous T2-weighted signal with respect to the spinal cord with flow voids occasionally visualized on the latter sequence.[11] These larger lesions show heterogeneous enhancement compared to their smaller counterparts. Large lesions may be visualized without contrast material, but small lesions are often isointense and thus difficult to differentiate from the spinal cord.[1] Associated syrinx and spinal cord edema are characteristic findings of this type of tumor, regardless of size. Vascular endothelial growth factor (VEGF) acting locally on the tumor or hydrodynamic forces, or both, within the abnormal tumor vasculature may drive fluid (plasma) extravasation. When these forces exceed the ability of surrounding tissue to reabsorb fluid, edema (with its associated increased interstitial pressure) and subsequent cyst formation occur (▶ Fig. 3.11 and ▶ Fig. 3.12).[19]

3.7 Myxopapillary Ependymoma

Myxopapillary ependymoma, a benign special variant of ependymoma, occurs almost exclusively in the conus medullaris and filum terminale of adults.[20] It is thought to originate from ependymocytes of the filum terminale, constitutes approximately 13% of all spinal ependymomas in this region, and is classified as a WHO grade I tumor.[20] It is found predominantly in children and young adults and there is a slight male preponderance. Most patients present with symptoms of chronic low back or neck pain, sensory deficits, motor weakness, or bowel or bladder dysfunction.[20] Myxopapillary ependymomas are generally slow-growing tumor, so they can become very large before diagnosis is made.[21] Associated scalloping of the vertebral body, scoliosis, and enlargement of the neural foramina may be seen. Hemorrhage may occur, which accounts for the sudden worsening of clinical symptoms.[21] Myxopapillary ependymoma can often be excised completely. With gross total resection, the prognosis is excellent, with 5-year survival of over 98% of cases.[22] Some sacral and presacral lesions behave aggressively and can become malignant and metastasize to lymph nodes, lung, and bone.[22] This is usually the case in children, where there is also a higher incidence of recurrence.[22]

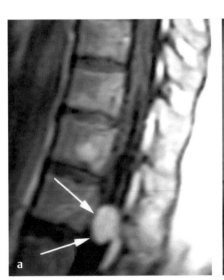
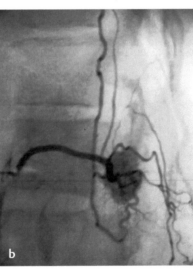

Fig. 3.11 Hemangioblastoma of the conus medullaris. **(a)** Contrast-enhanced sagittal T1-weighted magnetic resonance (MR) image demonstrates a well-circumscribed oval mass (*arrows*) with intense enhancement. **(b)** Spinal angiogram shows the hypervascular mass with a prominent feeding artery and draining vein. (Reproduced with permission from Koeller et al, p. 1738.[1])

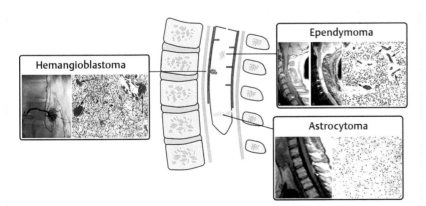

Fig. 3.12 Graphical representation of three primary intramedullary spinal cord tumors—hemangioblastoma, ependymoma, and astrocytoma—featuring their pattern of localization and proliferation within the spinal cord, common radiographic imaging findings, as well as histopathology.

3.7.1 Histopathology

Myxopapillary ependymomas are characteristically lobulated, soft, sausage-shaped masses that are often encapsulated.[22] The histologic hallmark of these tumors is the perivascular pseudorosette formation in which clear tumor cells align themselves, although true rosettes may be seen.[22] These tumors are quite distinctive due to their distribution of stromal mucin but their appearance can vary from case to case. The mucin is often located in the walls of vessels and is abundant. These tumors also contain small, round eosinophilic formations (PAS +) called "Balloons." Pseudorosettes are formed by papillary elements arranged radially around a hyalinized fibrovascular core that gives a "gland-like" appearance, but true papillae are not formed.[22] Just like ependymomas, myxopapillary ependymomas show the same immunophenotype: glial fibrillary acidic protein (GFAP), S-100, and vimentin positive (▶ Fig. 3.13).[22]

3.7.2 Imaging Characteristic

Unlike classical cellular ependymomas, myxopapillary ependymomas may present as hyperintense on T1 due to the presence of high mucin content, but most often, these tumors present as mass located in the caudal spinal cord/conus/filum terminale appearing isointense on T1 and highly intense on T2-weighted imaging.[21] Hemorrhage and calcification can also lead to regions of hyper- or hypointensity. Low intensity may be seen at the tumor margins because of hemorrhage (myxopapillary ependymomas are the subtype of ependymomas that are most prone to hemorrhage).[21] Calcification may also lead to regions of low

T2 signal.[21] Enhancement is virtually always seen after the intravenous administration of contrast material and, although intense, is somewhat nonhomogeneous (likely due to the presence of hemorrhage or cystic components) (▶ Fig. 3.14).[21]

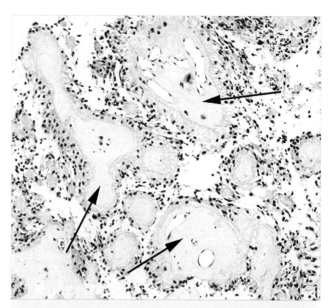

Fig. 3.13 Photomicrograph (original magnification, × 100; hematoxylin-eosin [H-E] stain) of a myxopapillary ependymoma reveals fibrovascular cores and mucoid material (*arrows*) in papillary formations lined with ependymal cells. (Reproduced with permission from Koeller et al, p. 1728.[1])

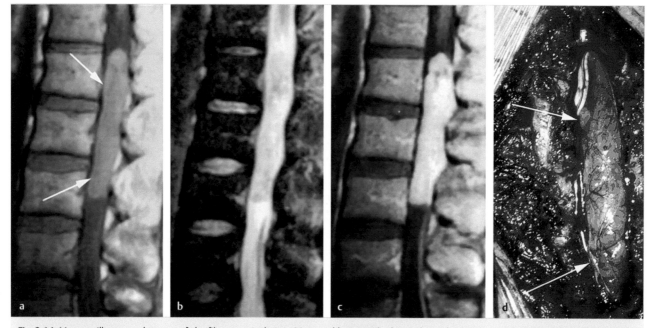

Fig. 3.14 Myxopapillary ependymoma of the filum terminale in a 39-year-old man with chronic lower back pain and right leg sciatica. **(a)** Sagittal T1-weighted magnetic resonance (MR) image shows a large intradural oval mass (*arrows*) extending from the conus medullaris to L3. It is isointense to slightly hyperintense relative to the spinal cord. **(b)** Sagittal T2-weighted MR image reveals mixed signal intensity within the mass. **(c)** Contrast-enhanced sagittal T1-weighted MR image demonstrates intense enhancement of the lesion. **(d)** Intraoperative photograph demonstrates the lobulated, oval intradural mass (*arrows*). An attachment to the filum terminale was noted at surgical resection. (Reproduced with permission from Koeller et al, p. 1729.[1])

3.8 Germ Cell Tumors

Germ cell tumors arise similar to the germinal cells of the genital organs, and they may sporadically arise in the CNS.[3,23] Germ cell tumors are very rare and account for 1% of all CNS tumors. They are more frequently seen in young adults in Japan (3%) and East Asia (12.5%).[23] Germinomas in the spine usually occur due to metastasis from intracranial primary germinoma; primary intramedullary spinal cord germinomas are exceedingly rare.[17] Germ cell tumors commonly involve the thoracic spine and patients generally present with combined sensory and motor deficits, often in the lower extremities, which can progress to gait dysfunction and urological dysfunction.[17] Often, they are associated with an increased serum level of betahuman chorionic gonadotropin (beta-hCG) with very high levels possibly indicating a particularly aggressive lesion and increased likelihood of earlier recurrence.[4] Treatment strategies have included radiation therapy alone, combination of radiation and chemotherapy, and adjuvant radiation and chemotherapy after surgical resection.[2,4]

3.8.1 Histopathology

Histologic examination reveals large, infiltrating epithelioid cells with abundant PAS + cytoplasm; large, round nuclei; and irregular and pleomorphic nuclei. They may exhibit small round lymphocytes infiltrating the stroma.[17] Immunohistologic staining is typically positive for placental alkaline phosphatase (PLAP), OCT3/4, and CD117, and negative for keratin, epithelial membrane antigen (EMA), hCG, and alpha-fetoprotein (AFP) (▶ Fig. 3.15).[17]

3.8.2 Imaging Characteristic

MRI findings for spinal germinomas are similar to spinal astrocytoma, appearing as hypointense or isointense mass on

T1-weighted imaging and hyperintense mass on T2-weighted imaging.[11] These tumors are just as likely to appear heterogenous as they are homogeneous upon contrast enhancement.[11] These tumors may have a mixed, solid, cystic-type appearance with the cystic components being hyperintense on T2-weighted imaging (▶ Fig. 3.16).[11]

3.9 Astrocytoma

Intramedullary astrocytomas arise from glial cells in the spinal cord and constitute the second most common spinal cord tumors.[11,24] Spinal cord astrocytomas represent 40% of IMSCTs and account for 60% of pediatric intramedullary tumors, making it the most common spinal neoplasm in children.[11,24] Spinal cord astrocytomas can be clinicopathologically divided into two distinct groups: diffuse or diffusely infiltrative astrocytomas and pilocytic astrocytomas.[25] Effort should be made to distinguish pilocytic and diffuse astrocytomas because the two tumor types differ in growth pattern, biological behavior, optimal therapy, and prognosis.[11,24]

Diffuse infiltrative astrocytomas are uncommon lesion that range from WHO grades II to IV.[25] A small percentage arise in association with neurofibromatosis or prior radiotherapy.[25] Spinal cord astrocytomas in almost 75% of adult patients are usually low-grade lesions (WHO grade I).[11,24] High-grade lesions appear in 10 to 15% of children and are mostly anaplastic astrocytoma.[11] Pilocytic astrocytoma is common in young children (WHO grade I) and is mostly found in the conus medullaris, but rare in adults.[25,26] Intramedullary astrocytomas are commonly found in the cervical spinal cord followed closely by the thoracic region and may extend along the entire length of the spinal cord (holocord presentation); however, lesions that extensive are rarely reported, and predominantly seen in children.[11] Most patients present with symptoms of back or neck pain, sensory deficits, motor weakness, or

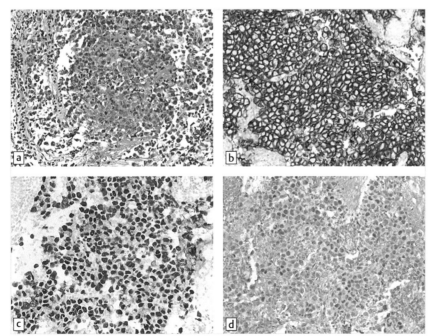

Fig. 3.15 Histological examination. (a) Hematoxylin and eosin stain demonstrating large round cells with large nuclei containing prominent nucleoli and granular chromatin. The cells are arranged in monomorphous sheets with background lymphocytes (100 ×). (b) Tumor cells are positive for C-KIT (100 ×). (c) Tumor cells are positive for SALL-4 (100 ×). (d) Tumor cells are weakly positive for OCT-4 (100 ×). (Reproduced with permission from Mehta et al, p. 478.e2.[23])

bowel or bladder dysfunction.[1] Due to the infiltrating nature of most astrocytomas, gross total resection is impossible without an unacceptable loss of neurological function; hence, they typically have worse prognosis.[2,24] Subtotal resection is usually the treatment of choice as it prevents excessive damage of normal spinal cord parenchyma.[2,24] Spinal cord astrocytomas in children are associated with a good prognosis, as neoplasms behave much like grade I pilocytic astrocytomas and displace neural tissue rather than infiltrate it, allowing for better resection.[2,24]

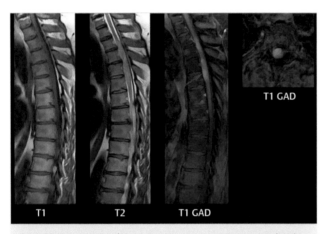

Fig. 3.16 Preoperative thoracic magnetic resonance imaging (MRI) shows three sagittal sequences (T1, T2, and T1 with gadolinium) on the left and an axial (T1 with gadolinium) on the right demonstrating an intramedullary mass between T2 and T5 (*arrow*). (Reproduced with permission from Loya et al, p. 3.[30])

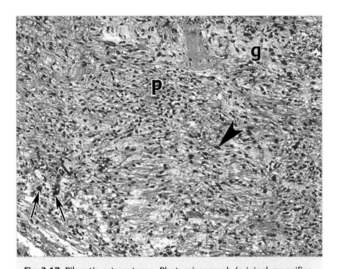

Fig. 3.17 Pilocytic astrocytoma. Photomicrograph (original magnification, × 40; hematoxylin-eosin [H-E] stain) of a classic pilocytic astrocytoma reveals a biphasic appearance with a loose glial component (*g*) with numerous microcysts and vacuoles and more compact piloid tissue (*p*) with elongated bipolar cells (*arrowhead*) showing fine fibrillary processes. Rosenthal fibers (*arrows*) are also noted. (Reproduced with permission from Koeller, Kelly K., and Elisabeth J. Rushing. From the archives of the AFIP: pilocytic astrocytoma: radiologic-pathologic correlation. RadioGraphics 2004; 24(6): 1693–1708.)

3.9.1 Histopathology

Astrocytomas are a heterogeneous group of infiltrating tumors characterized by ill-defined diffuse fusiform enlargement.[1,24] All astrocytomas are characterized by hypercellularity and the absence of a surrounding capsule.[1,24] Neoplastic astrocytes will extend along the "scaffold" of normal astrocytes, oligodendrocytes, and axons of the surrounding neural tissue in an infiltrative pattern.[1,24] As a result, astrocytomas are never circumscribed (with the exception of pilocytic astrocytomas). In the WHO classification, astrocytomas are graded from I to IV according to increasing degree of malignancy. Grade I astrocytomas, pilocytic astrocytomas, are often well-circumscribed, often cystic, composed of variable proportions of loose and compact tissues.[1,24] Pilocytic astrocytomas show a biphasic pattern with compact bipolar cells and loose-textured multipolar cells with microcysts and granular bodies.[1,24] Grade II corresponds to the fibrillary type and are the classic low-grade astrocytomas.[25] Diffuse astrocytomas arising in the spinal cord are more often well differentiated (grade II).[25] The cells of the grade II lesion vary from case to case.[25] In some, fibrillary astrocytes with naked, atypical, elongated, irregular, hyperchromatic nuclei embedded in a fibrillary background are seen. In others, the cytoplasm is more conspicuous, and cells are either fibrillary or gemistocytes.[25] Grade III, anaplastic astrocytomas, contains more pleomorphism, less differentiation, even more hypercellularity, and regions of necrosis compared with the lower grade lesions.[1,24,25,27] Grade IV lesions, or glioblastoma multiforme, are the most malignant type of astrocytomas and show evidence of endothelial proliferation at microscopic review.[1,24] Only 0.2 to 1.5% of astrocytomas of the spinal cord are classified as grade IV; they are distinctly uncommon in spinal cord (▶ Fig. 3.17, ▶ Fig. 3.18, ▶ Fig. 3.19, ▶ Fig. 3.20, ▶ Fig. 3.21, ▶ Fig. 3.22).[1,24,25,27]

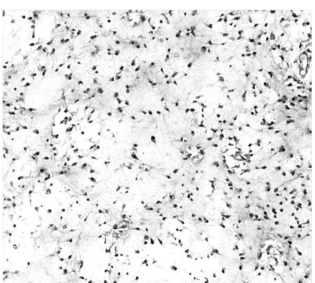

Fig. 3.18 Photomicrograph (original magnification, × 100; hematoxylin-eosin [H-E] stain) of a spinal cord astrocytoma reveals increased cellularity with mild nuclear pleomorphism. The lack of mitotic activity, endothelial proliferation, and necrosis support the histologic diagnosis of a grade II astrocytoma. (Reproduced with permission from Koeller et al, p. 1732.[1])

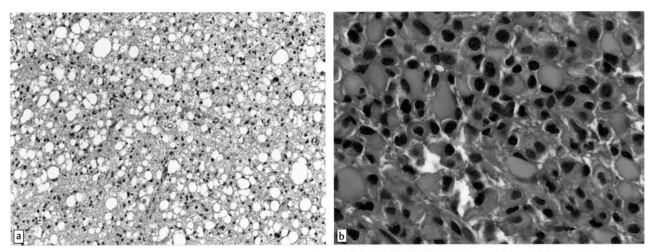

Fig. 3.19 (a) Histopathology specimen (FFPE) of a diffuse astrocytoma, WHO grade II, fibrillary type. The outline of the tumor is not clearly visible in scans, because the borders of the neoplasm tend to send out tiny microscopic fibrillary tentacles that spread into the surrounding brain tissue. (Reproduced with permission from Jensflorian. Histopathology specimen (FFPE) of a diffuse astrocytoma, WHO grade II, fibrillary type. Available at https://commons.wikimedia.org/wiki/File:Diffuse_astrocytoma_HE_stain.jpg; last accessed on 22 October 2015.) **(b)** Gemistocytic astrocytoma is a swollen, reactive astrocyte. They have a large cytoplasmic mass, long, branching processes, and increased cytoplasmic filaments (hematoxylin-eosin [H-E] stain, high magnification). (Reproduced with permission from Jensflorian. Histopathology specimen (FFPE) of a diffuse astrocytoma, WHO grade II, fibrillary type. Available at https://commons.wikimedia.org/wiki/File:Gemistocytic_astrocytoma.jpg; last accessed on 22 October 2015.)

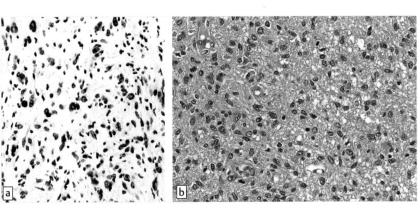

Fig. 3.20 (a) Anaplastic astrocytoma. Seen at low (left) and high (right) magnification. This degree of cellularity and pleomorphism warrants the diagnosis of anaplastic astrocytoma. **(b)** Astrocytoma with abundant mitoses despite low cell density (hematoxylin-eosin [H-E] stain, biopsy specimen). (Reproduced with permission from Jensflorian. Astrocytoma with abundant mitoses despite low cell density (HE stain, biopsy specimen). Libre Pathology (Creative Commons). Available at https://librepathology.org/wiki/File:Mitoses_astro_III.jpg; last accessed on 29 April 2018.)

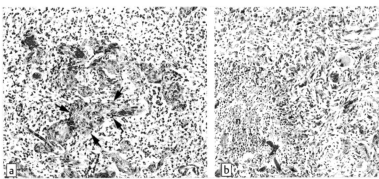

Fig. 3.21 (a) Photomicrograph (original magnification, ×200; hematoxylin-eosin [H-E] stain) of a spinal cord glioblastoma multiforme demonstrates a hypercellular pleomorphic neoplasm with endothelial proliferation (*arrows*). **(b)** Photomicrograph (original magnification, ×100; H-E stain) of a different field in the same tumor shows zones of necrosis (*n*) and mitotic activity (*arrowhead*). (Reproduced with permission from Koeller et al, p. 1733.[1])

3.9.2 Imaging Characteristic

MRI is the imaging technique of choice for the evaluation of spinal cord astrocytomas. MRI reveals neoplasms that are usually poorly defined from surrounding normal spinal cord and, just like ependymomas, are iso- to hypointense relative to the spinal cord on T1-weighted images and hyperintense on T2-weighted images.[1,24] Since astrocytomas arise from the cord parenchyma,

the location of astrocytomas within the spinal cord is variable and may be central or eccentric.[1] Tumor cysts are a common finding, and reactive cysts may be observed at the cranial and caudal ends.[24] Additionally, intramedullary astrocytomas may be associated with a syrinx.[1,24] The intravenous administration of gadolinium diethylenetriamine penta-acetic acid can help distinguish cyst from tumor and edema because cysts and areas of edema that contain no tumor will not enhance.[1,11,24] Pilocytic

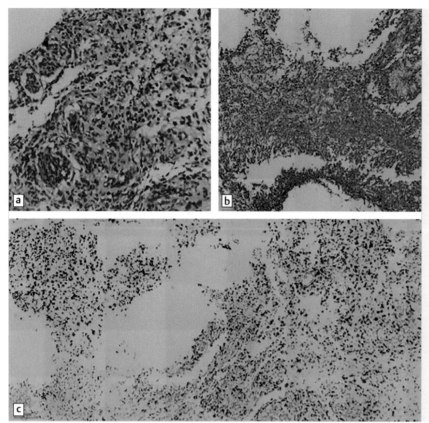

Fig. 3.22 Histopathological and immunochemical findings. **(a)** Hematoxylin and eosin stained section revealed that the tumor is composed of cells with prominent eosinophilic cytoplasm, nuclear atypia, and microvascular proliferation. **(b)** Immunohistochemical staining shows positivity for glial fibrillary acidic protein. **(c)** The proliferation index (anti-Ki67) is 60% (magnification [a] 200 ×, [b], and [c] 100 ×). (Reproduced with permission from Shen et al, p. 3.[31])

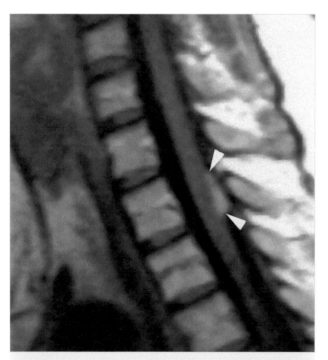

Fig. 3.23 Astrocytoma in a 35-year-old woman with lower extremity weakness and numbness. Contrast-enhanced sagittal T1-weighted magnetic resonance (MR) image demonstrates an irregularly enhancing intramedullary tumor with an enhancing exophytic component (*arrowheads*). (Reproduced with permission from Koeller et al, p. 1731.[1])

astrocytomas (WHO grade I) may enhance homogeneously or have patchy enhancement or no enhancement at all.[25] Virtually all cord astrocytomas show at least some enhancement following the intravenous administration of contrast material (▶ Fig. 3.23, ▶ Fig. 3.24, ▶ Fig. 3.25, ▶ Fig. 3.26, ▶ Fig. 3.27, ▶ Fig. 3.28).[24]

3.10 Melanoma

Primary spinal melanomas are exceptionally rare, highly malignant neoplasms, and may be intradural or extradural.[11] Melanomas arise from melanocytes or cells with the potential to become melanocytes. Primary CNS melanomas are thought to arise from the neural crest and account for approximately 1% of all melanomas.[11] According to the Hayward classification, the diagnosis of primary spinal cord melanoma is based on: (1) the absence of a melanoma outside the CNS; (2) involvement of the leptomeninges; (3) intramedullary spinal lesions; (4) hydrocephalus; (5) tumor in the pituitary pineal gland; and (6) a single intracerebral lesion.[28] These criteria along with a histologic confirmation of melanoma allow for a diagnosis of primary CNS melanoma. Differentiation of primary melanoma from metastatic disease must be accomplished as it holds important prognostic implication.[28,29] Primary intramedullary melanomas frequently involve the thoracic portion of the cord and present similarly to other IMSCTs, with symptoms like pain, weakness, and sensory and motor deficits, though due to the nature of these lesions the onset and progression of symptoms are much more aggressive.[17] Gross total surgical resection offers the most promising outcome for primary spinal cord melanoma, with

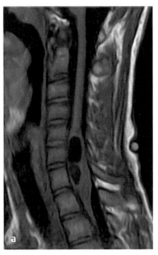
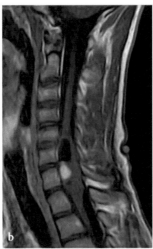
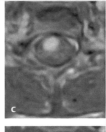
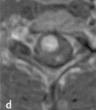

Fig. 3.24 A 17-year-old with intramedullary cervical pilocytic astrocytoma. Preoperative sagittal T1-weighted magnetic resonance (MR) images without (**a**) and with (**b**) contrast enhancement, and axial T1-weighted contrast-enhanced (**c, d**) MR images demonstrating a homogeneously enhancing lesion at the level of the C7 vertebral body. The lesion is intramedullary, located eccentrically in the right ventral spinal cord, and is associated with a large rostral cyst and a small caudal cyst. (Reproduced with permission from Ogden et al, pp. 253–257.[32])

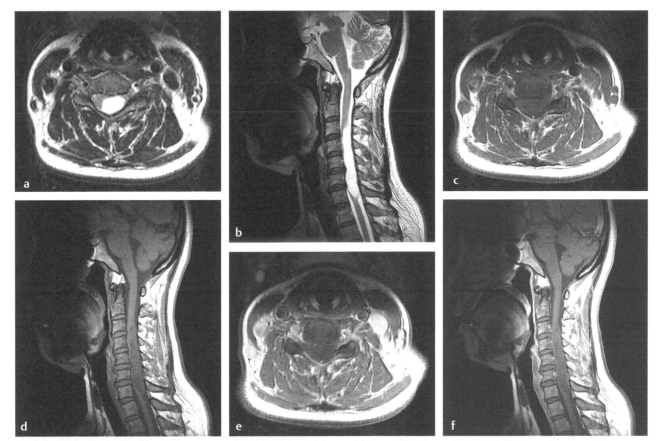

Fig. 3.25 A 50-year-old woman with nonenhancing WHO grade II diffuse astrocytoma. Her symptoms were progressive left-handed weakness, hypoesthesia, and lower right-legged paresthesia starting 5 months earlier. (**a, b**) Axial and sagittal T2-weighted magnetic resonance (MR) images show a well-demarcated hyperintense intramedullary mass at the cervical spinal cord. The mass is slightly eccentric to the left side from the spinal cord center on the axial image. There is no peritumoral edema, periapical cap, or hemorrhage. (**c, d**) The mass is hypointense on axial and sagittal T1-weighted images. (**e, f**) Contrast-enhanced T1-weighted images show that the mass is not enhanced at all. (Reproduced with permission from Seo et al, pp. 498–503.[33])

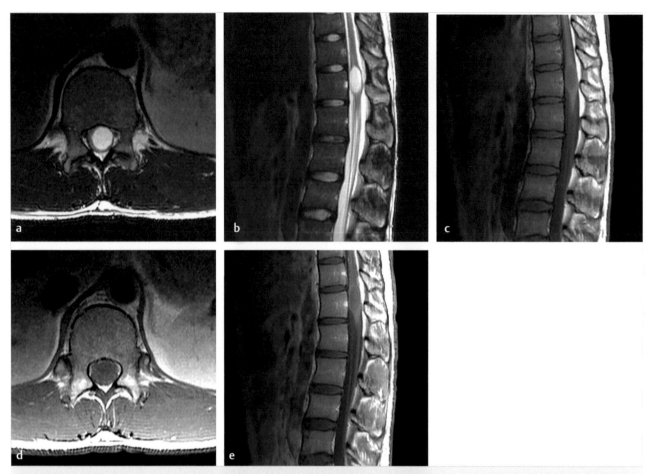

Fig. 3.26 A 19-year-old man with a nonenhancing WHO grade III anaplastic astrocytoma. His chief symptoms were left lower extremity weakness, hypoesthesia, and lower back pain starting 6 months earlier. (a, b) Axial and sagittal T2-weighted magnetic resonance (MR) images show a well-demarcated hyperintense mass at the center of the conus medullaris. (c) The mass is hypointense on the sagittal T1-weighted image. (d, e) Contrast-enhanced axial and sagittal T1-weighted images show that the mass is not enhanced at all. (Reproduced with permission from Seo et al, pp. 498–503.[33])

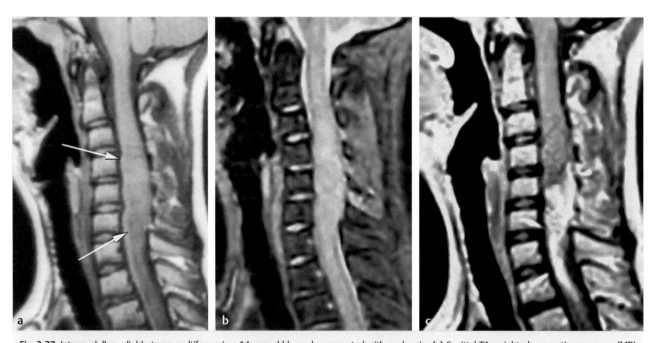

Fig. 3.27 Intramedullary glioblastoma multiforme in a 14-year-old boy who presented with neck pain. (a) Sagittal T1-weighted magnetic resonance (MR) image shows irregular expansion of the cervical spinal cord extending from C3 to C7 (arrows). The affected cord is slightly hypointense relative to the unaffected cord. Note expansion of the spinal canal secondary to bony remodeling. (b) Sagittal T2-weighted MR image reveals an abnormal area of high signal intensity throughout the expanded region. (c) Contrast-enhanced sagittal T1-weighted MR image displays irregular, intense, homogeneous enhancement of the inferior portion of the expanded cord from C5 through T1 (arrows). (Reproduced with permission from Koeller et al, p. 1734.[1])

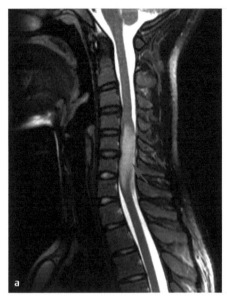
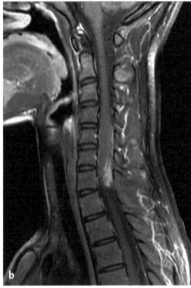

Fig. 3.28 Preoperative magnetic resonance imaging (MRI): **(a)** Sagittal T2-weighted MRI, which shows a high signal intramedullary lesion extending from C4 to C7, filling the involved spinal canal. **(b)** Postcontrast sagittal T1-weighted MRI showing a heterogeneous enhancement intramedullary lesion. *Red arrows* indicate the lesion. (Reproduced with permission from Shen et al.[31])

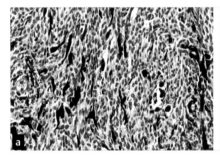
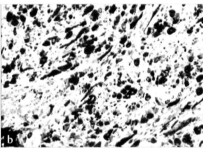

Fig. 3.29 Microscopic finding. **(a)** Photomicrograph shows atypical, bizarre cells with large pleomorphic nuclei, macronucleoli, and mitoses (hematoxylin-eosin [H-E], × 1250). **(b)** Immunohistochemical stains for human melanoma black-45 (HMB-45) reveals cytoplasmic reactivity (H-E, × 1250). (Reproduced with permission from Kim et al, pp. 157 161.[34])

adjuvant radiotherapy and chemotherapy (especially after inadequate resection) being recommended.[2,4]

3.10.1 Histopathology

Microscopic features include the formation of tight nests (reminiscent of whorls) surrounded by well-differentiated melanocytes with cytoplasm rich in melanin. Bland, oval nuclei with eosinophilic nucleoli may be seen.[29] Malignant melanoma has hypercellular sheets or nests of spindled or epithelioid cells, prominent nucleoli, and invasion of adjacent structures or necrosis may be seen.[29] Histopathologic confirmation is accomplished by demonstrating immunoreactivity for human melanoma black-45 (HMB-45) and S-100 protein (▶ Fig. 3.29).[29]

3.10.2 Imaging Characteristic

Characteristic imaging features on MRI are expansion of the spinal cord with an intramedullary mass that appears hyperintense on T1-weighted sequences, hypointense on T2-weighted

sequences, and homogeneous enhancement following infusion of gadolinium-based contrast agents.[11] These characteristics may vary from case to case depending on the melanocytic content and the intratumoral hemorrhage present (▶ Fig. 3.30).[11]

3.11 Conclusion

Primary spinal tumors are rare neoplasms which comprise about 15% of all central nervous system tumors and are divided into three groups based on their anatomical location: extradural, intradural-extramedullary, and intramedullary. Intramedullary spinal cord tumors (IMSCT) compromise about 2 to 5% of spinal tumors and arise inside the spinal cord itself. Ependymomas and astrocytomas account for 80 to 90% of all intramedullary tumors. Other intramedullary tumors are nerve sheath tumors (neuromas), lymphomas, gangliomas, hemangioblastomas, germ cell tumors, and metastases. In this chapter we will review the epidemiology, histopathology, imaging characteristics, and clinical presentation of IMSCT.

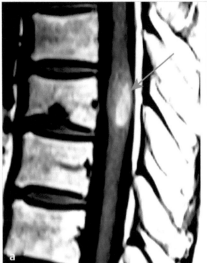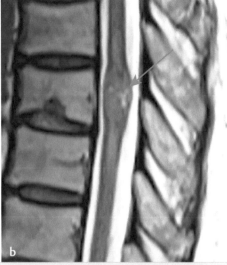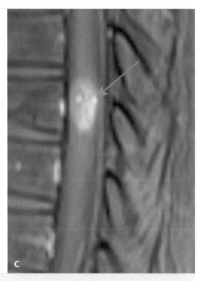

Fig. 3.30 Magnetic resonance imaging (MRI) of the thoracic spine showed an intramedullary mass at T8. The mass showed hyperintensity on T1 and T2 ([a], sagittal; [b], sagittal), moderate heterogeneous enhancement following gadolinium injection ([c], sagittal), lack of flow voids, mild surrounding edema, and cord expansion. Given the intramedullary location and signal characteristics, the primary consideration was for an ependymoma or astrocytoma; less likely consideration included hemangioblastoma or metastatic disease. Because of edema and cord expansion, hemorrhage and demyelinating processes were less likely. (Reproduced with permission from Wuerdeman et al, pp. 424–425.[28])

References

[1] Koeller KK, Rosenblum RS, Morrison AL. Neoplasms of the spinal cord and filum terminale: radiologic-pathologic correlation. Radiographics. 2000; 20 (6):1721–1749

[2] Tobin MK, Geraghty JR, Engelhard HH, Linninger AA, Mehta AI. Intramedullary spinal cord tumors: a review of current and future treatment strategies. Neurosurg Focus. 2015; 39(2):E14

[3] Hobbs JG, Desai B, Young JS, et al. Intramedullary spinal cord tumors: a review and discussion of surgical rationale. WSCJ. 2016; 7(2):65–83

[4] McGuire LS, Behbahini M, Das S, et al. Intramedullary amputation neuroma: a case report and review of the literature. Clin Neuropathol. 2017; 36(2):73–77

[5] Santagata S, Tuli S, Wiese DE , II, Day A, De Girolami U. Intramedullary neuroma of the cervicomedullary junction. Case report. J Neurosurg Spine. 2006; 5(4):362–366

[6] Schwannoma. The Spine Hospital at the Neurological Institute of New York. http://columbiaspine.org/condition/schwannoma/. Accessed May 14, 2018

[7] Conti P, Pansini G, Mouchaty H, Capuano C, Conti R. Spinal neurinomas: retrospective analysis and long-term outcome of 179 consecutively operated cases and review of the literature. Surg Neurol. 2004; 61(1):34–43, discussion 44

[8] Weedon D. 37—Neural and neuroendocrine tumors. In: Weedon's Skin Pathology. 3rd ed. Edinburgh: Churchill Livingstone; 2010:867–886.e18

[9] Baldassarre RL, Nakanote KA, Hughes TH. Imaging of peripheral neurogenic tumors. In: Handbook of Neuro-oncology Neuroimaging. Elsevier; 2016:777–796

[10] Butt AM. Macroglial lineages. In: Squire LR, ed. Encyclopedia of Neuroscience. Oxford: Academic Press; 2009:597–599

[11] Merhemic Z, Stosic-Opincal T, Thurnher MM. Neuroimaging of spinal tumors. Magn Reson Imaging Clin N Am. 2016; 24(3):563–579

[12] Guzey FK, Hıtay Y, Isler C. Primary spinal intramedullary lymphoma: a case report and review of the literature. 2015; 3:1049

[13] Algazi AP, Kadoch C, Rubenstein JL. Biology and treatment of primary central nervous system lymphoma. Neurotherapeutics. 2009; 6(3):587–597

[14] Herrlinger U, Weller M, Küker W. Primary CNS lymphoma in the spinal cord: clinical manifestations may precede MRI detectability. Neuroradiology. 2002; 44(3):239–244

[15] Bhushanam TV, Rajesh A, Linga VG, Uppin MS, Malik M. Primary intramedullary non-Hodgkin's lymphoma in an immunocompetent child. Spinal Cord. 2014; 52 Suppl 2:S21–S23

[16] Rossi A, Gandolfo C, Morana G, Tortori-Donati P. Tumors of the spine in children. Neuroimaging Clin N Am. 2007; 17(1):17–35

[17] Hirose T, Scheithauer BW, Lopes MBS, Gerber HA, Altermatt HJ, VandenBerg SR. Ganglioglioma: an ultrastructural and immunohistochemical study. Cancer. 1997; 79(5):989–1003

[18] Patel U, Pinto RS, Miller DC, et al. MR of spinal cord ganglioglioma. AJNR Am J Neuroradiol. 1998; 19(5):879–887

[19] Baggenstos MA, Butman JA, Oldfield EH, Lonser RR. Role of edema in peritumoral cyst formation. Neurosurg Focus. 2007; 22(5):E9

[20] Petersen D, Lystad RP. Spinal myxopapillary ependymoma in an adult male presenting with recurrent acute low back pain: a case report. Chiropr Man Therap. 2016; 24(1):11

[21] Kahan H, Sklar EML, Post MJD, Bruce JH. MR characteristics of histopathologic subtypes of spinal ependymoma. AJNR Am J Neuroradiol. 1996; 17(1):143–150

[22] Louis DN, Perry A, Reifenberger G, et al. The 2016 World Health Organization classification of tumors of the central nervous system: a summary. Acta Neuropathol. 2016; 131(6):803–820

[23] Mehta VA, Kretzer RM, Orr B, Jallo GI. Primary intramedullary spinal germ cell tumors. World Neurosurg. 2011; 76(5):478.e1–478.e6

[24] Smith AB, Soderlund KA, Rushing EJ, Smirniotopolous JG. Radiologic-pathologic correlation of pediatric and adolescent spinal neoplasms: Part 1, Intramedullary spinal neoplasms. AJR Am J Roentgenol. 2012; 198(1): 34–43

[25] Burger PC, Scheithauer BW, Vogel FS. Surgical Pathology of the Nervous System and Its Coverings. 4 ed. New York, NY: Churchill Livingstone; 2002

[26] Abul-Kasim K, Thurnher MM, McKeever P, Sundgren PC. Intradural spinal tumors: current classification and MRI features. Neuroradiology. 2008; 50(4): 301–314

[27] Dahlberg D, Halvorsen CM, Lied B, and Helseth E. Minimally invasive microsurgical resection of primary, intradural spinal tumours using a tubular retraction system. Br J Neurosurg. 2012; 26(4): 472–475.

[28] Wuerdeman M, Douglass S, Abda RB, Krasnokutsky M. A rare case of primary spinal cord melanoma. Radiol Case Rep. 2018; 13(2):424–426

[29] Sinha R, Rizvi TH, Chakraborti S, Ballal CK, Kumar A. Primary melanoma of the spinal cord: a case report. J Clin Diagn Res. 2013; 7(6):1148–1149

[30] Loya JJ, Jung H, Temmins C, Cho N, Singh H. Primary spinal germ cell tumors: a case analysis and review of treatment paradigms. Case Rep Med. 2013; 2013:798358

[31] Shen C-X, Wu J-F, Zhao W, Cai Z-W, Cai R-Z, Chen C-M. Primary spinal glioblastoma multiforme: A case report and review of the literature. Medicine (Baltimore). 2017; 96(16):e6634

[32] Ogden AT, Feldstein NA, McCormick PC. Anterior approach to cervical intramedullary pilocytic astrocytoma. Case report. J Neurosurg Spine. 2008; 9 (3):253–257

[33] Seo HS, Kim JH, Lee DH, et al. Nonenhancing intramedullary astrocytomas and other MR imaging features: a retrospective study and systematic review. AJNR Am J Neuroradiol. 2010; 31(3):498–503

[34] Kim MS, Yoon DH, Shin DA. Primary spinal cord melanoma. J Korean Neurosurg Soc. 2010; 48(2):157–161

4 Treatment of Intramedullary Spinal Cord Tumors

Nir Shimony, Cameron Brimley, Mari Groves, Mohammad Hassan A. Noureldine, and George I. Jallo

Summary

Intramedullary spinal cord tumors are rare entities in the pediatric population with significant morbidity. Presentation may be indolent and lead to delayed diagnosis and eventually large tumor burden or structural involvement when symptoms and signs occur. Therefore, a high index of suspicion must be maintained by all clinicians. Treatment and diagnosis include a combination of advanced imaging techniques, high surgical technique, and in some cases adjuvant oncological therapy. In the recent years we witnessed significant change in our understanding of the genetic parameters and the biologic behavior of these tumors. Some of these advancements led for change in treatment paradigm and most likely we will witness further change in the future. Today, surgical resection still holds a significant role in the treatment of spinal cord intramedullary tumors and demands high level of surgical techniques and strong multidisciplinary approach in the operating room and beyond. In this chapter we present the latest advancement in the treatment of intramedullary tumors, as well as our approach that was built after many years of experience.

Keywords: intramedullary, spinal cord, tumors, surgery monitoring, MRI

4.1 Introduction

Spinal tumors can be classified based on their anatomic location, either extradural, intradural-extramedullary, or intramedullary. This chapter will focus on intramedullary spinal cord tumors (IMSCTs) including details of relevant anatomy/embryology, epidemiology, tumor pathology and advances in genetic mutation/expression analysis, clinical presentation, diagnosis, and treatment.

The true history of spinal cord surgery is a little vague.[1,2,3] The first documented case of IMSCT resection was by Christian Fenger of Chicago in 1890.[3] Successful resections were done subsequently in the early 1900s by Anton von Eiselsberg and Charles Elseberg.[4] Additionally, Harvey Cushing reported first documented attempts at IMSCT resection at Johns Hopkins that he performed between 1908 and 1910.[3]

IMSCTs are fairly rare, yet they are generally associated with potential significant progressive morbidity and typically require treatment that involves surgical resection and in some cases adjuvant chemotherapy and radiotherapy. IMSCT symptoms can be similar to many other surgical and nonsurgical spine neurological pathologies, and frequently these group of tumors present in an indolent fashion with a delay in their ultimate diagnosis due to a progressive prodrome of nonspecific clinical findings. Therefore, a high index of suspicion must be maintained by all clinicians, including primary care physicians, general pediatricians, orthopedists, pain specialists, and neurosurgeons.[5]

4.2 Anatomy

Intramedullary tumors inherently compress or disrupt the spinal cord architecture. As such, it can disrupt the long spinal cord tracts' architecture and function. In some tumors the change they create in the gross microsurgical appearance of the spinal cord makes identification of landmarks difficult, while others are much better demarcated. Understanding spinal cord anatomy and being able to imagine and identify how the anatomy may be distorted around an intramedullary tumor are paramount to performing safe and successful surgery for IMSCTs.

The embryonal formation of the spinal cord begins after gastrulation with the notochord signaling the formation of the neural fold, which eventually forms the neural tube.[6,7,8] The neural tube starts as a single cell layer of germinal neuroepithelium. Cells migrate outward from this germinal matrix layer creating the intermediate zone, which will eventually become the spinal cord gray matter. These neurons send axons outward into the marginal zone, which becomes the white matter portion of the spinal cord. The ectoderm secretes bone morphogenetic protein (BMP) dorsally, inducing alar plate formation, while the notochord secretes Sonic hedgehog (SHH), inhibiting BMP and allowing the development of motor neurons within the basal plate.[6] The central canal is composed of remnants of the neural tube central cavity, is lined by ependymal cells, and is filled with cerebrospinal fluid (CSF). There are differential gradients of expression between the ventral SHH expression and BMPs in the dorsal ectoderm, which not only establishes a dorsoventral plane but also leads to the later establishment of distinct classes of neurons with the spinal cord, which potentially creates the platform for different specific tumors that rise from different cell lines.

Cross-sectional anatomy of the spinal cord shows the central butterfly-shaped gray matter with the efferent motor neuron cell bodies residing in the anterior horn, the autonomic neuron bodies in the lateral horn, and the afferent sensory neuron axons entering into the posterior horn. The majority of these neurons synapse with ascending and descending longitudinal white matter tracts connecting with the brain.

4.3 Pathology

4.3.1 Epidemiology

IMSCTs are rare and account for 2 to 4% of all central nervous system (CNS) lesions, which is essentially proportional to the tissue volume of the spinal cord, making up approximately 5% of the total CNS tissue.[9,10] Intramedullary tumors account for 20 to 30% of all spine tumors in adults and children.[11] Gliomas, predominantly astrocytomas and ependymomas, represent around 90% of IMSCTs.[12,13] Other types of intramedullary tumors include hemangioblastomas, gangliogliomas, lipomas, dermoid cysts, teratomas, and rarely intramedullary metastases. While ependymomas are the most common IMSCTs in adults, pediatric patients more commonly have astrocytomas.[13] For children under the age of 10, astrocytomas comprise approximately 80% of all intramedullary tumors and account for 60% of intramedullary neoplasms in adolescents.[13] Around the third decade of life, ependymomas become slightly more common than astrocytomas, while for patients greater than or equal to 40 years of age, they comprise close to 70% of all IMSCTs.[11,13]

IMSCTs most commonly arise in the cervical and thoracic spine. Specifically, approximately 60% of astrocytomas in children will develop in the cervical region and cervicothoracic junction.[14] Within the spinal cord, IMSCT growth patterns differ with astrocytomas appearing more eccentric, involving the white matter of the spinal cord, while ependymomas typically arise in the central region.[15]

Presentation depends upon the location of the lesion along the cephalic-caudal axis of the spinal cord, and upon the cross-sectional intramedullary location. Approximately 70% of patients present with motor weakness, 64% with sensory symptoms, and 38% with bladder dysfunction.[11] There is no apparent gender predilection for IMSCTs. Patients with neurofibromatosis type 1 (NF1) have a higher propensity to develop spinal astrocytomas and those with NF2 are at risk of developing ependymomas.[16]

4.3.2 Histology/Genetics

The most common pathology that is found in IMSCT comprises from either ependymomas or astrocytomas, as discussed above. Other types of IMSCTs include gangliogliomas, hemangioblastomas, dermoid cysts, lipomas, and others.

Astrocytomas are the most common IMSCTs in pediatric patients and a very common pathology among adults, as mentioned above. The astrocytomas that can be encountered in IMSCTs include pilocytic astrocytomas (WHO grade I; diffuse astrocytomas (WHO grade II; with infrequent encounters of malignant anaplastic astrocytomas) and glioblastomas (WHO grades III and IV, respectively) accounting for approximately 10 to 15% of pediatric astrocytic IMSCTs and up to 21.9% in a more recent SEER database review.[17,18,19] Astrocytomas commonly display infiltrative features without a clear plane separating tumor from normal neural structures. Histologically, low-grade astrocytic tumors appear hypercellular with mild nuclear atypia and few mitoses, while high-grade gliomas have a high rate of nuclear atypia and mitoses. Molecular subtype analysis has broadened our understanding of CNS tumors. Discoveries regarding the alterations of genes involved in the mitogen-activated protein kinase (MAPK) and BRAF pathways have been described in low-grade gliomas.[20,21,22,23,24,25] Other alterations that activate the MAPK pathway, such as mutations in NF1, RAF, RAS, and FGFR1, have also been identified.[26] In recent years, further understanding of the pathophysiological mechanisms of high-grade gliomas has included the discovery of a subcategory of midline tumors arising from the pons, thalamus, cerebellum, and to a lesser extent in the spinal cord. The characteristic mutation is in the complex of histone and includes the histone H3K27 M mutations that can be found commonly in the midline diffuse gliomas. These are characterized by point mutations within the chromatin modifiers H3 and are usually associated with poor clinical outcome, regardless of the WHO subtyping.[26,27]

Ependymomas of the spinal cord are typically WHO grade II. Classic ependymomas will display histopathological features of perivascular pseudorosettes, and are generally less cellular without vascular proliferation or significant mitoses. Genetic research has revealed significant molecular variation between ependymomas that grow in the different compartments of the CNS.[28] Whereas supratentorial ependymomas are commonly found to have a RELA fusion with increased NFkB signaling, spinal cord ependymomas (grades II and III) more commonly have NF2 mutation.[28,29] Subependymomas (WHO grade I) most commonly have been found to have a 6q deletion, while myxopapillary ependymomas (WHO grade I) are generally discussed separately since they commonly occur in the lumbar cistern and affect the conus medullaris and filum terminale.[29]

Hemangioblastomas are graded as WHO grade I and occur predominately in adults, with the peak incidence at the fourth decade for sporadic lesions and around the third decade of life for von Hippel–Lindau disease patients.[30] They are rare tumors and account for 2 to 6% of all spinal cord tumors, yet they are the third most common after astrocytomas and ependymomas.[31] They are generally well circumscribed and highly vascularized lesions that typically have a tumor nodule associated with a cystic structure.[32] Microscopically, they demonstrate capillary proliferation and are composed of both thin-walled vascular channels with interspersed intravascular tumor cells, known as stromal cells. These tumors do not exhibit necrosis and rarely have mitotic figures.[33] Approximately two-thirds occur spontaneously and around one-third are found in patients that have von Hippel–Lindau disease.[30] von Hippel–Lindau disease evolves from the autosomal dominant inheritance of the VHL gene on 3p25–26 with resultant increase in production of hypoxia-inducible factor (HIF). The metabolism shifts to anaerobic glycolysis and eventually stimulates secretion of factors that promote angiogenesis such as vascular endothelial growth factor (VEGF), platelet-derived growth factor (PDGF-β), erythropoietin (Epo), and transforming growth factor (TGF-α). This cascade affects the remodeling of the extracellular matrix and increases resistance to apoptosis and mobility of VEGF and erythropoietin, which create the tumor and the defective associated blood vessels.[34,35]

4.3.3 Radiology

On magnetic resonance imaging (MRI), IMSCTs normally appear as cord-expansile lesions. Commonly, these tumors are either isointense or hypointense on T1-weighted MRI, and hyperintense or isointense on T2-weighted imaging. In some cases, tumor-associated cysts may be present within or immediately rostral or caudal to the lesion. The presence of associate syringomyelia is common.[36] T2-weighted signal change in the surrounding spinal cord indicates edema associated with the tumor.

Astrocytomas are occasionally exophytic, with a portion of the tumor extending into the intradural extramedullary compartment component. As mentioned, astrocytomas typically have poorly defined margins, which may be apparent on imaging studies (▶ Fig. 4.1). Peritumoral edema is present in approximately 40% of cases, intratumoral cysts are present in about 20%, and peritumoral cysts are present in 15%.[37] Unlike ependymomas, hemorrhage is also uncommon and the enhancement pattern in astrocytomas is also a bit different and helps to differentiate it from other IMSCTs, since it is with a variable degree of contrast enhancement and with usual pattern of patchy enhancement.[37]

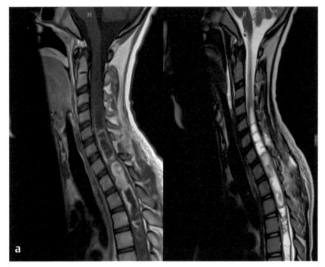

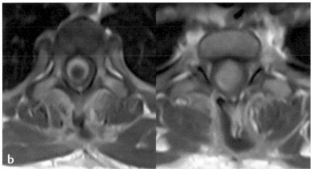

Fig. 4.1 Cervicothoracic spinal cord astrocytoma in **(a)** sagittal and **(b)** axial views. There is positive enhancement with poorly defined border. Adjacent cysts can be seen as well.

Ependymomas tend to be centrally located, growing from the ependymal cells lining the central canal. They are generally well circumscribed with homogenous contrast enhancement, although they do not have capsules (▶ Fig. 4.2). The typical imaging features differentiating astrocytomas from ependymomas are their location within the spinal cord (astrocytomas are eccentric while ependymomas are more central), presence of hemorrhage (more common in ependymomas), hemosiderin staining (more common for ependymomas), contrast enhancement (ependymomas demonstrate homogeneous enhancement, while astrocytomas are patchy), and presence of cysts (more common for ependymomas). Especially in T2-weighted imaging, peritumoral edema can be seen usually in 60% of cases and the more distinctive pattern is associated hemorrhage and hemosiderin staining that leads to the well-known "cap sign" (a hypointense hemosiderin rim) that can be visualized in up to one-third of the cases.[38,39]

Hemangioblastomas are well-circumscribed lesions presenting as a vividly enhancing nodule commonly associated with a cyst (▶ Fig. 4.3). Yet, although spinal hemangioblastomas usually appear as discrete nodules, there can be diffuse cord expansion as well as tumoral cyst, subarachnoid hemorrhage, or even hematomyelia.[38,40] The presence of syringomyelia is very common (50–100%).[38] They are slightly more common in the thoracic cord (50%) compared to the cervical cord (40%) and most commonly are eccentric and have an exophytic component.[41] Spinal hemangioblastomas can also present with "cap sign" due to their hemosiderin staining.[38,40]

4.4 Clinical Presentation

The duration and quality of clinical symptoms are highly variable with IMSCTs. Typically, IMSCTs exhibit indolent growth, which corresponds to their underlying slow and progressive clinical symptomatology. Therefore, it is not surprising that delays in diagnosis are fairly common and hence patients are

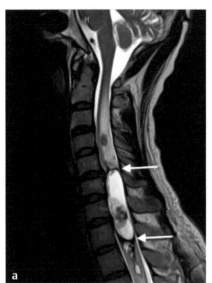
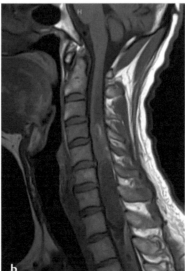
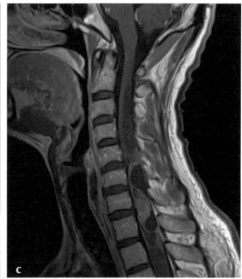

Fig. 4.2 Sagittal views of cervicothoracic ependymoma in **(a)** T2, **(b)** T1 with gadolinium and, **(c)** T1 without gadolinium. *White arrows* mark the "cap sign," which is the hypointense hemosiderin rim that can be commonly seen in ependymomas and in some hemangioblastomas as well.

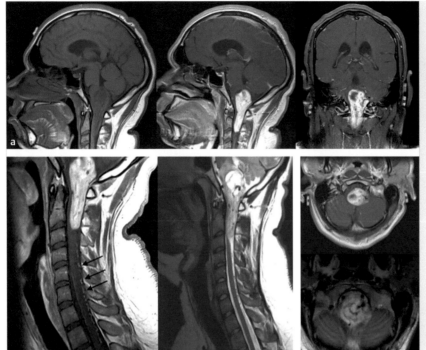

Fig. 4.3 Medullary cervical hemangioblastoma compressing the structures in the foramen magnum. Sagittal and coronal views **(a)** of contrast and noncontrast T1 sequences with vivid enhancement after administration of gadolinium. Sagittal views **(b)** of the cervical spine reveal engorgement of superficial veins common in spinal hemangioblastoma (*black arrows*). Axial views **(c)** of the tumor show the significant compression on the nearby structures.

eventually presented with big tumors with significant compromise of the spinal cord (▶ Fig. 4.4). Pain is the most frequent presenting symptom, often with axial back or neck pain and, occasionally, radicular pain due to nerve root impingement. Nocturnal pain can also be present related to the diurnal variation of endogenous steroid production. The expansile nature of IMSCTs can affect any of the traversing spinal cord tracts and structures in their vicinity. Weakness may occur due to corticospinal tract or lower motor neuron involvement. Sensory impairment, including numbness or paresthesia, may occur due to dorsal horn and spinothalamic tract impairment. Long tract impairment may result in gait ataxia and limb stiffness. Additionally, late-occurring findings can include bowel and bladder dysfunction, usually indicative of a more advanced disease state. Scoliosis is another possible presenting sign in children, a phenomenon likely occurring as a result of impaired innervation to the paraspinal musculature. Hence, it is a well-established practice that every kid who is diagnosed with scoliosis should have a spinal MRI in order to rule out spinal tumor or vascular lesion.[42]

Establishing baseline functionality is critical. The McCormick classification and Karnofsky performance scales are useful in defining the preoperative functional status of a patient.[43] Motor weakness and sensory impairment will typically be detected on examination, as well as long tract signs including positive Hoffman's and Babinski's signs, and general hyper-reflexia.

The reported average duration of symptoms prior to diagnosis of spinal cord tumors is between 8.1 and 17 months.[5,44] After identification and assessment, treatment with surgical resection is typically pursued to reduce the likelihood of symptom progression. Indications for surgical management include MRI findings of IMSCT in the setting of neurological symptoms localizable to the lesion, the presence of a cyst or

syrinx that is progressing or causing symptoms, and the need for pathological identification through tissue diagnosis. Occasionally, IMSCTs may be an incidental finding without any neurological symptoms, in which case conservative management may be considered.

4.5 Treatment

In some cases of clinically silent, incidentally found lesions, such as those discovered following trauma, serial monitoring and watchful waiting may be appropriate (▶ Fig. 4.4). However, for symptomatic or progressively enlarging lesions suspicious for IMSCTs, surgical intervention is the mainstay of treatment. The goals of surgery are to obtain a diagnosis and to decompress the spinal cord by performing a maximal tumor cytoreduction without causing a new permanent neurological deficit. Several groups have reported their experience with surgical resection of low-grade IMSCTs.[43,45,46,47] In experienced hands, gross total resection (GTR) can be achieved in a significant proportion of IMSCTs. Spinal ependymomas typically demonstrate clear surrounding tissue planes that facilitate tumor extirpation in their entirety. However, given the infiltrative nature of low-grade astrocytomas, tumor margins are often blurred and incorporated with normal neural structures, making total removal more challenging. The extent of resection for both ependymomas and astrocytomas was shown to be a significant prognostic factor.[11,48] Yet, a surgeon should always aim for maximal safe resection. Sending frozen section during surgery is important since in cases of high-grade gliomas, the surgeon should consider aiming for debulking only rather than gross total removal, although the last one is preferable when safely possible.[11,49]

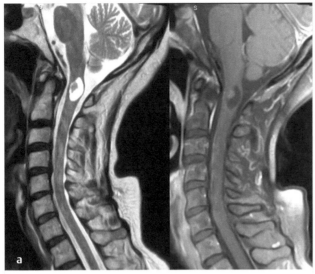

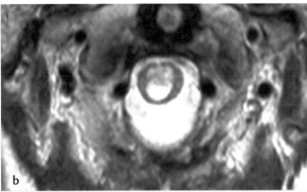

Fig. 4.4 (a, b) Cervical ependymoma that was diagnosed incidentally and was followed for 8 years without any change either in clinical symptoms or in signs or radiology parameters.

4.5.1 Surgical Intervention Nuances

- For cervical or high cervicothoracic IMSCTs, the head is placed in three-point fixation. When the lesion is mid or lower thoracic to upper lumbar, there is no need to fix the head in three-point fixation.
- Intraoperative neurophysiological monitoring is critical in providing the surgeon with real-time feedback regarding the functionality of longitudinal spinal cord tracts. This typically consists of somatosensory evoked potentials (SSEPs), motor-evoked potentials (MEPs), and epidural D-wave potentials, which are indicative of functioning corticospinal tract units below the level of resection.[50,51] Some advocate that for some cases surgery can be done without neuromonitoring, yet the authors believe that neuromonitoring should be part of the regular armamentarium for these surgeries.
- Midline skin incision and standard subperiosteal dissection are performed to expose the laminae of interest. Laminectomies or an osteoplastic laminoplasty can be performed to provide exposure of the thecal sac. Care should be taken not to disrupt the facet joints, which can lead to iatrogenic instability of the spinal column and future deformity. The bony exposure should extend above and below the lesion to allow adequate room for tumor resection

without significant spinal cord retraction or manipulation. Yet, exposure should be to an extent to suffice for safe and efficient intramedullary dissection without compromising unnecessary bony levels.

- Use of an osteoplastic laminoplasty, which allows for re-affixation of the posterior bony elements following tumor removal, has been shown to have some positive effect on decreasing the incidence of postoperative spinal deformity requiring fusion in the pediatric population. In addition, a trend toward a decreased rate of CSF leak has also been observed across age groups.[52,53]
- Following removal of the laminae, intraoperative ultrasound can provide further transdural tumor localization. At this time, the surgeon can also determine whether there is sufficient bone removal for tumor resection by identifying its upper and lower poles and augmenting the bony exposure if necessary.
- Epidural electrodes are subsequently placed for D-wave monitoring. For lower cervical and most of thoracic levels we advocate the use of both lower and upper D-wave. The later serves as control in case there is a loss of potentials (e.g., in case there is sharp decrease in D-wave potentials and the upper D-wave is down as well, it is more suggestive for artifact or even drop in mean arterial pressure rather than true injury at the surgical site).
- Use of an operating microscope is essential for IMSCT resection, typically brought into the field before or after dural opening, and before myelotomy.
- A midline durotomy is performed with placement of tenting sutures. Surrounding epidural cottonoids help to wick blood from the epidural space, preventing blood entry into the intradural space. Once the dura is opened sufficiently, it is important to survey the spinal cord and make note of irregularities such as rotation, focal prominence and bulging, or discoloration near the cord surface.
- Myelotomy is typically done at the midline at the dorsal median sulcus. Yet, it is important to consider tumor laterality, if any, when considering the location in which to perform the myelotomy. Special attention should be paid to surface veins, which dive inwards within the dorsal median sulcus, and the dorsolateral sulcus which can help orient the surgeon in cases of cord rotation and irregularity.
- Once the myelotomy is performed, retraction may cause diminished SSEPs due to dorsal column manipulation. The myelotomy should extend a sufficient length to have access to the tumor poles. The tumor typically lies several millimeters below the cord surface. Yet, care should be taken not to extend the myelotomy over normal cord just to have the tip of the pole in hand, since in a lot of cases once the core is decompressed the dissection over the poles is much easier and hence unnecessary normal cord dissection is avoided.
- Once the tumor substance is encountered, it may be useful to first obtain a few small specimens with a small tumor forceps for frozen section pathological examination to ensure a high likelihood of obtaining a definitive diagnosis. Following this, the remainder of the resection can be performed. Use of bipolar cautery should be limited as thermal injury can harm the surrounding normal neural structures, resulting in loss of function heralded by changes in neurophysiological monitoring. Effective resection can be achieved with gentle

tumor manipulation and dissection from surrounding structures. The surrounding plane between the tumor and spinal cord is sometimes easily discernible and in other situations, especially for infiltrative astrocytomas, it is less well defined. The presence of a syrinx may enhance resectability given the fluid filled space that, when decompressed, creates increased room for tumor manipulation.[54] For encapsulated lesions, tumor removal can be achieved by circumferential dissection of the lesion away from normal tissue. However, in many cases this is not possible and internal tumor debulking is necessary. Gentle suction and dissection can be effective in removing the tumor, but with firmer lesions an ultrasonic aspirating device or contact laser probe may be required for cytoreductive debulking.

- In some cases, GTR can be achieved, but in other instances this is not feasible without causing significant neurological deficit. Therefore, a surgeon's judgment is critical in determining when tumor resection should cease, regardless of whether remnant tumor is present. Neurophysiological monitoring should play an important role in this surgical decision. Evaluated together with MEPs, which are either present or absent (all-or-none), epidural D-wave monitoring provides valuable real-time feedback regarding the number of functional corticospinal tract units below the level of the lesion. This graded potential serves as a threshold at which a neurological deficit can be expected, and when interpreted in combination with MEPs, whether a deficit is likely to be transient or permanent.[55,56] Commonly, a D-wave threshold of 50% reduction is interpreted as a threshold at which tumor resection should cease. A drop of the MEPs in light of 50% reduction in D-wave potential will lead to postoperative transient deficit. If D-wave potential is decreased by more than 50% the postoperative deficit will be most likely permanent and should be avoided.
- Some groups advocate the use of dynamic monitoring with electrified ultrasonic aspirator or suction that allows approximation of the distance of the corticospinal tracts from the active resection site.[57]
- The intraoperative work is synchronized between the surgeon, the neuromonitoring team, and the anesthesiologist. Mean arterial pressure should be kept above 70 and in case of drop in potentials should be considered to be raised to a higher level in order to allow better perfusion to the spinal cord. The neuromonitoring team should advise the surgeon on any change and the surgeon in return should consider making a change at the specific site that is being manipulated, at the level of retraction or even to completely cease working until some recovery is noticed in the neuromonitoring.
- Once tumor resection is completed, meticulous hemostasis should be obtained with a variety of hemostatic agents, and if needed low-intensity bipolar cautery. The dura should be closed in a watertight fashion to decrease the likelihood of postoperative CSF leak. Use of a fibrin sealant may add additional protective effect against this complication following dural closure. We recommend waiting to remove the epidural D-wave electrodes until after dural closure is complete. If utilized, the laminoplasty should be re-affixed with miniplates, with special care taken to avoid epidural

compression of the thecal sac, and we tend to apply the bone back in such a way that the laminae and spinous process are a bit prominent and hence create a comparatively larger epidural space in case of postoperative swelling. The muscular fascia is closed in a watertight fashion and a layered superficial closure is preferred.

4.6 Surgical Outcome

The location, type, and size of the tumor affect the surgical outcome. An extensive tumor extending over multiple segments requires a more extensive myelotomy, which can disrupt the dorsal column tracts. With the use of intraoperative neuromonitoring, which allows the surgeon to be more aggressive, acute but transient postoperative decline is not unusual.[11] Up to one-third of patients will experience worsening of their neurologic status during their postoperative hospital course. Yet, approximately 25 to 41% of these patients who are acutely worse will revert back to at least their preoperative status within 6 months of surgery.[11,58] A good outcome following surgery is dependent on the preoperative functional status of the patient, the general tumor burden, the presence of surgical plane between the tumor and the normal structures, and the final pathology.

The resection of intramedullary astrocytomas presents unique challenges. A higher morbidity is associated with radical resection of astrocytomas in some reports. Clinical recurrence rates of partially excised astrocytomas are around 18 to 35%. Overall, GTR is possible for low-grade and high-grade astrocytomas in about 40 to 50% of cases regardless of tumor histology.[11,48,58,59,60,61] The ability to achieve GTR in spinal cord astrocytomas improved significantly in the last decades and progressed from quarter of the cases to almost half of the cases.[48] The resection of ependymomas poses a different challenge for the surgeon, since recurrence rates of ependymomas are dependent upon the extent of tumor resection.[62] Recent reports have cited a GTR rate of around 90 to 93% for ependymomas.[58]

Due to the low incidence of other IMSCTs, reports of clinical outcomes are much scarcer in comparison to other CNS tumors. In general, a radical resection for any IMSCT has been correlated with long-term survival.[63,64] Although in the past some studies suggested a low effect of GTR on progression-free survival and survival in general, recent data suggest that better extent of resection correlates with better results and correlates to the data we experienced in recent years with regard to brain gliomas.[10,11,19,48,65]

4.7 Adjuvant Therapy

Aggressive surgical intervention for IMSCTs has yielded excellent outcomes with minimal mortality and excellent quality of life.[66] Morbidity in the form of a new neurological deficit is often temporary and a postoperative decrease in more than one functional grade is rare.[46] Although radical tumor resection is the mainstay of treatment, adjuvant therapy may be applicable in some cases. Some groups have reported their experiences with an approach involving surgery for biopsy or partial resection followed by radiation therapy in cases of incomplete resection.[67,68] However, in recent years a better understanding of IMSCT led to advocating maximal safe resection rather than just biopsy. This is specifically true in pediatric cases, when controversy arises with possible radiation toxicity inducing growth retardation, secondary malignancy development, myelopathy, and spinal deformity requiring fusion. Radiation therapy is reserved as a last resort in the treatment of children with IMSCTs. Given that majority of the IMSCTs are low-grade lesions, the response to radiation is ambiguous. Additionally, if further intervention is required down the line, radiation can create difficulty discerning between tumor progression or radiation effect, as well as produce significant intraoperative challenges from scarring, potentially making second-look surgery hard to carry on. Although microsurgery may allow for GTR, microscopic cellular infiltration warrants continued monitoring over time. These cellular remnants may never progress, even over significant periods of time. If relapses or recurrences occur, repeat surgery or chemotherapy should be considered. In patients with lesions that are not surgically amenable, who do not tolerate chemotherapy, or those who have rapidly progressing malignant lesions, radiation therapy may play a role, although the benefit is not completely clear.[19]

The role of chemotherapy for IMSCTs is not clear-cut, as no randomized controlled trial has been performed evaluating its efficacy in this particular population of patients. Various chemotherapeutic and radiation therapy options have been utilized for spinal cord glioblastoma in an attempt to achieve even a small increase in survival in a dire patient population.[69] Carboplatin-based chemotherapy, typically used for intracranial low-grade gliomas, has been proposed as a possible adjunct treatment for IMSCTs, with some anecdotal evidence suggestive of satisfactory outcomes.[70]

Overall, the treatment approach for growing or symptomatic IMSCTs should be microsurgery with maximal safe tumor resection. If a satisfactory resection is achieved, interval monitoring can be applied. Even if small tumor remnants exist postoperatively, this can be carefully observed with serial imaging. With large recurrences, repeat surgery may be needed and for inoperable cases, adjuvant therapy, preferably with chemotherapy as a first-line intervention, is appropriate. In cases of high-grade lesions, postoperative treatment is warranted because of the high likelihood for microcellular spread that is beyond the obvious tumor, and since in many cases of infiltrative tumor GTR is not amenable as part of safe resection.

4.8 Conclusion

Spinal intramedullary tumors in the pediatric and the adult population are rare entities and are considered one of the complex entities for treatment in neurosurgery and neuro-oncology. For symptomatic patients or those who have impending radiographic images, maximal safe resection by an experienced surgeon should be the first step. The use of multi-modalities in the operative room as well as in the postoperative possible adjuvant treatment is important. The primary care physicians as well as pediatricians and neurologists should recognize the possibility for IMSCTs when assessing the patient with suspected new back pain or even new neurological deficit in order to prevent delayed diagnosis that will hamper the chances to get good clinical results for the patient.

References

[1] The diagnosis, localisation, and surgical treatment of tumours pressing on the spinal cord. Hospital (Lond 1886). 1892; 12(289):26–27

[2] Lloyd S. III. Chipault on the surgery of the spinal cord. Ann Surg. 1892; 16(6): 550–553

[3] Pendleton C, Rincon-Torroella J, Gokaslan ZL, Jallo GI, Quinones-Hinojosa A. Challenges in early operative approaches to intramedullary spinal cord tumors: Harvey Cushing's perspective. J Neurosurg Spine. 2015; 23(4):412–418

[4] Sciubba DM, Liang D, Kothbauer KF, Noggle JC, Jallo GI. The evolution of intramedullary spinal cord tumor surgery. Neurosurgery. 2009; 65(6) Suppl: 84–91, discussion 91–92

[5] Segal D, Lidar Z, Corn A, Constantini S. Delay in diagnosis of primary intradural spinal cord tumors. Surg Neurol Int. 2012; 3:52

[6] Copp AJ, Greene ND. Neural tube defects—disorders of neurulation and related embryonic processes. Wiley Interdiscip Rev Dev Biol. 2013; 2(2):213–227

[7] Jessell TM. Neuronal specification in the spinal cord: inductive signals and transcriptional codes. Nat Rev Genet. 2000; 1(1):20–29

[8] Copp AJ, Stanier P, Greene ND. Neural tube defects: recent advances, unsolved questions, and controversies. Lancet Neurol. 2013; 12(8):799–810

[9] Chamberlain MC, Tredway TL. Adult primary intradural spinal cord tumors: a review. Curr Neurol Neurosci Rep. 2011; 11(3):320–328

[10] Minehan KJ, Brown PD, Scheithauer BW, Krauss WE, Wright MP. Prognosis and treatment of spinal cord astrocytoma. Int J Radiat Oncol Biol Phys. 2009; 73(3):727–733

[11] Garcés-Ambrossi GL, McGirt MJ, Mehta VA, et al. Factors associated with progression-free survival and long-term neurological outcome after resection of intramedullary spinal cord tumors: analysis of 101 consecutive cases. J Neurosurg Spine. 2009; 11(5):591–599

[12] Babu R, Karikari IO, Owens TR, Bagley CA. Spinal cord astrocytomas: a modern 20-year experience at a single institution. Spine. 2014; 39(7):533–540

[13] Milano MT, Johnson MD, Sul J, et al. Primary spinal cord glioma: a surveillance, epidemiology, and end results database study. J Neurooncol. 2010; 98(1):83–92

[14] Cooper PR. Outcome after operative treatment of intramedullary spinal cord tumors in adults: intermediate and long-term results in 51 patients. Neurosurgery. 1989; 25(6):855–859

[15] Spain JA, Cressman S, Marin H, Patel SC, Corrigan JJ, Griffith B. Cord topographical anatomy and its role in evaluating intramedullary lesions. Curr Probl Diagn Radiol. 2018; 47(6):437–444

[16] Kresak JL, Walsh M. Neurofibromatosis: a review of NF1, NF2, and schwannomatosis. J Pediatr Genet. 2016; 5(2):98–104

[17] Binning M, Klimo P , Jr, Gluf W, Goumnerova L. Spinal tumors in children. Neurosurg Clin N Am. 2007; 18(4):631–658

[18] Allen JC, Aviner S, Yates AJ, et al. Children's Cancer Group. Treatment of high-grade spinal cord astrocytoma of childhood with "8-in-1" chemotherapy and radiotherapy: a pilot study of CCG-945. J Neurosurg. 1998; 88(2):215–220

[19] Luksik AS, Garzon-Muvdi T, Yang W, Huang J, Jallo GI. Pediatric spinal cord astrocytomas: a retrospective study of 348 patients from the SEER database. J Neurosurg Pediatr. 2017; 19(6):711–719

[20] Zhang J, Wu G, Miller CP, et al. St. Jude Children's Research Hospital–Washington University Pediatric Cancer Genome Project. Whole-genome sequencing identifies genetic alterations in pediatric low-grade gliomas. Nat Genet. 2013; 45(6):602–612

[21] Jones DT, Hutter B, Jäger N, et al. International Cancer Genome Consortium PedBrain Tumor Project. Recurrent somatic alterations of FGFR1 and NTRK2 in pilocytic astrocytoma. Nat Genet. 2013; 45(8):927–932

[22] Pfister S, Janzarik WG, Remke M, et al. BRAF gene duplication constitutes a mechanism of MAPK pathway activation in low-grade astrocytomas. J Clin Invest. 2008; 118(5):1739–1749

[23] Bar EE, Lin A, Tihan T, Burger PC, Eberhart CG. Frequent gains at chromosome 7q34 involving BRAF in pilocytic astrocytoma. J Neuropathol Exp Neurol. 2008; 67(9):878–887

[24] Sievert AJ, Jackson EM, Gai X, et al. Duplication of 7q34 in pediatric low-grade astrocytomas detected by high-density single-nucleotide polymorphism-based genotype arrays results in a novel BRAF fusion gene. Brain Pathol. 2009; 19(3):449–458

[25] Forshew T, Tatevossian RG, Lawson AR, et al. Activation of the ERK/MAPK pathway: a signature genetic defect in posterior fossa pilocytic astrocytomas. J Pathol. 2009; 218(2):172–181

[26] Chiang JC, Ellison DW. Molecular pathology of paediatric central nervous system tumours. J Pathol. 2017; 241(2):159–172

[27] Vettermann FJ, Neumann JE, Suchorska B, et al. K27 M midline gliomas display malignant progression by imaging and histology. Neuropathol Appl Neurobiol. 2017; 43(5):458–462

[28] Lee CH, Chung CK, Kim CH. Genetic differences on intracranial versus spinal cord ependymal tumors: a meta-analysis of genetic researches. Eur Spine J. 2016; 25(12):3942–3951

[29] Khatua S, Ramaswamy V, Bouffet E. Current therapy and the evolving molecular landscape of paediatric ependymoma. Eur J Cancer. 2017; 70:34–41

[30] Liu A, Jain A, Sankey EW, Jallo GI, Bettegowda C. Sporadic intramedullary hemangioblastoma of the spine: a single institutional review of 21 cases. Neurol Res. 2016; 38(3):205–209

[31] Mehta GU, Asthagiri AR, Bakhtian KD, Auh S, Oldfield EH, Lonser RR. Functional outcome after resection of spinal cord hemangioblastomas associated with von Hippel–Lindau disease. J Neurosurg Spine. 2010; 12(3):233–242

[32] Boström A, Hans FJ, Reinacher PC, et al. Intramedullary hemangioblastomas: timing of surgery, microsurgical technique and follow-up in 23 patients. Eur Spine J. 2008; 17(6):882–886

[33] Hussein MR. Central nervous system capillary haemangioblastoma: the pathologist's viewpoint. Int J Exp Pathol. 2007; 88(5):311–324

[34] Niu X, Zhang T, Liao L, et al. The von Hippel–Lindau tumor suppressor protein regulates gene expression and tumor growth through histone demethylase JARID1C. Oncogene. 2012; 31(6):776–786

[35] Haddad NM, Cavallerano JD, Silva PS. Von hippel–Lindau disease: a genetic and clinical review. Semin Ophthalmol. 2013; 28(5–6):377–386

[36] Jones BV. Cord cystic cavities: syringomyelia and prominent central canal. Semin Ultrasound CT MR. 2017; 38(2):98–104

[37] Seo HS, Kim JH, Lee DH, et al. Nonenhancing intramedullary astrocytomas and other MR imaging features: a retrospective study and systematic review. AJNR Am J Neuroradiol. 2010; 31(3):498–503

[38] Koeller KK, Rosenblum RS, Morrison AL. Neoplasms of the spinal cord and filum terminale: radiologic-pathologic correlation. Radiographics. 2000; 20(6):1721–1749

[39] Sun B, Wang C, Wang J, Liu A. MRI features of intramedullary spinal cord ependymomas. J Neuroimaging. 2003; 13(4):346–351

[40] Baker KB, Moran CJ, Wippold FJ , II, et al. MR imaging of spinal hemangioblastoma. AJR Am J Roentgenol. 2000; 174(2):377–382

[41] Chu BC, Terae S, Hida K, Furukawa M, Abe S, Miyasaka K. MR findings in spinal hemangioblastoma: correlation with symptoms and with angiographic and surgical findings. AJNR Am J Neuroradiol. 2001; 22(1):206–217

[42] Huisman TA. Pediatric tumors of the spine. Cancer Imaging. 2009; 9 Spec No A:S45–S48

[43] McCormick PC, Torres R, Post KD, Stein BM. Intramedullary ependymoma of the spinal cord. J Neurosurg. 1990; 72(4):523–532

[44] Grimm S, Chamberlain MC. Adult primary spinal cord tumors. Expert Rev Neurother. 2009; 9(10):1487–1495

[45] Kutluk T, Varan A, Kafalı C, et al. Pediatric intramedullary spinal cord tumors: a single center experience. Eur J Paediatr Neurol. 2015; 19(1):41–47

[46] Constantini S, Miller DC, Allen JC, Rorke LB, Freed D, Epstein FJ. Radical excision of intramedullary spinal cord tumors: surgical morbidity and long-term follow-up evaluation in 164 children and young adults. J Neurosurg. 2000; 93(2) Suppl:183–193

[47] McGirt MJ, Chaichana KL, Atiba A, Attenello F, Woodworth GF, Jallo GI. Neurological outcome after resection of intramedullary spinal cord tumors in children. Childs Nerv Syst. 2008; 24(1):93–97

[48] Azad TD, Pendharkar AV, Pan J, et al. Surgical outcomes of pediatric spinal cord astrocytomas: systematic review and meta-analysis. J Neurosurg Pediatr. 2018; 22(4):404–410

[49] Konar SK, Bir SC, Maiti TK, Nanda A. A systematic review of overall survival in pediatric primary glioblastoma multiforme of the spinal cord. J Neurosurg Pediatr. 2017; 19(2):239–248

[50] Sala F, Skinner SA, Arle JE, et al. Letter: guidelines for the use of electrophysiological monitoring for surgery of the human spinal column and spinal cord. Neurosurgery. 2018; 83(2):E82–E84

[51] Legatt AD, Emerson RG, Epstein CM, et al. ACNS guideline: transcranial electrical stimulation motor evoked potential monitoring. J Clin Neurophysiol. 2016; 33(1):42–50

[52] McGirt MJ, Chaichana KL, Atiba A, et al. Incidence of spinal deformity after resection of intramedullary spinal cord tumors in children who underwent laminectomy compared with laminoplasty. J Neurosurg Pediatr. 2008; 1(1):57–62

[53] McGirt MJ, Garcés-Ambrossi GL, Parker SL, et al. Short-term progressive spinal deformity following laminoplasty versus laminectomy for resection of intradural spinal tumors: analysis of 238 patients. Neurosurgery. 2010; 66(5):1005–1012

[54] Samii M, Klekamp J. Surgical results of 100 intramedullary tumors in relation to accompanying syringomyelia. Neurosurgery. 1994; 35(5):865–873, discussion 873

[55] Jallo GI, Freed D, Epstein F. Intramedullary spinal cord tumors in children. Childs Nerv Syst. 2003; 19(9):641–649

[56] Kothbauer K, Deletis V, Epstein FJ. Intraoperative spinal cord monitoring for intramedullary surgery: an essential adjunct. Pediatr Neurosurg. 1997; 26(5):247–254

[57] Barzilai O, Lidar Z, Constantini S, Salame K, Bitan-Talmor Y, Korn A. Continuous mapping of the corticospinal tracts in intramedullary spinal cord tumor surgery using an electrified ultrasonic aspirator. J Neurosurg Spine. 2017; 27(2):161–168

[58] Samartzis D, Gillis CC, Shih P, O'Toole JE, Fessler RG. Intramedullary spinal cord tumors: Part II-Management options and outcomes. Global Spine J. 2016; 6(2):176–185

[59] Nakamura M, Ishii K, Watanabe K, et al. Surgical treatment of intramedullary spinal cord tumors: prognosis and complications. Spinal Cord. 2008; 46(4):282–286

[60] Raco A, Piccirilli M, Landi A, Lenzi J, Delfini R, Cantore G. High-grade intramedullary astrocytomas: 30 years' experience at the Neurosurgery Department of the University of Rome "Sapienza." J Neurosurg Spine. 2010; 12(2):144–153

[61] Yang S, Yang X, Hong G. Surgical treatment of one hundred seventy-four intramedullary spinal cord tumors. Spine. 2009; 34(24):2705–2710

[62] Vijayakumar S, Estes M, Hardy RW , Jr, Rosenbloom SA, Thomas FJ. Ependymoma of the spinal cord and cauda equina: a review. Cleve Clin J Med. 1988; 55(2):163–170

[63] Jallo GI, Danish S, Velasquez L, Epstein F. Intramedullary low-grade astrocytomas: long-term outcome following radical surgery. J Neurooncol. 2001; 53(1):61–66

[64] Jallo GI, Freed D, Epstein FJ. Spinal cord gangliogliomas: a review of 56 patients. J Neurooncol. 2004; 68(1):71–77

[65] Raco A, Esposito V, Lenzi J, Piccirilli M, Delfini R, Cantore G. Long-term follow-up of intramedullary spinal cord tumors: a series of 202 cases. Neurosurgery. 2005; 56(5):972–981, discussion 972–981

[66] Schneider C, Hidalgo ET, Schmitt-Mechelke T, Kothbauer KF. Quality of life after surgical treatment of primary intramedullary spinal cord tumors in children. J Neurosurg Pediatr. 2014; 13(2):170–177

[67] Minehan KJ, Shaw EG, Scheithauer BW, Davis DL, Onofrio BM. Spinal cord astrocytoma: pathological and treatment considerations. J Neurosurg. 1995; 83(4):590–595

[68] O'Sullivan C, Jenkin RD, Doherty MA, Hoffman HJ, Greenberg ML. Spinal cord tumors in children: long-term results of combined surgical and radiation treatment. J Neurosurg. 1994; 81(4):507–512

[69] Hernández-Durán S, Bregy A, Shah AH, Hanft S, Komotar RJ, Manzano GR. Primary spinal cord glioblastoma multiforme treated with temozolomide. J Clin Neurosci. 2015; 22(12):1877–1882

[70] Hassall TE, Mitchell AE, Ashley DM. Carboplatin chemotherapy for progressive intramedullary spinal cord low-grade gliomas in children: three case studies and a review of the literature. Neuro-oncol. 2001; 3(4):251–257

5 Electrophysiological Testing for Intramedullary Spinal Tumor Surgery

Tito Vivas-Buitrago, Luca Ricciardi, William Clifton III, Anteneh M. Feyissa, Karim ReFaey, and Alfredo Quinones-Hinojosa

Summary

Intramedullary spinal cord tumors (IMSCTs) represent about 20% of all intraspinal tumors and 2 to 4% of the tumors in the central nervous system, with low-grade ependymomas (more frequent in adults) and low-grade astrocytomas (in children) being the most commonly found. Surgical resection is the first line of treatment and is currently the most effective one, but still represents a high risk for transient or permanent postoperative neurologic complications associated with spinal cord injury during the procedure. Intraoperative neurophysiologic monitoring (IONM) may help decrease postoperative deficits by detecting variations in neurophysiologic function (NF) during surgery. Early identification of NF changes may guide surgeons during the surgical resection, providing feedback that allows appropriate modifications in their strategy and in some cases interrupt the ongoing surgery before the damage becomes irreversible. In this chapter, we describe the fundamental monitoring techniques utilized during the resection of intramedullary tumors including somatosensory and motor evoked potentials, D-waves, dorsal column mapping, and spontaneous electromyography.

Keywords: intramedullary tumors, somatosensory evoked potentials, motor evoked potentials, D-waves, dorsal column mapping, spontaneous electromyography, H-waves

5.1 IONM Types

5.1.1 Somatosensory Evoked Potentials (SSEPs)

SSEPs provide information from the sensory pathways by applying electric stimulation in a peripheral nerve which is then conducted throughout the nervous pathway up to the cortex and recorded for intraoperative functionality monitoring.[1,2,3,4,5] Distal stimulated nerves are usually the posterior tibial nerve (L4–S2), with electrode placement at the medial malleolus, and the median or ulnar nerve (C5–T1) using the wrist as the electrode location.[6] Registration sites include the skin at the plexuses levels (peripheral nerves), the cervical spine (dorsal columns), and the contralateral hemi-scalp (somatosensory cortex).[7] ▶ Fig. 5.1 shows an example of SSEPs' monitoring. Recordings can be obtained throughout the surgical procedure since there is no risk of involuntary patient movement. Signal changes can occur in amplitude and/or latency, and its interpretation may be controversial in some situations. However, a significant decrease in amplitude by more than 50% or an increase in latency above 10% of the readings at baseline should be considered as a high risk for postoperative deficits, with higher correlation for sensory deficits such as proprioception.[8,9] It has been reported that SSEPs can identify insults to the spinal cord with a sensitivity of 92% and a specificity of 98.9%.[10] SSEPs are not intended to reliably provide information status from the motor pathways and assuming so has led to "false negatives" reported by several studies in which patients developed a postoperative motor deficit despite normal intraoperative SSEPs monitoring.[11,12,13,14,15] Strict anesthetic level cutoff values are not necessary when running SSEPs, but levels must be low enough to allow a strong and stable signal.

5.1.2 Motor Evoked Potentials (MEPs)

Having a dedicated motor function monitoring technique is essential given the SSEPs' difficulties to monitor the anterior cord, which is the anatomical location of the motor structures. MEPs stimulate the upper motor neurons and conduct the electric input throughout the pyramidal tract, all the way to the muscles where the stimulus is recorded, allowing monitoring and assessment of the descending corticospinal motor pathways. This technique was approved by the FDA in 2002.[7,16,17,18,19] Stimulation of the primary motor cortex can be implemented by applying electrical impulses through electrodes placed at the scalp.[9,20,21] Techniques to record MEPs after transcranial stimulation include myogenic recorded MEPs (mTc-MEPs) with percutaneous electrodes placed in the upper and lower extremities, and D-wave recordings from electrodes at the epidural or subdural space, placed rostral and caudal to the tumor location (▶ Fig. 5.1).

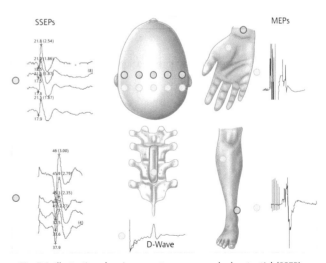

Fig. 5.1 Illustration showing somatosensory evoked potential (SSEP) regions of stimulation at the upper and lower extremities, and scalp regions of signal recording represented with *blue points*. Transcranial motor evoked potential (MEP) stimulation areas in the scalp, and muscle group recording sites at the upper and lower extremities are represented with *yellow points*.

5.1.3 Myogenic Tc-MEPs (mTc-MEPs)

mTc-MEPs monitor the muscular action potentials, and if present indicate the functionality of the motor system. They also provide more specific data for muscle groups status, which are of special help when assessing for lateralized weakness at the upper or lower extremities.[9,22,23,24] Common muscles used for recording are the tibialis anterior and abductor hallucis in the lower extremities, and the abductor pollicis and extensor digitorum in the upper extremities.[4,10] ▶ Fig. 5.1 shows an example of mTc-MEPs monitoring. Readings can be affected by commonly used neuromuscular blocking agents like halogenated anesthetics.[25,26,27] mTc-MEPs are not collected continuously but an on-demand stimulation is performed based on the surgeon's judgment and demand since stimulation often provokes involuntary muscle movements that pose a risk for injury during the dissection/resection. mTc-MEP signals can be categorized as polyphasic, biphasic, and absent, where a degradation from polyphasic to biphasic signal can predict a decrease of one to two points in the Medical Research Council (MRC) motor score, and absence of evocable response implicates irreversible neurological compromise.[4,24,28] Decreased or nonnoticeable potentials allow surgeons to correct their surgical strategy in order to minimize postsurgical deficit risk. Recommended strategies in the presence of signal changes are illustrated in ▶ Table 5.1.

5.1.4 D-wave

D-wave monitoring identifies corticospinal action potentials initiated by activation of fast axonal fibers with higher sensitivity in detecting early injury to the spine.[29,30] D-wave readings are obtained through electrodes placed in the spinal epidural or subdural space, rostral and caudal to the tumor.[9,24,31] The rostral electrode serves as the control because it detects signals from the cortex before being transmitted through the distorted tumor environment. Recordings from the caudal electrode are then compared with the rostral, and changes in the peak-to-peak amplitude of D-waves by 50% or increase in latency by 10% are considered abnormal.[7,32,33] Stable mTc-MEPs and D-waves during surgery allow the surgeon to continue the

tumor resection with more confidence. However, in cases when there is a change or loss of signal in mTc-MEPs or D-waves, actions may be necessary to avoid permanent motor deficits. These corrective measures are illustrated in ▶ Table 5.1.[22] In addition, neuromuscular blocking agents used during surgical procedures do not affect recordings. D-wave monitoring is not reliable below T12 since there are not enough corticospinal fibers. This technique does not provide information regarding the status of specific muscle groups.[22]

5.1.5 Dorsal Column Mapping (DCM)

Identification of the medial dorsal median sulcus is critical when performing the myelotomy to access IMSCT. This is the region of the column with less to no physiological electrical conductivity and is commonly found in the midline. DCM is of particular help in cases of IMSCT where the tumor distorts the spinal cord anatomy. Mapping is carried out with the implantation of thin needle electrodes in the lower extremities to record the impulses from adjacent peripheral nerves, followed by stimulation of the dorsal column with a lateral to medial orientation using a bipolar probe until the zone with the lowest amplitude or no response is identified.[17,34]

5.1.6 Hoffmann's Reflex

H-reflex monitoring emerged recently due to the SSEPs' and MEPs' limitation to provide a continuous monitoring of the motor function during spinal surgery.[35,36] Although not the gold standard in IONM, it is mainly used when SSEPs or MEPs cannot be obtained due to pre-existing neurological alterations.[36] In the H-reflex, an electrical afferent activation originates from the muscle's large 1a nerve fibers which is conducted to the dorsal horn of the spinal cord where it synapses with the motor neurons, followed by an efferent response that involves orthodromic motor conduction through the motor fibers at the same level as the afferent pathway.[37] The electrical activity involved in this reflex is then recorded by electromyography to detect H-waves and assess the circuitry integrity at the targeted level in a continuous manner.[36,38] The gastrocnemius and flexor carpi

Table 5.1 Combined motor evoked potentials data interpretation and suggested corrective measures

D-wave	Muscle MEPs	Corrective measures	Predicted outcome
Unchanged	Present	None	Unchanged
Unchanged or decrease by more than 50%	Present with minor changes (decreased amplitude or increased threshold)	Transiently move to a different area; warm irrigation; correct hypotension	Unchanged
Unchanged or decrease by less than 50%	Unilaterally or bilaterally lost	All of the above, then transiently stop surgery and/or improve spinal cord blood flow (local irrigation with papaverine). If mMEPs do not reappear, terminate surgery in selective cases; as a rule, surgery can continue.	Transient motor deficit (affecting the involved extremity)
Decrease by more than 50%	Bilaterally lost	Stop surgery immediately. If D-waves do not recover, terminate surgery.	Permanent motor deficit
Unmonitorable	Bilaterally lost	All of the above. If mMEPs do not recover, terminate surgery.	Cannot differentiate between transient and permanent motor deficit

Abbreviations: MEP, motor evoked potential; mMEP, myotonic motor evoked potential.
Source: Adapted from Sala et al,[7] with permission from Oxford University Press.

Table 5.2 Comparison of the characteristics of various spinal cord monitoring techniques

Modality	Speed Response	Anatomic sensitivity	Anesthesia	Criteria for abnormality	Comments
Tc-MEP (Muscle-MEP)	++++	Corticospinal tract Anterior horn cell	TIVA optimal Nitrous oxide and halogenated inhalational agents reduce amplitudes Neuromuscular blockade reduces responses	Many 1. 100 V increase in threshold 2. Absence 3. Various levels of amplitude decline 4. Simplification of waveform	Well established
Tc-MEP (D-wave)	++	Corticospinal tract	Minimal anesthesia effects	50% decline in amplitude	Well established
SSEP	+	Dorsal column sensory pathways	Cortical potentials reduced with high concentrations of halogenated anesthetic agents	Generally accepted: 1. 50% decline in amplitude 2. 10% increase in latency Varies with surgical procedure and anesthesia	Well established
H-reflex	++	Propriospinal motor pathways Corticospinal tract Spinal gray matter Anterior horn cell	TIVA optimal Neuromuscular blockade reduces responses	Variable	Awaiting additional studies

* + Indicates the time.
Source: Adapted from Stecker.[42]

radialis muscles are usually used for recording.[35] Some studies suggest that a sustained intraoperative suppression > 90% of the H-reflex amplitude correlates with postoperative deficits.[16, 36,39,40] H-reflexes are less affected by halogenated anesthetics when compared to Tc-MEPs.[40,41] A summary with a comparison of some of the abovementioned IONM techniques is available in ► Table 5.2.[42]

5.1.7 Electromyography (EMG)

Depolarization and subsequent muscle contraction can be determined by direct nerve compression or manipulation. A simple intramuscular needle may detect those stimulations far better than skin electrodes. However, complete neurotmesis may occur without any noticeable variation in EMG. The "free-run" or "continuous" EMG is most commonly used in intraoperative monitoring, allowing surgeons to notice variations in real time, although "triggered" EMG could be useful in peripheral nerve identification or during instrumented spinal surgeries to estimate proximity to nerve roots. The main limitation in some regions is the feasibility of placing an intramuscular electrode for recording.[17,34]

5.2 Case Illustration

A 17-year-old female presented with an 18-month history of intermittent numbness in the anterior upper thigh and inguinal region, as well as mild lumbar pain. Neurological examination revealed normal upper and lower bilateral extremity strength: + 3 right knee and ankle reflex compared to + 2 left knee/ankle, negative Hoffman's and Babinski's reflex, and negative ankle clonus. Decreased sensation to touch on the upper thigh and inguinal regions. A magnetic resonance imaging (MRI) scan revealed a nonenhancing, intramedullary lesion centered to the right of midline extending from upper T10 to T12 vertebral level, measuring 1.6 cm by 6.0 cm in transverse and craniocaudal dimensions, respectively (► Fig. 5.2).

5.2.1 Surgical Procedure and IONM

The patient was kept under general endotracheal anesthesia. Postinduction SSEPs baseline responses were well defined and reproducible with normal latencies and morphology from bilateral ulnar and posterior tibial nerves. mTc-MEPs displayed compound muscle action potentials with excellent morphology and repeatability from upper and lower extremities bilaterally. Thoracic vertebrae levels 9th, 10th, and 11th were identified under fluoroscopy guidance. Skin incision and paraspinal muscles dissection were carried out, followed by a laminoplasty of the 9th, 10th, and 11th vertebrae. Dura was exposed and intact. Ultrasound was used to identify the tumor margins followed by the dural opening. DCM was performed, and the medial dorsal sulcus was found at midline. A myelotomy was carried out in this location. There was no identifiable plane between the tumor and the spinal cord. The tumor was very vascular (► Fig. 5.3a).

Preliminary intraoperative report from the frozen specimen was consistent with a low-grade glioma. An ultrasonic aspirator was used for tumor debulking. After resection of approximately 80% of the tumor, SSEPs signal decreased by more than 50% in the right popliteal nerve. MEPs were requested and showed a decrement greater than 90% in the right leg and foot response amplitude (► Fig. 5.3c). The procedure was stopped momentarily, warm irrigation was applied, and mean arterial pressure was increased by 10 to 15 torr without signal recovery. Surgery was terminated, and the dura was closed. There was no significant loss of Tc-MEPs response amplitudes by more than 90%, no sharp rise in thresholds greater than 100 V, and no acute and sustained change in polyphasic to biphasic morphology of the responses from the left lower or right upper extremities during the procedure. The decrease in right posterior tibial somatosensory responses and the right lower extremity MEPs persisted during closing.

Postoperatively, the patient presented with right leg and foot weakness: Right hip flexion 4/5, able to raise leg off the bed and

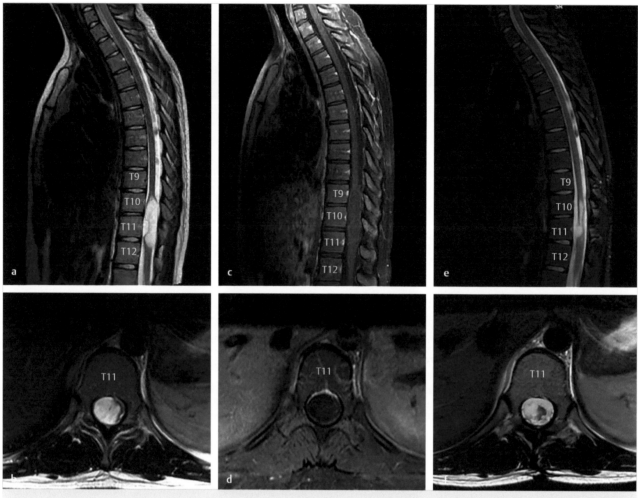

Fig. 5.2 Preoperative T2-weighted sagittal **(a)** and axial **(b)**, and T1-weighted with contrast sagittal **(c)** and axial **(d)** magnetic resonance imaging (MRI) scans, showing the patient's large intramedullary mass extending from T10 to T12. Postoperative T2-weighted sagittal **(e)** and axial **(f)** MRI scan showing the residual tumor.

provide some resistance, 4 + /5 leg adduction and abduction, 4 + /5 dorsi and plantar flexion. The patient showed decreased sensation to light touch in both lower extremities: R 25% and L 35% (leg). The final pathology report was consistent with an astrocytoma (WHO grade II). After 3 months of intense physical therapy the patient showed complete recovery.

5.3 Discussion

The evidence-based role of the diagnostic ability of IONM (SSEPs, Tc-MEPs, and D-wave) to predict postoperative deficits have been well established. D-waves have demonstrated to be the most predictive marker of postsurgical deficits. EMG seems to anticipate mTc-MEPs deterioration in case of pathway injuries. In cases in which D-waves monitoring is not available, EMG implementation to mTc-MEPs may result effectively in detecting early and continuous signal changes. This has been established by levels I and II evidence-based studies.[43]

The prognostic implications of intraoperative monitoring changes have not been as clearly established. There has been no high level (I or II) evidence to suggest that the use of IONM improves postoperative deficits or intraoperative neurologic deterioration.[43] This has been studied both in cases of spinal cord tumor resection as well as complex scoliosis surgery. A recent publication by Harel et al delineated a retrospective review of patients undergoing resection of intramedullary spinal cord tumors compared to historical controls without the use of monitoring.[44] The result was a statistically insignificant difference in the rates of the new postoperative neurological deficits between the two groups. The remainder of the literature is composed of lower evidence-based studies (III) that have created more questions than answers with variable results.[43] It is clear that the diagnostic value of IONM has been well proven by high levels of evidence; however, how the intraoperative findings and changes in monitoring translated into patient outcomes and improved care has yet to be thoroughly studied.

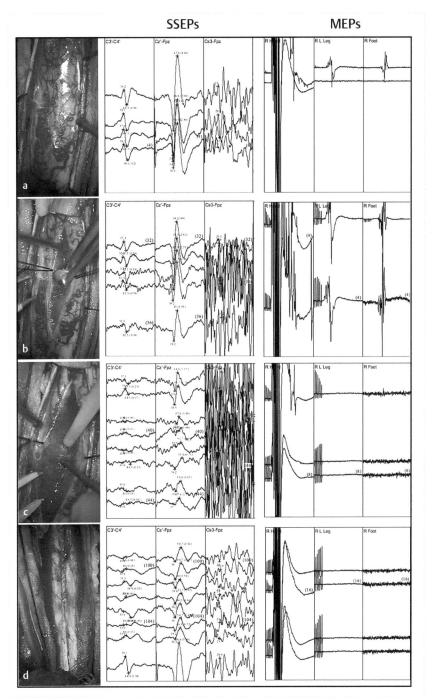

Fig. 5.3 Intraoperative microscopic view of the intramedullary spinal cord tumor. Increased vascularization at the level of the tumor is noticed **(a)**. Myelotomy and biopsy are performed after identification of the medial dorsal sulcus **(b)**. Tumor debulking with the aid of an ultrasonic aspirator; a decrease greater than 50% in somatosensory evoked potentials (SSEPs) and greater than 90% for Tc-MEP is observed in the right leg during resection of the tumor **(c)**. Dural closure after interruption of the procedure due to decreased SSEP and motor evoked potential (MEP) signals and no response to recovery maneuvers **(d)**.

5.4 Conclusion

IONM is a commonly used tool to assist neurologic surgeons in the resection of intramedullary spinal cord tumors. The diagnostic value of this tool is instrumental in predicting postoperative deficits following spinal cord surgery. However, the prognostic and therapeutic implications of intraoperative changes have yet to be established. The treating neurosurgeon must understand the benefits and limitations of this tool in order to provide the highest level of care to patients with intramedullary tumors. Although not currently a standard of care, further studies investigating the therapeutic implications of this tool may continue to shape the field and increase the usefulness of this technology.

References

[1] Macon JB, Poletti CE. Conducted somatosensory evoked potentials during spinal surgery. Part 1: control conduction velocity measurements. J Neurosurg. 1982; 57(3):349–353

[2] Macon JB, Poletti CE, Sweet WH, Ojemann RG, Zervas NT. Conducted somatosensory evoked potentials during spinal surgery. Part 2: clinical applications. J Neurosurg. 1982; 57(3):354–359

[3] Nuwer MR, Aminoff M, Desmedt J, et al. International Federation of Clinical Neurophysiology. IFCN recommended standards for short latency

somatosensory evoked potentials. Report of an IFCN committee. Electroencephalogr Clin Neurophysiol. 1994; 91(1):6–11

[4] Cheng JS, Ivan ME, Stapleton CJ, Quinones-Hinojosa A, Gupta N, Auguste KI. Intraoperative changes in transcranial motor evoked potentials and somatosensory evoked potentials predicting outcome in children with intramedullary spinal cord tumors. J Neurosurg Pediatr. 2014; 13(6):591–599

[5] Verla T, Fridley JS, Khan AB, Mayer RR, Omeis I. Neuromonitoring for intramedullary spinal cord tumor surgery. World Neurosurg. 2016; 95: 108–116

[6] Owen JH. The application of intraoperative monitoring during surgery for spinal deformity. Spine. 1999; 24(24):2649–2662

[7] Sala, F., Palandri, G., Basso, E., Lanteri, P., Deletis, V., Faccioli, F., & Bricolo, A. Motor evoked potential monitoring improves outcome after surgery for intramedullary spinal cord tumors: a historical control study. Neurosurgery. 2006; 58(6), 1129–1143.

[8] Dawson EG, Sherman JE, Kanim LE, Nuwer MR. Spinal cord monitoring. Results of the Scoliosis Research Society and the European Spinal Deformity Society survey. Spine. 1991; 16(8) Suppl:S361–S364

[9] Kothbauer K, Deletis V, Epstein FJ. Intraoperative spinal cord monitoring for intramedullary surgery: an essential adjunct. Pediatr Neurosurg. 1997; 26(5): 247–254

[10] Nuwer MR, Dawson EG, Carlson LG, Kanim LE, Sherman JE. Somatosensory evoked potential spinal cord monitoring reduces neurologic deficits after scoliosis surgery: results of a large multicenter survey. Electroencephalogr Clin Neurophysiol. 1995; 96(1):6–11

[11] Lesser RP, Raudzens P, Lüders H, et al. Postoperative neurological deficits may occur despite unchanged intraoperative somatosensory evoked potentials. Ann Neurol. 1986; 19(1):22–25

[12] Ginsburg HH, Shetter AG, Raudzens PA. Postoperative paraplegia with preserved intraoperative somatosensory evoked potentials. Case report. J Neurosurg. 1985; 63(2):296–300

[13] Kelleher MO, Tan G, Sarjeant R, Fehlings MG. Predictive value of intraoperative neurophysiological monitoring during cervical spine surgery: a prospective analysis of 1055 consecutive patients. J Neurosurg Spine. 2008; 8(3):215–221

[14] Pelosi L, Jardine A, Webb JK. Neurological complications of anterior spinal surgery for kyphosis with normal somatosensory evoked potentials (SEPs). J Neurol Neurosurg Psychiatry. 1999; 66(5):662–664

[15] Zornow MH, Grafe MR, Tybor C, Swenson MR. Preservation of evoked potentials in a case of anterior spinal artery syndrome. Electroencephalogr Clin Neurophysiol. 1990; 77(2):137–139

[16] Deletis V, Sala F. Intraoperative neurophysiological monitoring of the spinal cord during spinal cord and spine surgery: a review focus on the corticospinal tracts. Clin Neurophysiol. 2008; 119(2):248–264

[17] Quiñones-Hinojosa A, Lyon R, Zada G, et al. Changes in transcranial motor evoked potentials during intramedullary spinal cord tumor resection correlate with postoperative motor function. Neurosurgery. 2005; 56(5): 982–993, discussion 982–993

[18] Choi I, Hyun SJ, Kang JK, Rhim SC. Combined muscle motor and somatosensory evoked potentials for intramedullary spinal cord tumour surgery. Yonsei Med J. 2014; 55(4):1063–1071

[19] Quiñones-Hinojosa A, Lyon R, Du R, Lawton MT. Intraoperative motor mapping of the cerebral peduncle during resection of a midbrain cavernous malformation: technical case report. Neurosurgery. 2005; 56(2) Suppl:E439–, discussion E439 discussion E

[20] Gugino LD, Romero JR, Aglio L, et al. Transcranial magnetic stimulation coregistered with MRI: a comparison of a guided versus blind stimulation technique and its effect on evoked compound muscle action potentials. Clin Neurophysiol. 2001; 112(10):1781–1792

[21] Calancie B, Harris W, Broton JG, Alexeeva N, Green BA. "Threshold-level" multipulse transcranial electrical stimulation of motor cortex for intraoperative monitoring of spinal motor tracts: description of method and comparison to somatosensory evoked potential monitoring. J Neurosurg. 1998; 88(3):457–470

[22] Sala F, Palandri G, Basso E, et al. Motor evoked potential monitoring improves outcome after surgery for intramedullary spinal cord tumors: a historical control study. Neurosurgery. 2006; 58(6):1129–1143, discussion 1129–1143

[23] Sala F, Lanteri P, Bricolo A. Motor evoked potential monitoring for spinal cord and brain stem surgery. Adv Tech Stand Neurosurg. 2004; 29:133–169

[24] Morota N, Deletis V, Constantini S, Kofler M, Cohen H, Epstein FJ. The role of motor evoked potentials during surgery for intramedullary spinal cord tumors. Neurosurgery. 1997; 41(6):1327–1336

[25] Taniguchi M, Schramm J. Motor evoked potentials facilitated by an additional peripheral nerve stimulation. Electroencephalogr Clin Neurophysiol Suppl. 1991; 43:202–211

[26] Kalkman CJ, Drummond JC, Patel PM, Sano T, Chesnut RM. Effects of droperidol, pentobarbital, and ketamine on myogenic transcranial magnetic motor-evoked responses in humans. Neurosurgery. 1994; 35(6):1066–1071

[27] Kalkman CJ, Drummond JC, Ribberink AA, Patel PM, Sano T, Bickford RG. Effects of propofol, etomidate, midazolam, and fentanyl on motor evoked responses to transcranial electrical or magnetic stimulation in humans. Anesthesiology. 1992; 76(4):502–509

[28] Herdmann J, Lumenta CB, Huse KO. Magnetic stimulation for monitoring of motor pathways in spinal procedures. Spine. 1993; 18(5):551–559

[29] Park JH, Hyun SJ. Intraoperative neurophysiological monitoring in spinal surgery. World J Clin Cases. 2015; 3(9):765–773

[30] Macdonald DB, Skinner S, Shils J, Yingling C, American Society of Neurophysiological Monitoring. Intraoperative motor evoked potential monitoring—a position statement by the American Society of Neurophysiological Monitoring. Clin Neurophysiol. 2013; 124(12):2291–2316

[31] Jallo GI, Kothbauer KF, Epstein FJ. Intrinsic spinal cord tumor resection. Neurosurgery. 2001; 49(5):1124–1128

[32] Muramoto A, Imagama S, Ito Z, et al. The cutoff amplitude of transcranial motor evoked potentials for transient postoperative motor deficits in intramedullary spinal cord tumor surgery. Spine. 2014; 39(18):E1086–E1094

[33] Forster MT, Marquardt G, Seifert V, Szelényi A. Spinal cord tumor surgery—importance of continuous intraoperative neurophysiological monitoring after tumor resection. Spine. 2012; 37(16):E1001–E1008

[34] Mehta AI, Mohrhaus CA, Husain AM, et al. Dorsal column mapping for intramedullary spinal cord tumor resection decreases dorsal column dysfunction. J Spinal Disord Tech. 2012; 25(4):205–209

[35] Leppanen RE. Intraoperative applications of the H-reflex and F-response: a tutorial. J Clin Monit Comput. 2006; 20(4):267–304

[36] Feyissa AM, Tummala S. Intraoperative neurophysiologic monitoring with Hoffmann reflex during thoracic spine surgery. J Clin Neurosci. 2015; 22(6): 990–994

[37] Misiaszek JE. The H-reflex as a tool in neurophysiology: its limitations and uses in understanding nervous system function. Muscle Nerve. 2003; 28(2): 144–160

[38] Cottrell JE, Young WL. Cottrell and Young's Neuroanesthesia. Elsevier Health Sciences; 2016

[39] Leis AA. Physiology of acute spinal cord injury (SCI) in humans. I. Behavior of the H-reflex and F-wave immediately following injury to rostral spinal cord in humans. J Clin Neurophysiol. 1997; 14(4):347

[40] Leis AA, Kronenberg MF, Stětkárová I, Paske WC, Stokić DS. Spinal motoneuron excitability after acute spinal cord injury in humans. Neurology. 1996; 47(1):231–237

[41] Zhou HH, Mehta M, Leis AA. Spinal cord motoneuron excitability during isoflurane and nitrous oxide anesthesia. Anesthesiology. 1997; 86(2):302–307

[42] Stecker MM. A review of intraoperative monitoring for spinal surgery. Surg Neurol Int. 2012; 3 Suppl 3:S174–S187

[43] Hadley MN, Shank CD, Rozzelle CJ, Walters BC. Guidelines for the use of electrophysiological monitoring for surgery of the human spinal column and spinal cord. Neurosurgery. 2017; 81(5):713–732

[44] Harel R, Schleifer D, Appel S, Attia M, Cohen ZR, Knoller N. Spinal intradural extramedullary tumors: the value of intraoperative neurophysiologic monitoring on surgical outcome. Neurosurg Rev. 2017; 40(4):613–619

6 Intramedullary Spinal Cord Tumors: Current Research and Potential Therapeutics

Nikki M. Barrington, Tania M. Aguilar, James S. Ryoo, and Ankit I. Mehta

Summary

Although intramedullary spinal cord tumors are auspiciously rare, their scarcity in patient populations makes them challenging to study and develop adequate treatment paradigms. Nevertheless, a variety of surgical and nonsurgical treatment options are presently in use, with many novel treatment modalities currently under study in animal models that may emerge as promising human therapies in the coming years. The mainstay of treatment for virtually all intramedullary spinal cord tumors is gross total resection, and as such many studies have focused on the efficacy and safety of a variety of intraoperative imaging modalities and intraoperative monitoring techniques that allow for safer and more complete resection of tumors, some of which were previously considered inoperable. In addition to operative therapies, adjuvant radiation therapy and chemotherapy are used in the treatment of intramedullary spinal cord tumors, and recent research has focused on improving the precision of radiotherapies and advances in targeted irradiation of tumor tissues. Chemotherapies, historically limited by challenges of tissue penetration and systemic toxicity, have recently emerged as promising treatment options alongside a variety of targeted drug delivery systems, from tumor genotype-specific therapies to nanomedicine-based therapies, all of which aim to increase chemotherapeutic efficacy while minimizing toxic side effects. Taken together, these budding therapeutic advances suggest that individualized, targeted, and localized therapies represent the future of intramedullary spinal cord tumor treatment.

Keywords: intraoperative imaging, augmented reality, localized drug delivery

6.1 Epidemiology of Intramedullary Spinal Cord Tumors

Intramedullary spinal cord tumors are considered rare, comprising only 2 to 4% of all central nervous system (CNS) tumors.[1,2] The most common types of intramedullary spinal cord tumors are ependymomas and astrocytomas, both of which are considered gliomas. Ependymomas are the most common intramedullary spinal cord tumor type among adults, while astrocytomas are more common among children and adolescents.[1,2,3] Astrocytomas more commonly present as low-grade tumors (WHO grade I or II). Other less-common intramedullary spinal cord tumor types include hemangioblastomas, gangliogliomas, paragangliomas, primary CNS lymphomas, melanomas, and epidermoid cysts.[1,2,3] Hemangioblastomas are tumors derived from mesenchymal stem cells of CNS vascular structures and are most commonly seen in the cerebellum, but 13% appear in the spinal cord.[1,2] Gangliogliomas, although rare, are most commonly found in the pediatric population and are derived from both glial and ganglion cells as the name implies.[1,2] Lastly, intramedullary spinal cord metastases are exceedingly rare, representing 1 to 3% of all intramedullary spinal cord tumors and typically originating from lung cancers, breast cancers, or lymphoma (▶ Table 6.1).[1,2,4,5]

6.2 Diagnosis of Intramedullary Spinal Cord Tumors

Intramedullary spinal cord tumors can represent a diagnostic challenge because they can present with a variety of symptoms, the most common of which is diffuse back pain, but other presenting symptoms can include paresthesias, loss of vibratory or proprioception, spasticity, and weakness.[1,6] Diagnosis of intramedullary spinal cord tumors in the pediatric population can be particularly challenging as these tumors typically present with nonspecific symptoms.[1] Magnetic resonance imaging (MRI) can be used to reliably diagnose specific types of intramedullary spinal cord tumors as each type exhibits unique characteristics. MRI qualities and signal characteristics for intramedullary spinal cord tumor types have been well described.[1,3]

A recent retrospective chart review study[7] found that 89% of preoperative diagnoses were correct. The authors describe a

Table 6.1 Intramedullary spinal cord tumors

Tumor	Incidence	Location	Prognosis
Ependymoma	Most common (50–60% of IMSCTs)	Cervical > thoracic > lumbar	Good
Myxopapillary ependymoma	Rare	Filum terminale and conus medullaris	Excellent
Astrocytoma	Second most common	Cervical > thoracic > lumbar	Poor
Hemangioblastoma	Very rare; increased incidence in VHL disease patients	Cervical > thoracic > lumbar	Excellent
GCT	Very rare	Cervical > thoracic > lumbar	Good
Ganglioglioma	Rare	Cervical > thoracic > lumbar	Good
CNS lymphoma	Rare	Cervical > thoracic > lumbar	Poor
Melanoma	Very rare	Cervical > thoracic > lumbar	Poor

Abbreviations: CNS, central nervous system; GCT, giant cell tumor; IMSCTs, intramedullary spinal cord tumors; VHL, von Hippel-Lindau.
Source: Reproduced with permission from Tobin et al.[2]

Table 6.2 Simplified intramedullary spinal cord tumor diagnostic paradigm

	Spinal cord swelling	Contrast effect	Homogenous contrast effect	Central on axial imaging
Ependymoma	✓	✓		✓
Astrocytoma	✓			
Hemangioblastoma	✓	✓	✓	
Other disease				

Source: Adapted from Arima et al.[7]

simplified diagnostic paradigm based on four MRI characteristics that can be used to accurately diagnose intramedullary spinal cord tumors including spinal cord swelling, contrast effect, homogeneity of contrast effect, and central location on axial imaging (▶ Table 6.2).

6.3 Current Research and Potential Surgical Therapies for Intramedullary Spinal Cord Tumors

6.3.1 Introduction

Gross total resection (GTR) is the primary treatment for both ependymomas and astrocytomas; however, ependymomas are typically more amenable to GTR given their clear plane of dissection,[2] while astrocytomas tend to be more infiltrative in nature and therefore more difficult to resect. Astrocytomas with higher tumor grade and infiltrative tumor pathology as well as those that are treated via subtotal resection (STR) have been associated with worse prognosis.[8] Due to these challenges, astrocytomas were historically more likely to be managed with biopsy and medical therapies[6]; however, GTR has been shown to be successful, particularly with low-grade astrocytomas.[9] More recent research on the management of ependymomas and astrocytomas suggests that GTR improves overall survival in all tumor grades; however, radiation only improves overall survival in high-grade tumors.[10] Surgical management may improve survival due to advances in microsurgical techniques, intraoperative imaging modalities, and intraoperative neurophysiological monitoring, which have allowed for increased safety and efficacy in the operative management of intramedullary spinal cord tumors that were previously less amenable to resection.[11] With regard to the less common intramedullary spinal cord tumor types, the primary treatment is surgical resection for virtually all tumors including hemangioblastoma, germ cell tumors, gangliogliomas, and melanoma.[2] In the case of metastatic disease, clinical improvement has been seen in approximately half of the patients treated surgically, while conservative treatment maintains neurological status in most patients.[4] The following discussion elaborates on current research and recent advances in the surgical treatment of intramedullary spinal cord tumors.

6.3.2 Therapeutic Advances

Minimally Invasive Surgical Techniques

Minimally invasive surgical techniques for the resection of intramedullary spinal cord tumors have been in development for many years. These techniques were originally applied to intradural extramedullary tumors and then adapted to intramedullary tumors, with one of the first case reports describing resection of a thoracic intramedullary ependymoma using a muscle-splitting extended hemilaminar approach with a positive outcome.[12] Additional techniques have been developed over time, such as unilateral multilevel interlaminar fenestration (UMIF) for intraspinal lesions, including cervical intramedullary tumors.[13,14] As of 2014, research investigating the outcomes of minimally invasive approaches in intramedullary spinal cord tumors continued to be sparse as these techniques were still emerging; however, a minimally invasive approach for resecting these tumors had been described in detail.[15] More recently, a retrospective study evaluated outcomes of minimally invasive surgery for resection of spinal hemangioblastoma and found that all patients exhibited complete tumor resection on postoperative MRI with no perioperative or postoperative complications.[16] Though more outcomes-based studies are clearly necessary to fully evaluate minimally invasive surgical techniques for intramedullary spinal cord tumors, the available evidence suggests that these techniques are safe and effective.

Intraoperative Raman Spectroscopy

One of the challenges neurosurgeons face in resecting intramedullary spinal cord tumors is differentiating cancerous from normal tissue, and intraoperative imaging is a powerful tool that can allow surgeons to obtain more complete tumor resection. Raman spectroscopy has recently emerged as a noninvasive method by which to differentiate between diseased and normal tissues. In Raman spectroscopy spectra that result from the inelastic scattering of incident light can be used to rapidly identify various molecular species within a given tissue, including proteins, lipids, nucleic acids, and carbohydrates.[17,18,19] Though the physics of Raman spectroscopy is beyond the scope of this chapter, this technology has been used in recent years for intraoperative detection of brain tumor cells. One study of a handheld intraoperative Raman spectroscopy device reported 93% sensitivity and 91% specificity for detection of cancer cells in patients with grade II to grade IV gliomas.[17] This modality has several potential uses including superior assessment of tumor margins intraoperatively, without the need to wait for specimen evaluation by a pathologist.[18] Though Raman spectroscopy data can be complex, advanced analytical techniques such as feature engineering have recently been applied to improve molecular profiling of glioma.[20] As of this writing, intraoperative Raman spectroscopy has yet to be studied in the resection of intramedullary spinal cord tumors. However, given the infiltrative nature of certain tumor types such as

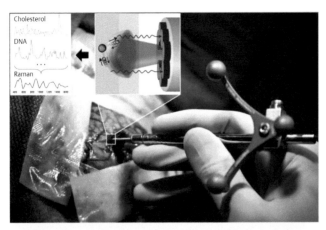

Fig. 6.1 A handheld contact fiber optic probe for Raman spectroscopy (Emvision, LLC) shown interrogating brain tissue during surgery. The diagram shows how excitation of various molecules (*blue* and *green*) via laser light (red) produces Raman scattering (*purple*), resulting in distinct spectra in cancerous tissue relative to normal brain tissue. (From Jermyn et al.[17] Reprinted with permission from AAAS.)

astrocytoma, Raman spectroscopy is a promising imaging modality by which neurosurgeons might improve the efficacy and safety of surgical resection for intramedullary spinal cord tumors in the future (▶ Fig. 6.1).

Intraoperative Fluorescence Imaging with 5-Aminolevulinic Acid

5-Aminolevulinic acid (5-ALA) is a precursor of hemoglobin that subsequently breaks down into fluorescent porphyrins in tumor tissue, particularly malignant glioma tissue, making it a useful agent for intraoperative imaging of intramedullary spinal cord tumors for many years.[21] In a randomized controlled multicenter phase III trial, investigators found that among patients with malignant glioma, 65% of patients randomly assigned to 5-ALA fluorescence imaging compared to 36% of patients randomly assigned to white light experienced complete resection, ultimately leading to increased survival in these patients.[21] In a case study of cordectomy as palliative treatment for intramedullary malignant glioma, intraoperative 5-ALA fluorescence imaging was found to be useful in assessing tumor invasion.[22] 5-ALA fluorescence can typically be detected using standard operating microscopes fitted with optical filters. Strong fluorescence using this method has been correlated with greater fluorescence using spectroscopy, and conversely weak fluorescence visualized on the operating microscope has been correlated with weaker fluorescence using spectroscopy.[23] Tumors with strong fluorescence have been shown to correspond with solid proliferation and high cell densities, whereas tumors with weak fluorescence have been shown to correspond with infiltrating tumor and medium cell densities. Furthermore, 5-ALA fluorescence imaging appears to be more effective in revealing residual tumor than contrast enhancement on MRI.[23] 5-ALA fluorescence may be more effective in detecting certain intramedullary spinal cord tumor types. In one study of 52 patients, 5-ALA fluorescence imaging detected all ependymomas, meningiomas, hemangiopericytomas, and metastases of primary

CNS tumors, but failed to detect any neurinomas, carcinoma metastases, or primary spinal gliomas (including a grade II astrocytoma and a grade III anaplastic oligoastrocytoma), in contrast to previous studies suggesting efficacy in detection of malignant spinal gliomas.[24] This discrepancy is further elucidated in a recent review of 5-ALA fluorescence-guided intraoperative imaging, which concluded that 5-ALA fluorescence imaging is most reliable and most commonly used in the setting of high-grade gliomas. In the context of low-grade gliomas, standard operating microscopes have a low detection rate for 5-ALA fluorescence. The authors propose that augmenting 5-ALA fluorescence with superior detection modalities such as spectrographic probes, confocal imaging, or scanning fiber endoscopes, all of which have been attempted with encouraging findings, may expand 5-ALA fluorescence imaging toward reliable detection of low-grade gliomas in the future.[25]

Other Intraoperative Imaging Modalities

Intraoperative angiography via near-infrared indocyanine green videoangiography (ICG-VA) has previously been used in vascular and tumor surgery to allow for evaluation of vascular flow. This imaging modality involves intravenous injection of indocyanine green immediately before each image is captured. This technique has been applied to intramedullary tumor resection in recent years in patients with a variety of intramedullary tumor types including ependymoma, astrocytoma, hemangioblastoma, and cavernous malformation.[26] ICG-VA allowed for successful visualization of spinal vascular anatomy including arteries and veins and most importantly allowed for differentiation of arteries feeding into tumors and veins draining from tumors from the tumor tissue itself.[26] This particular imaging modality allows for greater precision in intramedullary tumor resection and may be particularly useful in resection of highly vascular tumors.

Diffusion tensor imaging (DTI) and diffusion tensor-fiber tracking (DT-FT), otherwise known as tractography, are additional modalities that have been used for preoperative visualization of intramedullary spinal cord tumors to aid in surgical planning. DTI and DT-FT allow for evaluation of the direction of white matter tracts and have traditionally been used in the brain but can also be used in the spinal cord to determine the extent of tumor infiltration. DTI has been studied in pediatric populations with intramedullary spinal cord tumors and has been found to better define tumor margins and the location of tumor tissue relative to the white matter tracts of the spinal cord.[27] Certain characteristics including splaying and displacement of fiber tracts indicate tumor margins and can help determine the feasibility of surgical resection, whereas visualization of infiltration into white matter tracts suggests that biopsy may be a more ideal treatment method.[27]

Intraoperative magnetic resonance imaging (iopMRI), available for many years, has traditionally been used in the visualization of cranial tumors, particularly cerebral gliomas and pituitary adenomas.[28] Intraoperative MRI has improved over the years thanks to high-field magnets that have resulted in improved image quality. More recently, attempts have been made to use iopMRI in the resection of intramedullary spinal cord tumors. In a case series of two patients with diffuse cervical intramedullary glioma, high-field iopMRI was successfully utilized to visualize residual tumor; however, several difficulties were encountered in terms of adapting the iopMRI setup to cervical spine surgery and achieving ideal patient positioning.[28] This case report suggests that iopMRI may be a useful tool in intramedullary spinal cord tumor resection when adequately adapted to the unique challenges of spine surgery. That being said, some of the imaging modalities previously discussed, such as Raman spectroscopy, may ultimately allow for superior detection of tumor margins and/or residual tumor in the future.

Intraoperative Monitoring

Intraoperative monitoring (IOM) has been used in neurosurgical cases including intramedullary spinal cord tumor resections for decades. Originally this monitoring was only available in the form of somatosensory evoked potentials (SEPs), changes in which presumably reflected spinal cord dysfunction. However, SEPs are not directly representative of motor pathways and as such some patients with no changes in SEPs might experience postoperative motor deficits.[29] Conversely, it is also possible that patients with changes in SEPs may not experience postoperative motor deficits, potentially resulting in an unnecessarily terminated or incomplete tumor resection in patients who would have otherwise experienced a successful outcome.[29] These challenges limited the usefulness of IOM in intramedullary spinal cord surgeries. More recently, motor evoked potentials (MEPs) have been monitored in combination with SEPs, especially in the context of intramedullary spine surgery. Following transcranial electrical stimulation (TES), both muscle (mMEPs) and epidural MEPs (D-wave) are monitored to ensure the functional integrity of corticospinal pathways, particularly during the most critical components of the operation. Changes in mMEPs and D-waves allow the surgeon to make decisions in real time about whether or not to proceed with tumor debulking based on the risk of causing a transient or permanent motor deficit.[29] Changes in MEP waveform, loss of the MEP waveform, and decreased duration of the MEP in response to TES have been significantly associated with motor loss.[30] In addition to these IOM modalities, more recently both spontaneous and triggered electromyography have been used in conjunction with SEPs and MEPs to help detect nerve root injuries, known as combined multimodal intraoperative neuromonitoring.[31] Electromyography has also been used in conjunction with microstimulation of motor fibers via a bipolar probe and subsequent monitoring of corresponding muscle groups to map corticospinal tracts intraoperatively. This technique allows for the differentiation of motor pathways from tumor tissue while resecting intramedullary tumors, and was successful in preserving motor tracts in the case of a patient with cervicomedullary junction cystic ependymoma.[32] Combining IOM modalities has also been shown to be useful in resection of intramedullary tumors in the pediatric population. One retrospective study determined that intraoperative transcranial MEPs and SEPs can predict postoperative motor deficits following intramedullary spinal cord tumor resection in pediatric patients.[33,34] This study noted that these modalities can be combined with dorsal column mapping, particularly for high-risk tumor locations such as the upper cervical spinal cord. As surgical approaches to intramedullary spinal cord tumor resection typically involve an incision in the dorsal median raphe between the two dorsal columns, dorsal column mapping utilizes neurophysiologic monitoring, such as amplitude changes in SEPs,[34] to differentiate between the median raphe and dorsal columns prior to incision. Taken together, the varied IOM modalities that have emerged as mainstays in intramedullary spinal cord tumor surgery over the past decade have allowed for safer tumor resection and resection of tumors that previously would not have been amenable to surgical treatment.

Genotype-Targeted Local Intraoperative Therapies

Individualized therapies based on tumor genotype continue to emerge as novel treatment strategies, particularly for intramedullary spinal cord gliomas. Recent advances in rapid genotyping tools have allowed for rapid intraoperative genotyping and subsequent targeting of tumors harboring mutations, making them susceptible to certain therapies. More specifically, Shankar et al[35] utilized intraoperative genotyping to identify tumors with isocitrate dehydrogenase 1 (IDH1) or IDH2 metabolic enzyme mutations, which are common in low-grade gliomas and make these tumors susceptible to certain chemotherapeutic agents. In addition to individualizing therapies based on tumor genotype, the authors developed a microparticle drug delivery system consisting of a drug compound encapsulated in a biodegradable copolymer to allow for sustained release and reduced systemic toxicity. This microparticle drug delivery system delivered a nicotinamide phosphoribosyltransferase (NAMPT) inhibitor (GMX-1778) targeting tumor cells with IDH mutations and subsequently demonstrated prolonged survival in a mouse model of spinal cord glioma. These results suggest that changes might be made to typical intraoperative workflows such that rapid genotyping of an initial surgical biopsy is completed during tumor resection. Following resection, the genotyping results indicating the tumor's chemotherapeutic susceptibilities subsequently determine the specific localized therapy applied to ensure tumor eradication, particularly at surgical margins. Fortunately, research on intramedullary spinal cord tumor therapeutics has begun to focus on identifying tumor mutations that may represent treatment targets. A recent study of spinal cord gliomas found NF2 mutations in 15.7% of tumors, RP1 mutations in 5.9% of tumors, and ESX1 mutations in 5.9% of tumors.[36] Though this particular study focused on gliomas, the concept of genotype-targeted local therapies could be readily applied to other intramedullary tumor types and drug compounds targeting other mutations.

Augmented Reality in Spinal Tumor Surgery

In addition to targeted intraoperative therapies, augmented reality implemented on the heads-up displays of operating microscopes, though available for many years, has only recently been studied in the context of spinal tumor surgery, though it has previously been used in cranial surgeries (▶ Fig. 6.2). A recent study[37] examining the safety of augmented reality in intradural spinal tumor surgery, including patients with a variety of tumor types (ependymoma, glioma, hemangioblastoma, meningioma, metastasis), found that operating microscope-based augmented reality can be applied reliably to spinal surgery and can assist with visualization of the tumor and surrounding

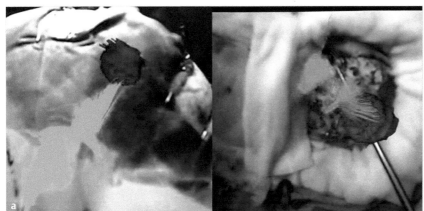

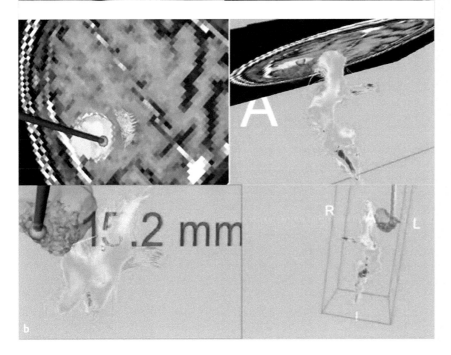

Fig. 6.2 (a) Augmented reality navigation monitor using a handheld web camera. A tumor (*red*) and motor tractography (*green*) were superimposed onto the patient's head before disinfection and after dural incision. (b) Upper: Dual three-dimensional (3D) layout display in 3D slicer. Lower: Distance between the bipolar tip and motor tractography was measured. (Reproduced with permission from Inoue D, Cho B, Mori M et al. Preliminary study on the clinical application of augmented reality neuronavigation. Journal of Neurological Surgery Part A Central European Neurosurgery 2013; 74(2): 071–076.)

structures. As discussed with regard to intraoperative imaging and monitoring, this technique may improve the GTR of challenging tumor types such as high-grade astrocytoma and other infiltrative tumors.

6.4 Current Research and Potential Systemic and Nonsurgical Therapies for Intramedullary Spinal Cord Tumors

6.4.1 Introduction

Although surgery continues to represent the foundation of treatment for intramedullary spinal cord tumors, both radiotherapy and chemotherapy have historically been used as adjuvant therapies in cases of subtotal resection, recurrence, or tumors that are considered inoperable due to extensive infiltration into nearby eloquent tissue.[2,3] In these cases, adjuvant radiotherapy is more commonly used than chemotherapy in the treatment of almost all intramedullary spinal cord tumors.[2]

Radiotherapy options include photon beam conformal radiotherapy (traditional radiation therapy) and proton beam radiotherapy, but therapeutic advances such as stereotactic radiosurgery have made radiation therapy much more precise, resulting in decreased radiation burden to normal tissues. One notable exception to adjuvant radiotherapy is CNS lymphoma presenting in the intramedullary spinal cord, in which case the primary treatment is intrathecal chemotherapy.[2,3] Additionally, the deleterious long-term side effects of radiation therapy in the pediatric population have historically resulted in the use of combination chemotherapeutic regimens including platinum and alkylating agents in these populations.[3] Such agents also have a role in the treatment of certain tumor types such as spinal germinomas, which can be treated with agents such as cisplatin, bleomycin, vinblastine, and etoposide.[6] For other tumor types such as astrocytoma and hemangioblastoma, chemotherapeutic regimens have employed antiangiogenic drugs and alkylating agents, both alone and in combination.[6] In the past, chemotherapeutic options were limited by both systemic toxicity and the challenge of drug penetration through the blood–spinal cord barrier. However, recent advances in personalized medicine and nanomedicine have made localized chemotherapy a promising treatment option for intramedullary spinal cord tumors, the details of which are presented in the discussion that follows.

6.4.2 Therapeutic Advances

Clinical Drug Trials

There are numerous completed and ongoing Phase 1 and Phase 2 clinical drug trials for intramedullary spinal cord tumors, particularly ependymoma and astrocytoma (▶ Table 6.3). The vast majority of these trials have studied combination chemotherapeutic regimens, but unfortunately most have not yet published results beyond Phase 1 maximum tolerated dosages and pharmacokinetic parameters. As many of these trials have studied combination therapies using antiangiogenic agent bevacizumab and/or alkylating agent temozolomide as part of therapy, further discussion of recent research on these therapies follows.

Bevacizumab and Temozolomide

In recent years, adjuvant temozolomide has become a more frequently used therapy in spinal cord gliomas. In a case report[49] of a 26-year-old woman with cervical intramedullary glioblastoma multiforme, the patient was treated with GTR, radiotherapy, and temozolomide, with subsequent survival significantly longer than average at 33 months postoperatively. The authors postulate that this combination of therapies may have contributed to the prolonged survival seen in this case. Another study of temozolomide therapy in spinal cord glioma found that temozolomide treatment during and after radiation therapy might improve survival in some patients.[50] Bevacizumab has also been evaluated in a small cohort of patients with recurrent spinal cord glioblastoma[51] who had previously failed temozolomide treatment. This study reported that 51% of patients experienced stable disease, 34% experienced partial responses, and 17% showed progressive disease following bevacizumab treatment, with three grade 3 toxicities during the duration of the study. A more recent study[52] evaluated the use of temozolomide in combination with bevacizumab in a rat model of intramedullary spinal cord glioma and found that a combination of these drugs reduced tumor volume and resulted in improved neurological outcomes in terms of hind limb motor function.

Radiation Therapy

The primary radiation methods utilized for adjuvant treatment of intramedullary spinal cord gliomas include traditional photon beam conformal radiotherapy and more recently, proton beam therapy. Proton beam therapy has the advantage of allowing for dose concentration in the target tissue while avoiding normal tissues, making it an attractive adjuvant therapy option for tumors surrounded by eloquent tissue.[53] In pediatric cranial ependymoma, proton beam therapy was found to reduce the average dose of radiation required by 28 to 64% compared to traditional photon beam conformal radiotherapy, with the decreased dose allowing for reduced systemic toxicity and less exposure of normal brain tissue to radiation.[53] Similar findings have previously been shown in pediatric medulloblastoma, with proton beam craniospinal irradiation resulting in decreased doses of radiation to normal tissues.[54] In adults with medulloblastoma, patients receiving proton beam therapy

experienced less morbidity in the course of treatment relative to patients receiving photon beam therapy, specifically experiencing less gastrointestinal and hematologic toxicity.[55] However, in patients with spinal cord gliomas, the type of radiation (photon beam versus proton beam) has been associated with overall survival, with proton beam treated patients experiencing worse survival than photon beam treated patients,[56] in contrast to the results of the pediatric ependymoma study discussed. Interestingly, the cohort of patients undergoing proton beam radiation therapy in this study actually had more favorable demographics and prognostic indications, such as younger age and more complete surgical resections prior to radiation; however, these patients nevertheless experienced worse outcomes compared to their photon beam treated counterparts.[56] In addition to traditional radiation therapies, targeted radiation therapies have been combined with image guidance to treat certain types of recurrent intramedullary spinal cord tumors. In one case report describing a unique application of intracavitary irradiation, a patient with recurrent pilocytic astrocytoma was treated with computed tomography (CT)-guided intracavitary irradiation with rhenium-186. This treatment was successful in stabilizing the cystic component of the tumor, thereby relieving the patient's neurological symptoms with limited side effects.[57]

Stereotactic Spine Radiosurgery

Stereotactic radiosurgery (SRS) has emerged over the past decade as an alternative to traditional radiotherapy that allows for the delivery of large cumulative doses of radiation to target tissues with high precision. As with proton beam radiotherapy in contrast to photon beam conformal radiotherapy, SRS reduces the volume of nontumor tissue exposed to radiation and therefore allows for both increased efficacy and reduced toxicity.[58] This therapy has specifically been applied to the spine in the form of stereotactic spine radiosurgery (SSR) and has been used successfully in the treatment of intramedullary ependymomas, hemangioblastomas, arteriovenous malformations, and metastases.[58] SRS may be particularly useful in cases of intramedullary metastasis, where one study reported complete response in 22% of patients receiving SRS for intramedullary metastasis as well as partial response in 33%, stable disease in 33%, and progressive disease in 11% of patients.[59] In these cases, there was no clinically detectable radiation toxicity seen during the follow-up period, suggesting that SRS and specifically SSR may have reasonable efficacy and low toxicity in the treatment of intramedullary spinal cord tumors, particularly those that arise as a result of metastatic disease.

Localized Nonviral Gene Delivery

Given the limitations of both radiotherapy and chemotherapy as adjuvant therapies in the treatment of intramedullary spinal cord tumors, gene therapy has emerged in recent years as a promising subject of research in preclinical models of spinal cord tumors. Pennant et al[60] utilized a nonviral gene carrier PAM-RG4, a highly branched dendrimer macromolecule with high transfection efficiency, to introduce the apoptosis-inducing gene apoptin in a rat model of spinal cord glioma. The apoptin protein produced by this gene has previously been shown to induce apoptosis specifically in transformed and malignant human cells, but not in normal human cells, and as such can selectively

Table 6.3 Completed and ongoing clinical drug trials accepting patients with intramedullary spinal cord tumors (ependymoma and astrocytoma)

	Drug	Mechanism	Study type	Results	Age; n	Endpoint (clinical)	Associated references
1	Temozolomide + lapatinib (NCT00826241)	Alkylating agent, tyrosine kinase inhibitor	Phase 2, open label	All-cause mortality and adverse events reported; clinical endpoints not yet reported	18–65, ≥65; 58	Time-to-progression (volumetric increase of ≥25% was defined as progression)	None
2	Marizomib (NCT03727841)	Proteasome inhibitor	Phase 2, open label	None	18 +; ongoing	Progression-free survival at 6 months	[38,39,40]
3	Carboplatin + bevacizumab (NCT01295944)	Alkylating agent, antiangiogenic agent	Phase 2, open label	None	18 +; ongoing	Progression-free survival at 1 year	None
4	Bevacizumab + irinotecan (NCT00381797)	Antiangiogenic agent, topoisomerase inhibitor	Phase 2, open label	Adverse events reported; clinical endpoints not yet reported	<18, 18–65; 15	Complete response defined as complete disappearance of all enhancing tumor or partial response as a ≥50% reduction in tumor size	[41]
5	Vorinostat + temozolomide (NCT01076530)	HDAC inhibitor, alkylating agent	Phase 1, open label	5-day cycles of vorinostat + TMZ were well tolerated in children with recurrent CNS malignancies; myelosuppression is the dose-limiting toxicity	1–21; 27	Maximum tolerated dose and pharmacokinetic parameters	[42]
6	Cediranib (NCT00326664)	Antiangiogenic agent	Phase 1, open label	None	1–21; 55	Maximum tolerated dose	None
7	Ispinesib (NCT00363272)	Kinesin spindle protein inhibitor	Phase 1, open label	None	1–21; 30	Maximum tolerated dose	None
8	Temozolomide + veliparib (NCT00946335)	Alkylating agent, PARP inhibitor	Phase 1, open label	None	1–21; 31	Maximum tolerated dose, acute toxicities, chronic toxicities, plasma drug concentrations, and pharmacokinetic parameters	None
9	Romidepsin (NCT00053963)	Antibiotic	Phase 1, open label	None	1–21; 30	Maximum tolerated dose	None
10	Tamoxifen, carboplatin, topotecan (NCT00541138)	Estrogen receptor blocker, alkylating agents	Phase 2, open label	None	18 +; 50	Toxicity profile, response rate determined via RECIST criteria, reason for going off-study, progression, survival	None
11	Nivolumab (NCT03173950)	Anti-PD-1 antibody	Phase 2, open label	None	18 +; ongoing	Rate of achieving a complete response or partial response confirmed by imaging 1 month later, rate of durable stable disease lasting at least 6 months	[43,44,45]
12	Vorinostat, temozolomide, or bevacizumab with RT, then bevacizumab + temozolomide (NCT01236560)	HDAC inhibitor, alkylating agent, antiangiogenic agent	Phase 2/3, open label	None	3–21 years; 101	Maximum tolerated dose, event-free survival at 1 year	None
13	Temozolomide + lomustine + RT	Alkylating agents	Phase 2, open label	None	3–21; 118	1-year overall survival, occurrence of death attributable to complications of protocol therapy during therapy or within 30 days of therapy termination	[46,47,48]

Abbreviations: CNS, central nervous system; HDAC, histone deacetylase; PARP, poly (adenosine diphosphate-ribose) polymerase; RECIST, response evaluation criteria in solid tumors; RT, radiotherapy.

target tumor cells.[61] The authors demonstrated that introduction of the apoptin gene in their C6 glioma intramedullary rat tumor model resulted in slowed tumor progression, thereby preserving hindlimb function in the rats, and ultimately demonstrated reduction in tumor volume on histopathological analysis. The apoptin gene holds promise as a potential therapeutic for intramedullary spinal cord tumors; however, further study will be needed to elucidate the ideal delivery method and potential synergistic effects with chemotherapeutic agents.

Magnetic Nanoparticle Localized Therapies

Though nanomedicine has broadened the landscape of potential therapeutics for intramedullary spinal cord tumors, most applications have continued to rely on systemic administration and subsequent accumulation of compounds of interest in target tissues rather than guided drug delivery. Venugopal et al[63] developed and evaluated a superparamagnetic drug delivery platform employing gold-coated magnetite nanoparticles injected intrathecally and an external magnetic stimulus to guide nanoparticles to the target tissue. This study found that the accumulation of magnetic nanoparticles near the target site could be visualized using MRI following intrathecal injection directly into the cerebrospinal fluid in rats, and further confirmed localization of nanoparticles via histology. In another study exploring magnetic drug targeting, Kheirkhah et al[62]

demonstrated successful localization of magnetic nanoparticles bound to chemotherapeutic agent doxorubicin in a rat model of spinal cord glioma. The doxorubicin-loaded gold-coated magnetite nanoparticles were injected into the intrathecal space and subsequently localized to the site of the tumor via a neodymium magnet implanted in the fascia overlying the tumor site (▶ Fig. 6.3). The authors demonstrated localization of both the magnetic nanoparticles and their conjugated doxorubicin to the tumor site as well as apoptosis of tumor cells in the spinal cord. This proof-of-concept study demonstrated how magnetic nanoparticle technology represents a novel drug delivery method with the potential to increase the efficacy and reduce the systemic toxicity of traditional chemotherapeutic agents.

Localized Intratumoral Drug Delivery with Biodegradable Vehicles

To combat the challenges of poor penetration and systemic toxicity, Tyler et al[64] studied the efficacy and safety of paclitaxel delivered via biodegradable gel depot delivery system in a rat model of intramedullary gliosarcoma. This study found that OncoGel (the specific gel depot delivery system utilized in this study) was safe for intramedullary injection in rats and furthermore extended median survival as well as functional motor outcomes as

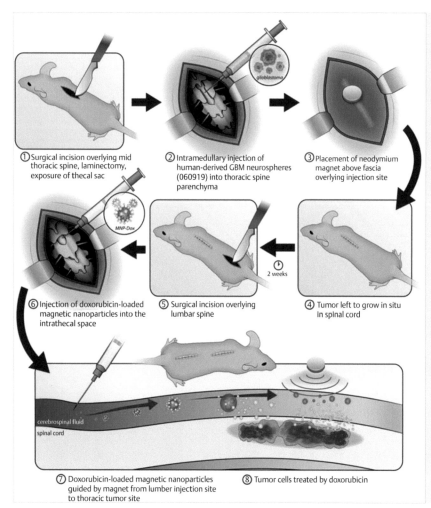

① Surgical incision overlying mid thoracic spine, laminectomy, exposure of thecal sac

② Intramedullary injection of human-derived GBM neurospheres (060919) into thoracic spine parenchyma

③ Placement of neodymium magnet above fascia overlying injection site

④ Tumor left to grow in situ In spinal cord

⑤ Surgical incision overlying lumbar spine

2 weeks

⑥ Injection of doxorubicin-loaded magnetic nanoparticles into the intrathecal space

MNP-Dox

cerebrospinal fluid
spinal cord

⑦ Doxorubicin-loaded magnetic nanoparticles guided by magnet from lumber injection site to thoracic tumor site

⑧ Tumor cells treated by doxorubicin

Fig. 6.3 Schematic of experimental design. In this study, an initial thoracic incision and laminectomy were performed followed by implantation of glioblastoma cells and subdermal placement of a neodymium magnet. Tumor cells were left to grow in situ, after which magnetic nanoparticles conjugated to doxorubicin were introduced into the lumbar intrathecal space. The previously implanted magnet then guided the nanoparticles to the tumor site. (Reproduced with permission from Kheirkhah et al.[62] From Creative Commons, http://creativecommons.org/licenses/by/4.0/.)

Table 6.4 Local antiangiogenic treatment studies for glioma

Type of study	Animal	Drug/treatment	Delivery vehicle	Delivery mechanism	Effect of the treatment
In vivo [66]	Rat	Endostatin	Encapsulation of endostatin-producing cells by sodium alginate	Local stereotactic injection	84% longer survival of treatment group compared to the control
In vitro and in vivo [67,68]	Rat	Synthetic endostatin; BCNU	Bis-[carboxyphenoxy-propane]-sebacic-acid (pCPP:SA) polymer	Local implant	Local endostatin + systemic BCNU had significantly improved ($p < 0.001$) long-term survival when compared to control groups and either treatment alone
In vivo [69]	Mouse	AZD2171 (cediranib)	PLGA microspheres	Local subcutaneous injection	Significantly less vascularized tumors, tumors with more defining edges, and halted growth of tumors when compared to the control group
In vivo [70]	Rat	Imatinib mesylate	PLGA microspheres	Local stereotactic injection	Subcutaneous model: Significant inhibition of glioblastoma cells, 88% suppression of tumor volume, and 77% reduction of tumor weight; Intracranial model: Significant (79%) reduction in tumor volume and significant increase in apoptosis
In vivo [71]	Rat	Heparin; cortisone	Biodegradable polyanhy-dride polymer matrix	Local subcutaneous injection	Local delivery of heparin + cortisone: 4.5-fold reduction in growth of glioma; local delivery of cortisone: 2.3-fold reduction in growth of glioma
In vivo [72]	Rat	Minocycline; BCNU	pCPP:SA	Local implant	Local minocycline + systemic BCNU had significantly increased median survival (42 days) compared to systemic BCNU alone (23 days), intracranial minocycline alone (19 days), and control group (14 days)
In vivo [73]	Rat	Minocycline; temozolomide (TMZ); radiotherapy	pCPP:SA	Local implant	Minocycline locally heightened the effects of radiotherapy and oral temozolomide in increasing the length of survival
In vivo [74,75]	Mouse	Bevacizumab; irinotecan (CPT-11)	None	Convection-enhanced delivery	Monotherapy: 30% longer survival rate of mice treated with local bevacizumab compared to IV bevacizumab; combination therapy: nearly double survival time of mice treated with local bevacizumab + CPT-11 when compared to IV bevacizumab + CPT-11
In vivo [75]	Mouse	Bevacizumab-coding gene AAVrh.10BevMab	Adeno-associated virus	Local stereotaxic injection	Increased survival, redacted tumor volume, and reduced tumor blood vessel density
In vivo [76]	Rat	BCNU	Microbubbles	Intravenous drug delivery and BBB disruption with focused ultrasound	BCNU-loaded microbubbles followed by FUS resulted in weakened blood–brain barrier, tumor-specific activity, enhanced delivery, and improved median survival time

Abbreviations: BBB, Basso–Beattie–Bresnahan; BCNU, bis-chloroethylnitrosourea; FUS, focused ultrasound surgery; PLGA, poly lactic-co-glycolic acid.
Source: Reprinted by permission from Springer Nature, from Arnone et al.[65]

evidenced by increased scores on the Basso–Beattie–Bresnahan (BBB) scale. As with gene therapies, this localized drug delivery system has only been evaluated in animal models and will require extensive further study to evaluate efficacy, toxicity, and optimal combination with radiotherapy or other systemic therapies (▶ Table 6.4).

Localized Targeted Antiangiogenic Drug Therapy

As discussed previously, the antiangiogenic agent bevacizumab has been used systemically in the treatment of spinal cord glioma with mixed results.[51,52] As with other chemotherapeutic agents, efficacy is limited by penetration through the blood–brain barrier or blood–spinal cord barrier. To combat this,

recent research has shifted focus to various drug delivery systems for antiangiogenic treatment of gliomas. To date, virtually all of these studies have evaluated animal models of cranial gliomas using a variety of antiangiogenic agents[65]; however, many of these concepts could readily be applied to spinal cord gliomas. ▶ Table 6.4 describes the results of these studies, all of which had some level of success in terms of prolonging survival and/or curtailing tumor growth.

6.5 Conclusion

Over the past decade, advances in operative techniques, intraoperative imaging, and IOM alongside nonoperative, targeted, localized, and personalized therapies have revolutionized the treatment of intramedullary spinal cord tumors.

These advances have improved the safety and efficacy of surgical resection and allowed previously inoperable tumors to become amenable to resection. In the future, intraoperative imaging modalities such as Raman spectroscopy and augmented reality will allow neurosurgeons to achieve exceptional surgical outcomes in resecting intramedullary spinal cord tumors. Furthermore, personalized medicine via intraoperative tumor genotyping will allow for selection and placement of patient-specific, high-efficacy adjunctive therapies before the patient even leaves the operating room. As with surgical therapies, radiation therapies for intramedullary spinal cord tumors have become much more targeted and precise via stereotactic spine radiosurgery, thereby increasing efficacy and reducing toxic side effects. Though the results of numerous clinical drug trials for various chemotherapeutic regimens remain inconclusive, recent advances in drug delivery, from magnetic nanoparticles to biodegradable vesicles, have shown promise in animal models and may allow for targeted delivery of chemotherapeutic drugs in the future, overcoming the challenges of CNS penetration and limiting toxicity. Future research should focus on studying drug delivery models used in cranial tumors in animal models of intramedullary spinal cord tumors, and most importantly translating these animal models to human studies. Together, these therapies hold great promise for the future of intramedullary spinal cord tumor treatment, allowing patient care to be individualized and optimized more than ever before.

References

[1] Shah AH, Niazi TN. Intradural Extramedullary and Intramedullary Spinal Cord Tumors. In Ellenbogen, RG, Sekhar, LN, & Kitchen, N, eds. Principles of Neurological Surgery, Fourth Edition, pp. 500–509. Elsevier Inc; 2018

[2] Tobin MK, Geraghty JR, Engelhard HH, Linninger AA, Mehta. AI. Intramedullary spinal cord tumors: a review of current and future treatment strategies. 2015; 39(2):E14

[3] Post NH, Cooper PR. Management of intramedullary spinal cord tumors. In: Rees J, Wen PY, eds. Blue Books of Neurology. Vol. 36. Elsevier Inc.; 2010

[4] Sung WS, Sung MJ, Chan JH, et al. Intramedullary spinal cord metastases: a 20-year institutional experience with a comprehensive literature review. World Neurosurg. 2013; 79(3–4):576–584

[5] Kalita O. Current insights into surgery for intramedullary spinal cord metastases: a literature review. Int J Surg Oncol. 2011; 2011:989506

[6] Juthani RG, Bilsky MH, Vogelbaum MA. Current management and treatment modalities for intramedullary spinal cord tumors. Curr Treat Options Oncol. 2015; 16(8):39

[7] Arima H, Hasegawa T, Togawa D, et al. Feasibility of a novel diagnostic chart of intramedullary spinal cord tumors in magnetic resonance imaging. Spinal Cord. 2014; 52(10):769–773

[8] Khalid S, Kelly R, Carlton A, et al. Adult intradural intramedullary astrocytomas: a multicenter analysis. J Spine Surg. 2019; 5(1):19–30

[9] Epstein FJ, Farmer JP, Freed D. Adult intramedullary astrocytomas of the spinal cord. J Neurosurg. 1992; 77(3):355–359

[10] Hamilton KR, Lee SS, Urquhart JC, Jonker BP. A systematic review of outcome in intramedullary ependymoma and astrocytoma. J Clin Neurosci. 2019; 63: 168–175

[11] Shrivastava RK, Epstein FJ, Perin NI, Post KD, Jallo GI. Intramedullary spinal cord tumors in patients older than 50 years of age: management and outcome analysis. J Neurosurg Spine. 2005; 2(3):249–255

[12] Ogden AT, Fessler RG. Minimally invasive resection of intramedullary ependymoma: case report. Neurosurgery. 2009; 65(6):E1203–E1204, discussion E1204

[13] Koch-Wiewrodt D, Wagner W, Perneczky A. Unilateral multilevel interlaminar fenestration instead of laminectomy or hemilaminectomy: an alternative surgical approach to intraspinal space-occupying lesions. Technical note. J Neurosurg Spine. 2007; 6(5):485–492

[14] Xie T, Qian J, Lu Y, et al. Unilateral multilevel interlaminar fenestration: a minimally invasive approach for cervical intramedullary lesions. J Clin Neurosci. 2014; 21(7):1196–1204

[15] Tredway TL. Minimally invasive approaches for the treatment of intramedullary spinal tumors. Neurosurg Clin N Am. 2014; 25(2):327–336

[16] Krüger MT, Steiert C, Gläsker S, Klingler JH. Minimally invasive resection of spinal hemangioblastoma: feasibility and clinical results in a series of 18 patients. J Neurosurg Spine. 2019; 31:1–10

[17] Jermyn M, Mok K, Mercier J, et al. Intraoperative brain cancer detection with Raman spectroscopy in humans. Sci Transl Med. 2015; 7(274):274ra19

[18] Brusatori M, Auner G, Noh T, Scarpace L, Broadbent B, Kalkanis SN. Intraoperative Raman spectroscopy. Neurosurg Clin N Am. 2017; 28(4):633–652

[19] Auner GW, Koya SK, Huang C, et al. Applications of Raman spectroscopy in cancer diagnosis. Cancer Metastasis Rev. 2018; 37(4):691–717

[20] Lemoine É, Dallaire F, Yadav R, et al. Feature engineering applied to intraoperative in vivo Raman spectroscopy sheds light on molecular processes in brain cancer: a retrospective study of 65 patients. Analyst (Lond). 2019; 144 (22):6517–6532

[21] Stummer W, Pichlmeier U, Meinel T, Wiestler OD, Zanella F, Reulen HJ,, ALA-Glioma Study Group. Fluorescence-guided surgery with 5-aminolevulinic acid for resection of malignant glioma: a randomised controlled multicentre phase III trial. Lancet Oncol. 2006; 7(5):392–401

[22] Ewelt C, Stummer W, Klink B, Felsberg J, Steiger HJ, Sabel M. Cordectomy as final treatment option for diffuse intramedullary malignant glioma using 5-ALA fluorescence-guided resection. Clin Neurol Neurosurg. 2010; 112(4): 357–361

[23] Stummer W, Tonn JC, Goetz C, et al. 5-Aminolevulinic acid-derived tumor fluorescence: the diagnostic accuracy of visible fluorescence qualities as corroborated by spectrometry and histology and postoperative imaging. Neurosurgery. 2014; 74(3):310–319, discussion 319–320

[24] Millesi M, Kiesel B, Woehrer A, et al. Analysis of 5-aminolevulinic acid-induced fluorescence in 55 different spinal tumors. Neurosurg Focus. 2014; 36(2):E11

[25] Hendricks BK, Sanai N, Stummer W. Fluorescence-guided surgery with aminolevulinic acid for low-grade gliomas. J Neurooncol. 2019; 141(1):13–18

[26] Takami T, Yamagata T, Naito K, Arima H, Ohata K. Intraoperative assessment of spinal vascular flow in the surgery of spinal intramedullary tumors using indocyanine green videoangiography. Surg Neurol Int. 2013; 4:135

[27] Choudhri AF, Whitehead MT, Klimo P, Jr, Montgomery BK, Boop FA. Diffusion tensor imaging to guide surgical planning in intramedullary spinal cord tumors in children. Neuroradiology. 2014; 56(2):169–174

[28] Giordano M, Gerganov VM, Metwali H, et al. Feasibility of cervical intramedullary diffuse glioma resection using intraoperative magnetic resonance imaging. Neurosurg Rev. 2013; 37:139–146

[29] Sala F, Bricolo A, Faccioli F, Lanteri P, Gerosa M. Surgery for intramedullary spinal cord tumors: the role of intraoperative (neurophysiological) monitoring. Eur Spine J. 2007; 16 Suppl 2:S130–S139

[30] Quiñones-Hinojosa A, Lyon R, Zada G, et al. Changes in transcranial motor evoked potentials during intramedullary spinal cord tumor resection correlate with postoperative motor function. Neurosurgery. 2005; 56(5): 982–993, discussion 982–993

[31] Lall RR, Lall RR, Hauptman JS, et al. Intraoperative neurophysiological monitoring in spine surgery: indications, efficacy, and role of the preoperative checklist. Neurosurg Focus. 2012; 33(5):E10

[32] Gandhi R, Curtis CM, Cohen-Gadol AA. High-resolution direct microstimulation mapping of spinal cord motor pathways during resection of an intramedullary tumor. J Neurosurg Spine. 2015; 22(2):205–210

[33] Cheng JS, Ivan ME, Stapleton CJ, Quinones-Hinojosa A, Gupta N, Auguste KI. Intraoperative changes in transcranial motor evoked potentials and somatosensory evoked potentials predicting outcome in children with intramedullary spinal cord tumors. J Neurosurg Pediatr. 2014; 13(6):591–599

[34] Nair D, Kumaraswamy VM, Braver D, Kilbride RD, Borges LF, Simon MV. Dorsal column mapping via phase reversal method: the refined technique and clinical applications. Neurosurgery. 2014; 74(4):437–446, discussion 446

[35] Shankar GM, Kirtane AR, Miller JJ, et al. Genotype-targeted local therapy of glioma. Proc Natl Acad Sci USA. 2018; 115(36):E8388–E8394

[36] Zhang M, Iyer RR, Azad TD, et al. Genomic landscape of intramedullary spinal cord gliomas. Sci Rep. 2019; 9(1):18722

[37] Carl B, Bopp M, Saß B, Pojskic M, Nimsky C. Augmented reality in intradural spinal tumor surgery. Acta Neurochir (Wien). 2019; 161(10):2181–2193

[38] Wu J, Armstrong TS, Gilbert MR. Biology and management of ependymomas. Neuro-oncol. 2016; 18(7):902–913

[39] Harrison SJ, Mainwaring P, Price T, et al. Phase I clinical trial of marizomib (NPI-0052) in patients with advanced malignancies including multiple myeloma: Study NPI-0052-102 final results. Clin Cancer Res. 2016; 22(18): 4559-4566

[40] Di K, Lloyd GK, Abraham V, et al. Marizomib activity as a single agent in malignant gliomas: ability to cross the blood-brain barrier. Neuro-oncol. 2016; 18(6):840-848

[41] Han K, Peyret T, Quartino A, et al. Bevacizumab dosing strategy in paediatric cancer patients based on population pharmacokinetic analysis with external validation. Br J Clin Pharmacol. 2016; 81(1):148-160

[42] Hummel TR, Wagner L, Ahern C, et al. A pediatric phase 1 trial of vorinostat and temozolomide in relapsed or refractory primary brain or spinal cord tumors: a Children's Oncology Group phase 1 consortium study. Pediatr Blood Cancer. 2013; 60(9):1452-1457

[43] Gilbert MR, Ruda R, Soffietti R. Ependymomas in adults. Curr Neurol Neurosci Rep. 2010; 10(3):240-247

[44] Okada H, Weller M, Huang R, et al. Immunotherapy response assessment in neuro-oncology: a report of the RANO working group. Lancet Oncol. 2015; 16(15):e534-e542

[45] Daud AI, Loo K, Pauli ML, et al. Tumor immune profiling predicts response to anti-PD-1 therapy in human melanoma. J Clin Invest. 2016; 126(9):3447-3452

[46] Pollack IF, Hamilton RL, Sobol RW, et al. Children's Oncology Group. IDH1 mutations are common in malignant gliomas arising in adolescents: a report from the Children's Oncology Group. Childs Nerv Syst. 2011; 27(1): 87-94

[47] Pollack IF, Hamilton RL, Burger PC, et al. Children's Oncology Group. Akt activation is a common event in pediatric malignant gliomas and a potential adverse prognostic marker: a report from the Children's Oncology Group. J Neurooncol. 2010; 99(2):155-163

[48] Pollack IF, Hamilton RL, Sobol RW, et al. Children's Oncology Group. Mismatch repair deficiency is an uncommon mechanism of alkylator resistance in pediatric malignant gliomas: a report from the Children's Oncology Group. Pediatr Blood Cancer. 2010; 55(6):1066-1071

[49] Tseng HM, Kuo LT, Lien HC, Liu KL, Liu MT, Huang CY. Prolonged survival of a patient with cervical intramedullary glioblastoma multiforme treated with total resection, radiation therapy, and temozolomide. Anticancer Drugs. 2010; 21(10):963-967

[50] Kim WH, Yoon SH, Kim CY, et al. Temozolomide for malignant primary spinal cord glioma: an experience of six cases and a literature review. J Neurooncol. 2011; 101(2):247-254

[51] Chamberlain MC, Johnston SK. Recurrent spinal cord glioblastoma: salvage therapy with bevacizumab. J Neurooncol. 2011; 102(3):427-432

[52] Gwak SJ, An SS, Yang MS, et al. Effect of combined bevacizumab and temozolomide treatment on intramedullary spinal cord tumor. Spine. 2014; 39(2):E65-E73

[53] Mizumoto M, Oshiro Y, Takizawa D, et al. Proton beam therapy for pediatric ependymoma. Pediatr Int. 2015; 57(4):567-571

[54] Howell RM, Giebeler A, Koontz-Raisig W, et al. Comparison of therapeutic dosimetric data from passively scattered proton and photon craniospinal irradiations for medulloblastoma. Radiat Oncol 2012;7(1):116.

[55] Brown AP, Barney CL, Grosshans DR, et al. Proton beam craniospinal irradiation reduces acute toxicity for adults with medulloblastoma. Int J Radiat Oncol Biol Phys. 2013; 86(2):277-284

[56] Kahn J, Loeffler JS, Niemierko A, Chiocca EA, Batchelor T, Chakravarti A. Long-term outcomes of patients with spinal cord gliomas treated by modern conformal radiation techniques. Int J Radiat Oncol Biol Phys. 2011; 81(1): 232-238

[57] Colnat-Coulbois S, Klein O, Braun M, Thouvenot P, Marchal JC. Management of intramedullary cystic pilocytic astrocytoma with rhenium-186 intracavitary irradiation: case report. Neurosurgery. 2010; 66(5):E1023-E1024, discussion E1024

[58] Park H-K, Chang J-C. Review of stereotactic radiosurgery for intramedullary spinal lesions. Korean J Spine. 2013; 10(1):1-6

[59] Shin DA, Huh R, Chung SS, Rock J, Ryu S. Stereotactic spine radiosurgery for intradural and intramedullary metastasis. Neurosurg Focus. 2009; 27(6):E10

[60] Pennant WA, An S, Gwak SJ, et al. Local non-viral gene delivery of apoptin delays the onset of paresis in an experimental model of intramedullary spinal cord tumor. Spinal Cord. 2014; 52(1):3-8

[61] Van Oorschot AA, Fischer DF, Grimbergen JM, et al. Apoptin induces apoptosis in human transformed and malignant cells but not in normal cells. Proc Natl Acad Sci USA 1997;94(11): 5843-5847

[62] Kheirkhah P, Denyer S, Bhimani AD, et al. Magnetic drug targeting: a novel treatment for intramedullary spinal cord tumors. Sci Rep. 2018; 8(1):11417

[63] Venugopal I, Habib N, Linninger A. Intrathecal magnetic drug targeting for localized delivery of therapeutics in the CNS. Nanomedicine (Lond). 2017; 12 (8):865-877

[64] Tyler BM, Hdeib A, Caplan J, et al. Delayed onset of paresis in rats with experimental intramedullary spinal cord gliosarcoma following intratumoral administration of the paclitaxel delivery system OncoGel. J Neurosurg Spine. 2012; 16(1):93-101

[65] Arnone GD, Bhimani AD, Aguilar T, Mehta AI. Localized targeted antiangiogenic drug delivery for glioblastoma. J Neurooncol. 2018; 137(2):223-231

[66] Read TA, Sorensen DR, Mahesparan R, et al. Local endostatin treatment of gliomas administered by microencapsulated producer cells. Nat Biotechnol. 2001; 19(1):29-34

[67] Cattaneo MG, Pola S, Francescato P, Chillemi F, Vicentini LM. Human endostatin-derived synthetic peptides possess potent antiangiogenic properties in vitro and in vivo. Exp Cell Res. 2003; 283(2):230-236

[68] Pradilla G, Legnani FG, Petrangolini G, et al. Local delivery of a synthetic endostatin fragment for the treatment of experimental gliomas. Neurosurgery. 2005; 57(5):1032-1040, discussion 1032-1040

[69] Shivinsky A, Bronshtein T, Haber T, Machluf M. The effect of AZD2171- or sTRAIL/Apo2L-loaded polylactic-co-glycolic acid microspheres on a subcutaneous glioblastoma model. Biomed Microdevices. 2015; 17(4):69

[70] Benny O, Menon LG, Ariel G, et al. Local delivery of poly lactic-co-glycolic acid microspheres containing imatinib mesylate inhibits intracranial xenograft glioma growth. Clin Cancer Res. 2009; 15(4):1222-1231

[71] Tamargo RJ, Leong KW, Brem H. Growth inhibition of the 9 L glioma using polymers to release heparin and cortisone acetate. J Neurooncol. 1990; 9(2): 131-138

[72] Frazier JL, Wang PP, Case D, et al. Local delivery of minocycline and systemic BCNU have synergistic activity in the treatment of intracranial glioma. J Neurooncol. 2003; 64(3):203-209

[73] Bow H, Hwang LS, Schildhaus N, et al. Local delivery of angiogenesis-inhibitor minocycline combined with radiotherapy and oral temozolomide chemotherapy in 9 L glioma. J Neurosurg. 2014; 120(3):662-669

[74] Wang W, Sivakumar W, Torres S, et al. Effects of convection-enhanced delivery of bevacizumab on survival of glioma-bearing animals. Neurosurg Focus. 2015; 38(3):E8

[75] Hicks MJ, Funato K, Wang L, et al. Genetic modification of neurons to express bevacizumab for local anti-angiogenesis treatment of glioblastoma. Cancer Gene Ther. 2015; 22(1):1-8

[76] Fan CH, Ting CY, Liu HL, et al. Antiangiogenic-targeting drug-loaded microbubbles combined with focused ultrasound for glioma treatment. Biomaterials. 2013; 34(8):2142-2155

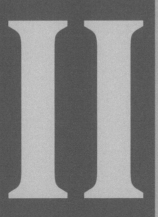

7 Intradural Extramedullary Spinal Tumors: Histopathology and Radiology

Sean M. Barber, Jared S. Fridley, John E. Donahue, Jeffrey M. Rogg, and Ziya L. Gokaslan

Summary

Intradural extramedullary spinal tumors (IESTs) are relatively rare lesions, although they may confer considerable morbidity due to compression of adjacent neurovascular anatomy. IESTs are more common (80% of intraspinal tumors in adults, 65–70% of intraspinal tumors in children) than intramedullary spinal tumors, and although a large majority of intradural intramedullary spinal tumors are glial in origin, the differential for IESTs is relatively broad. This chapter will summarize the histologic and radiographic findings in IESTs.

Keywords: intradural extramedullary spinal tumors, histology, radiology, meningioma, schwannoma, neurofibroma, paraganglioma

7.1 Nerve Sheath Tumors

Schwannomas are the most common intradural extramedullary spinal tumors (IESTs) in adults, accounting for 25 to 30% of cases.[1,2,3,4,5] Neurofibromas, in contrast, are rarely seen within the spinal canal, except in association with neurofibromatosis type 1 (NF1). Schwannomas and neurofibromas are both benign tumors (WHO grade I) and are together known as nerve sheath tumors due to their origin from the outer coverings of peripheral nerves. Rarely, malignant peripheral nerve sheath tumors (MPNSTs) may arise from the dedifferentiation of a peripheral nerve sheath tumor (most commonly from plexiform neurofibromas in patients with neurofibromatosis) or de novo from peripheral nerves.[5]

The peak incidence for schwannomas occurs between the fourth and fifth decades of life, with an equal incidence in males and females, while neurofibromas affect all ages and sexes without discrimination.[4] A large majority of schwannomas are solitary and sporadic (90%), although a small percentage (4%) arise in association with neurofibromatosis type 2 (NF2) and may present in multiples (schwannomatosis).[5]

Clinically, peripheral cutaneous/subcutaneous neurofibromas are often discovered as a painless, palpable mass, but neurofibromas associated with a spinal nerve root may cause radicular pain or myelopathy if spinal cord compression is present. Similarly, schwannomas may be discovered incidentally, as a palpable mass (when subcutaneous), due to hearing loss (in patients with vestibular schwannomas), or due to radicular or myelopathic symptoms from nerve root or spinal cord compression (when intraspinal). Intraspinal and paraspinous schwannomas occur more commonly in the cervical and lumbar regions.[1,6] Since schwannomas favor sensory (dorsal) nerve roots, motor deficits are uncommon.[5]

7.1.1 Nerve Sheath Tumor Radiology

On magnetic resonance imaging (MRI), schwannomas (▶ Fig. 7.1 and ▶ Fig. 7.2) appear as well-circumscribed masses with a variable cystic component (40%).[7] They enhance strongly and homogenously in the majority of cases[7] and often displace the spinal cord, conus medullaris, and/or cauda equina laterally and ventrally as they frequently arise from dorsal roots.[1,8] The solid portion is typically isointense to spinal cord on T1-weighted images (70% of cases) and heterogeneously isointense-to-hyperintense on T2-weighted images. "Target sign" may be seen—though more common with neurofibromas—with central T2 hypointensity and increased postcontrast enhancement on T1-weighted images. When intraspinal schwannomas become large enough, they extend into the neural foramina and paraspinous space resulting in a "dumbbell" appearance (15–25% of cases, particularly in the cervical spine).[6] Over time, schwannomas may also enlarge and remodel nearby foraminal bone or cause erosion and scalloping of the posterior aspect of the vertebral body, a finding more easily visualized on computed tomography (CT) or X-ray.[1]

Neurofibromas (▶ Fig. 7.3, ▶ Fig. 7.4, ▶ Fig. 7.5) appear as rounded or fusiform masses on MRI. Like schwannomas, they are often isointense on T1 and hyperintense on T2 and may lead to remodeling or scalloping of adjacent bone, but they typically enhance only mildly.[1,7] "Target sign" is a common feature of neurofibromas, though it may also be present with schwannomas, where central hypointensity may be seen on T2-weighted images. Although schwannomas tend to displace nerves, neurofibromas may remain confined to the epineurium, resulting in nerve enlargement. Neurofibromas are often small and multiple, particularly in patients with NF1, and may be mistaken for leptomeningeal metastases. When neurofibromas are solitary, they are almost indistinguishable from schwannomas.[9]

7.1.2 Nerve Sheath Tumor Histology

Schwannomas are composed entirely of neoplastic Schwann cells with moderate eosinophilic cytoplasm and indistinct cell borders, histologically appearing in two distinct patterns: highly cellular, compact areas (Antoni A) with variable nuclear palisading (Verocay bodies) and hypocellular areas of loosely organized cells (Antoni B) with ill-defined processes and lipidization (▶ Fig. 7.6).[5] Vasculature is often thick walled and hyalinized, with frequent associated hemorrhage. Nuclear pleomorphism and occasional mitoses can be seen, but malignant transformation of conventional schwannomas is rare. Tumor cells will strongly express S-100 and SOX10 proteins, and may also express Leu-7, calretinin, and focal glial fibrillary acidic protein (GFAP). Schwannoma cells will exhibit a pericellular reticulin pattern related to their surface basement membranes, and membranes will stain for collagen IV and laminin.[5] Several variants of schwannoma have been described, including cellular schwannoma (which consists primarily of Antoni A areas), plexiform schwannoma (typically involving nerve plexuses; seen in skin in subcutaneous tissue), and melanotic schwannoma (grossly pigmented, reactive for melanoma markers).

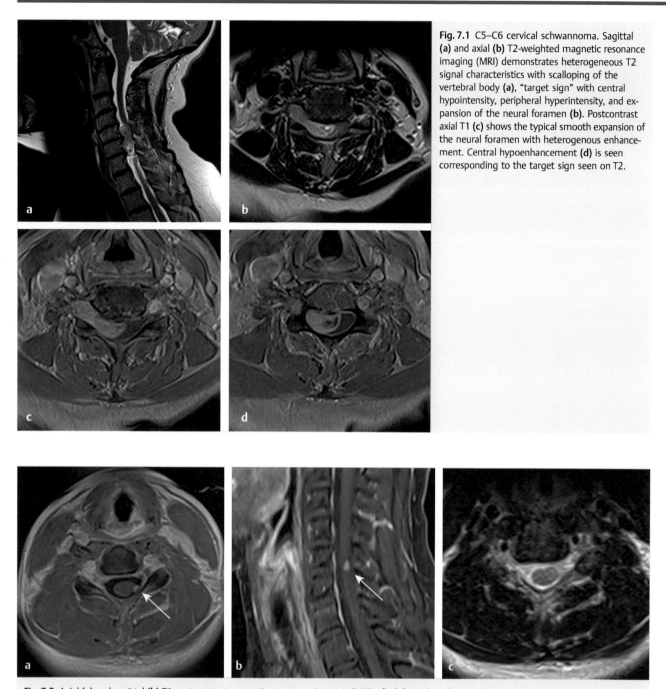

Fig. 7.1 C5–C6 cervical schwannoma. Sagittal (a) and axial (b) T2-weighted magnetic resonance imaging (MRI) demonstrates heterogeneous T2 signal characteristics with scalloping of the vertebral body (a), "target sign" with central hypointensity, peripheral hyperintensity, and expansion of the neural foramen (b). Postcontrast axial T1 (c) shows the typical smooth expansion of the neural foramen with heterogenous enhancement. Central hypoenhancement (d) is seen corresponding to the target sign seen on T2.

Fig. 7.2 Axial (a) and sagittal (b) T1 postcontrast magnetic resonance imaging (MRI) of a left C6 dorsal root schwannoma (*arrow*). The mass is poorly defined on axial T2 (c) because of its poor signal discrimination from cerebrospinal fluid (CSF).

Neurofibromas are histologically composed of Schwann cells and fibroblasts in a matrix of collagen fibers on a myxoid background (▶ Fig. 7.7). The Schwann cells in neurofibroma are, however, smaller than those seen in schwannomas. Collagen fiber matrices may be present in dense bundles said to resemble "shredded carrots." Neurofibroma vasculature, unlike that of schwannomas, tends to lack hyalinization.[5] Neurofibromas will stain for S-100, SOX10, and basement membrane markers—albeit less diffusely than schwannomas. Residual axons are also often seen coursing through neurofibromas as positive immunoreactivity for neurofilament proteins.

7.2 Meningiomas

Meningiomas are the second-most common IESTs (25%).[1,6] These are meningothelial (arachnoidal) tumors that arise from the inner surface of the dura mater. Conventional meningiomas occur more commonly in middle-aged and elderly females (female:male, 1.7:1) with a peak incidence in the sixth and seventh decades of life,[5,10] while atypical and anaplastic meningiomas have a male preponderance.[11] Spinal meningiomas exhibit an even more exaggerated female predominance (90% of cases) and tend to occur in the thoracic spine (80% of cases).[5,7]

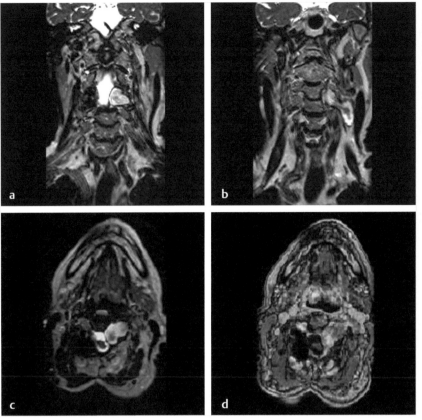

Fig. 7.3 Magnetic resonance imaging (MRI) of a left C4 "dumbbell"-shaped intradural and extradural neurofibroma. Coronal (a, b) and axial (c) T2-weighted images demonstrate an expanded and scalloped neural foramen with a T2 hyperintense rim and central hypointensity ("target sign"). The mass demonstrates heterogenous enhancement characteristics on axial T1 postcontrast image (d).

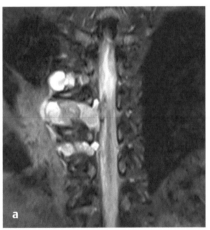
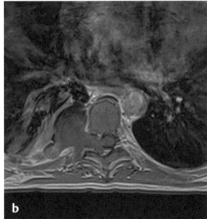

Fig. 7.4 Magnetic resonance imaging (MRI) of multilevel midthoracic neurofibromas in a patient with neurofibromatosis type 1 (NF1). Coronal T2-weighted (a) and axial T1 postcontrast images (b) demonstrate typical smooth scalloped expansion of the neural foramen with intradural, extradural, and extraforaminal extension.

Spinal atypical and anaplastic meningiomas are extremely rare. Clinically, spinal meningiomas typically present with local or radicular pain (21–83%), gait difficulty (57.5%), and motor (50–83%) or sensory deficits (36–81.3%) due to compression of spinal cord and/or nerve roots.[12,13] They may also be discovered incidentally on imaging studies or at autopsy.

7.2.1 Meningioma Radiology

Meningiomas (▶ Fig. 7.8 and ▶ Fig. 7.9) are solid, well-circumscribed extra-axial masses with a broad attachment to the dura and variable calcification and cystic components. They are predominantly isointense-to-hypointense to spinal cord on both T1- and T2-weighted MRI, often with homogenous gadolinium

enhancement, though typically less intense than in schwannomas.[7] Intraspinal meningiomas occur most commonly in the thoracic spine (80%),[7] where they often arise dorsally, causing spinal cord compression with myelopathy. Dural "tails" are less commonly seen in spinal meningiomas than in their cranial counterparts.[7,8]

7.2.2 Meningioma Histology

The histological appearance of meningiomas varies widely, with 13 morphologic variants having been described. The most common subtypes overall are meningothelial and transitional, while psammomatous and clear-cell meningiomas are the most common subtypes found in the spine. Most subtypes have a

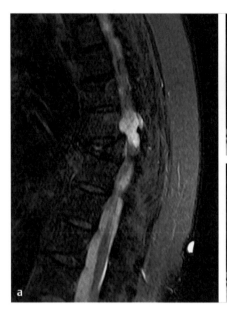
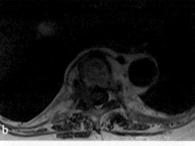
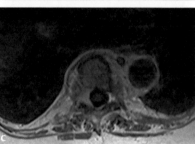

Fig. 7.5 Magnetic resonance imaging (MRI) of a midthoracic neurofibroma. Axial T2 image **(a)** demonstrates typical T2 hyperintensity. Axial precontrast **(b)** and postcontrast **(c)** images show a uniform, intense contrast enhancement and an enlarged, scalloped neural foramen with intradural, extradural, and extraforaminal extension.

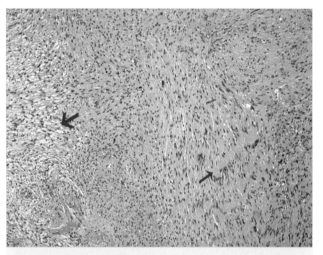

Fig. 7.6 Schwannoma. More densely cellular areas of Antoni A tissue containing Verocay bodies (*thin arrow*) can be seen adjacent to more loosely cellular areas of Antoni B tissue (*thick arrow*).

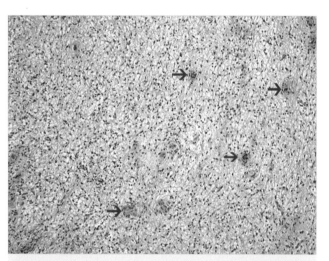

Fig. 7.7 Neurofibroma. The tumor consists mostly of loosely organized cellular tissue. Multiple axons (*arrows*) can be seen coursing through the tumor in cross section.

similar, benign clinical course, although the clear cell, chordoid, papillary, and rhabdoid subtypes are classified as WHO grade II or III and are thus more likely to recur and metastasize. Of these higher grade subtypes, only clear-cell subtype is usually seen in the spinal region.[14] Most meningiomas stain for epithelial membrane antigen (EMA) and vimentin. S-100 and cytokeratin staining is variable.

Meningothelial (or syncytial) meningiomas (▶ Fig. 7.10) are composed of lobules of uniform cells with the appearance of arachnoid cap cells: oval nuclei and variable central clearing or intranuclear inclusions. The lobules of cells may be separated by thin collagenous septae. Tumor cell processes are interlaced, making cells difficult to distinguish from one another and giving the cells the false appearance of a syncytium.

Fibrous meningiomas (▶ Fig. 7.11) are less common, but features of these are seen in other, more common meningiomas. Fibrous meningiomas are composed of spindle cells in parallel, star-shaped, and interwoven bundles over a collagen-rich background. Tumor cells form wide bundles with variable abundance of intercellular collagen.

Transitional meningiomas (▶ Fig. 7.12) are relatively common, and "transition" histologically between meningothelial and fibrous subtypes. Collagen, seen in abundance in the fibrous variant, cuts the lobules of uniform cells in the meningothelial variant, creating the classic cellular whorls that are often described as being associated with meningiomas. When these whorls calcify over time, they become concentric, lamellated psammoma bodies.

Psammomatous meningiomas (▶ Fig. 7.13) are those containing a large proportion of these psammoma bodies. They may accumulate to such a degree that they become confluent, forming larger calcified structures. The neoplastic cells themselves are often of a mixed meningothelial and fibrous appearance. Psammomatous meningiomas are commonly found in the

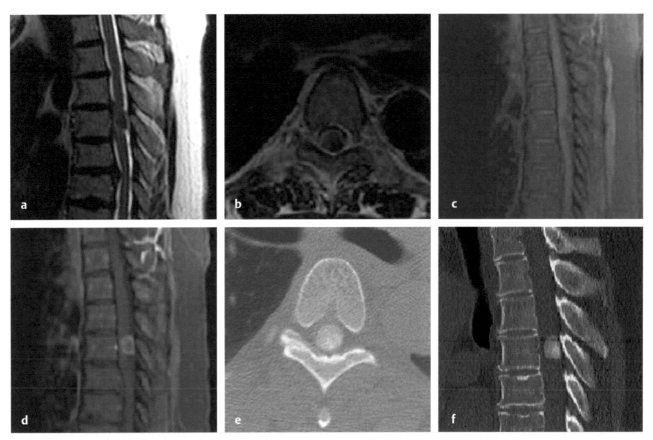

Fig. 7.8 A midthoracic dorsal meningioma. Sagittal **(a)** and axial **(b)** T2-weighted images demonstrate a dural-based, hypointense mass. Sagittal precontrast **(c)** and postcontrast **(d)** T1-weighted imaging demonstrates uniform enhancement. Central hypoenhancement on T1-weighted postcontrast images relates to the dense, central calcification seen on axial **(e)** and sagittal **(f)** computed tomography (CT) images. Note the severe spinal cord compression on axial series.

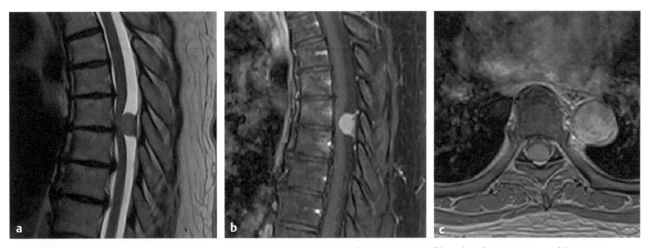

Fig. 7.9 Classic appearance of a midthoracic meningioma. Sagittal T2 **(a)**, sagittal T1 postcontrast **(b)**, and axial T1 postcontrast **(c)** magnetic resonance imaging (MRI) sequences demonstrate a dural-based mass causing expansion of the intradural extramedullary space with spinal cord compression. The meningioma is T2 hypointense **(a)** and demonstrates uniform contrast enhancement with adjacent dural enhancement **(b)**. Severe compression of the spinal cord is seen on axial T1 postcontrast images **(c)**.

thoracic spinal canal in middle-aged women,[5] and among all the meningioma subtypes, they are overrepresented in the spinal meninges as compared to the brain.[14]

Clear-cell meningiomas (▶ Fig. 7.14) tend to occur in the lumbar spine region, which is a rare site for any other meningioma subtype.[14] They are composed of polygonal cells with periodic

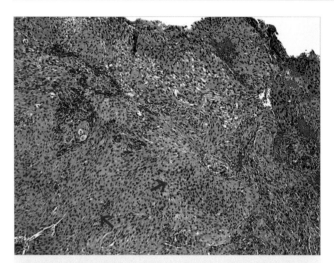

Fig. 7.10 Meningothelial (syncytial) meningioma. Lobules of uniform cells (*arrows*) comprise this tumor.

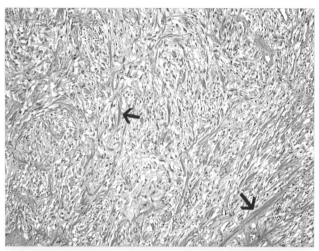

Fig. 7.11 Fibrous meningioma. The tumor cells have been divided into lobules by copious amounts of collagen (*arrows*) present within the tumor.

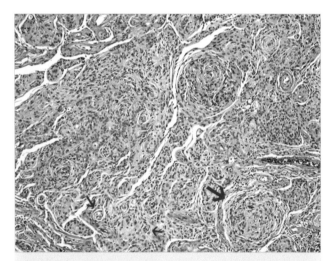

Fig. 7.12 Transitional meningioma. Many large (*large arrows*) and small (*small arrows*) concentric cellular whorls are seen throughout the tumor.

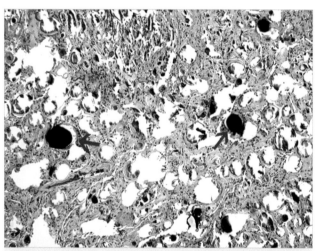

Fig. 7.13 Psammomatous meningioma. Numerous psammoma bodies (*arrows*) are present within this tumor. Many have been displaced from the plane of section due to the difficulty of cutting calcified structures.

acid-Schiff (PAS)-positive, diastase-sensitive cytoplasmic clearing related to accumulation of intracytoplasmic glycogen. Clear-cell meningiomas exhibit high rates of recurrence and seeding of cerebrospinal fluid (CSF), and are thus considered WHO grade II. Other grade II (atypical) and grade III (anaplastic/malignant) meningiomas are extremely rare in the spinal meninges.[14]

7.3 Paragangliomas

Paragangliomas are neoplasms arising from neuroendocrine cells of neural crest origin that are associated with the autonomic nervous system. A majority of paragangliomas occur within the adrenal gland (e.g., pheochromocytomas) or in the head and neck. Spinal paragangliomas are rare (3.4–3.8% of cauda equina tumors),[5,15,16] often benign (WHO grade I) neoplasms that are found in the intradural, extramedullary

compartment, most commonly in the region of the conus medullaris, cauda equina, and filum terminale.[17,18] Spinal paragangliomas are seldom "functional," and the symptoms seen with catecholamine-secreting paragangliomas (e.g., flushing, tachycardia, hypertension) have been reported only rarely with spinal paragangliomas.[19,20,21]

Spinal paragangliomas often present with back pain or radiculopathy, although they may rarely cause spinal cord compression, leading to myelopathic symptoms.[22,23,24] Adults are most commonly affected (peak incidence, fourth–sixth decades), and a slight male predominance is seen (male:female, 1.4:1).[5]

7.3.1 Paraganglioma Radiology

The radiographic features of paragangliomas are largely nonspecific, and differentiating spinal paragangliomas from other

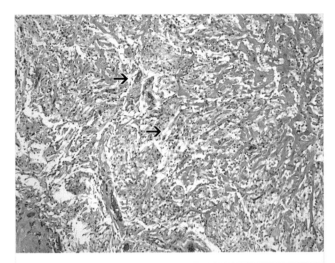

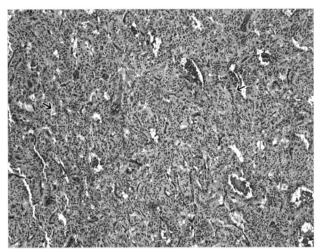

Fig. 7.15 Paraganglioma. The tumor consists of nests ("Zellballen") of neuroendocrine cells separated by fine fibrovascular septa (*arrows*).

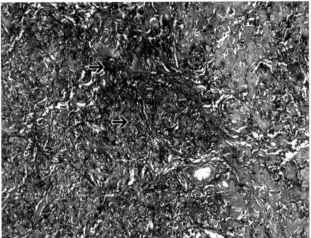

Fig. 7.14 Clear-cell meningioma. Top: Cells with clear cytoplasm (*arrows*) on hematoxylin and eosin (H&E) stain can be seen in the midst of a collagenous meshwork. Bottom: These cells are filled with glycogen, which stains strongly with periodic acid-Schiff (PAS) (*arrows*).

more common tumors in the cauda equina region (e.g., schwannomas) can be difficult based on radiographic criteria alone. On MRI, spinal paragangliomas will appear as well-circumscribed mass lesions with a variable cystic component, most commonly in the lumbosacral region.[25] The solid portion is often hypointense to isointense on T1-weighted sequences, and hyperintense on T2 with strong postgadolinium enhancement. Paragangliomas are highly vascular tumors, and ectatic, serpentine vessels may be seen on T2-weighted MRI.[26] A T2 hypointense rim ("cap sign") may also be seen, and may provide a clue as to the diagnosis.[5]

7.3.2 Paraganglioma Histology

Histologically, paragangliomas (▶ Fig. 7.15) consist of two distinct cell populations: chief (type I) cells arranged in nests or lobules (Zellballen), surrounded by a single layer of sustentacular (type II) cells. Chief cells are round or polygonal with central nuclei, finely stippled chromatin, small nucleoli, and clear-to-eosinophilic, granular cytoplasm. Sustentacular cells are spindle-shaped with long processes that stain for S-100 protein.[5] Mature ganglion cells may also be seen. Hemorrhagic and necrotic foci as well as scattered mitoses may be present, but carry no prognostic significance.

Chief cells will stain for neuron-specific enolase (NSE), synaptophysin, and chromogranin, in addition to neurofilament proteins. In addition to staining for S 100, sustentacular cells will variably stain for GFAP.[5]

7.4 Myxopapillary Ependymomas

Myxopapillary ependymomas are slow-growing, benign (WHO grade I) ependymal gliomas that occur almost exclusively in the conus medullaris, cauda equina, and filum terminale (and they account for the large majority of tumors occurring in this region).[5,27] They are rare tumors, occurring with an incidence of 0.08 (male) or 0.05 (female) per 100,000 person/year and present at a median age of 36, often with a history of back pain and variable sphincter dysfunction and motor, sensory, and gait disturbances.[5,28]

These tumors are thought to originate from the ependymal glia of the filum terminale, which accounts for their tendency to be found in the lumbar canal, although cases of myxopapillary ependymomas arising in the cervicothoracic spinal cord, ventricular system, and brain parenchyma have been reported.[29,30,31] Despite their benign histology and low-grade designation, myxopapillary ependymomas can locally invade and recur in up to 41% of patients, making capsule integrity and complete resection a priority.[28]

7.4.1 Myxopapillary Ependymoma Radiology

Myxopapillary ependymomas (▶ Fig. 7.16 and ▶ Fig. 7.17) appear as well-circumscribed masses within the lumbar intradural compartment. Although often considered intramedullary, they have

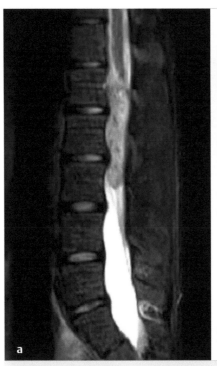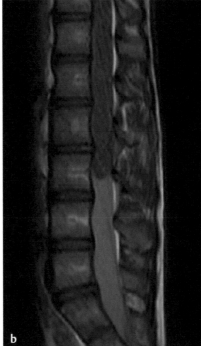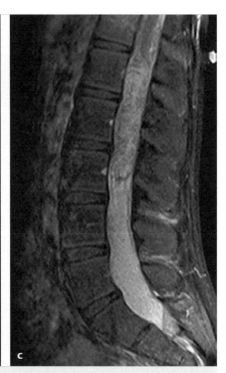

Fig. 7.16 Large myxopapillary ependymoma arising caudal to the conus demonstrating heterogeneous T2 hyperintense signal (a) with uniform enhancement seen between precontrast and postcontrast imaging (b, c). The mass fills the intradural space causing scalloping of the vertebral bodies. Obstruction to cerebrospinal fluid (CSF) flow results in T1 hyperintense CSF on precontrast images below the mass because of increased protein content.

been reported as extramedullary masses on occasion.[32] If they become sufficiently large, they, like schwannomas, may expand the spinal canal and cause vertebral body scalloping or foraminal enlargement. On MRI, myxopapillary ependymomas are often isointense to spinal cord, with variable areas of T1 signal intensity resulting from mucinous components, hemorrhage, or calcification. They are often high-intensity on T2-weighted images and often enhance strongly and homogeneously.[1,5]

7.4.2 Myxopapillary Ependymoma Histology

Histologically, myxopapillary ependymomas (▶ Fig. 7.18) exhibit GFAP-positive cuboidal tumor cells radially arranged (i.e., in a papillary manner) around vascularized cores with mucoid degeneration, loosely resembling the perivascular pseudorosettes seen in classic ependymoma. A myxoid matrix will sometimes be seen between tumor cells and vasculature which is Alcian blue positive. In addition to GFAP, tumor cells will show positivity for S-100 and vimentin, but will typically not stain for cytokeratins.[5]

7.5 Leptomeningeal Metastases

Leptomeningeal metastasis/carcinomatosis occurs when the pia, arachnoid, and CSF become seeded with malignant cells, either from primary CNS tumors or other systemic neoplasms. Leptomeningeal metastases are diagnosed in 1 to 5% of patients with solid tumors, 5 to 15% of patients with leukemia/lymphoma, and 1 to 2% of patients with primary CNS tumors and are most commonly seen in the basal cisterns of the brain, the dorsal aspect of the spinal cord, and the cauda equina.[33,34,35,36] Of the systemic tumors metastasizing to the leptomeninges, adenocarcinomas are the most frequent, and breast, lung, and melanoma are the most common primary tumors.[33] Tumor cells may reach the leptomeninges via hematogenous spread (arterial or via Batson's plexus), direct extension, or through perineural or perivascular migration,[33] whereafter further dissemination may occur through bulk CSF flow.

Patients with spinal leptomeningeal metastases may present with radicular symptoms, myelopathy, bladder/bowel dysfunction, or axial pain.[34] The diagnosis is often made through a combination of imaging findings and CSF cytology.

7.5.1 Leptomeningeal Metastases Radiology

When leptomeningeal metastases are suspected, gadolinium-enhanced MRI of the entire neuraxis is the study of choice. Imaging should be obtained prior to lumbar puncture so as to prevent false positives, as dural-arachnoid enhancement may occur as a result of CSF drainage in the absence of leptomeningeal disease. Dural and perineural enhancement along with

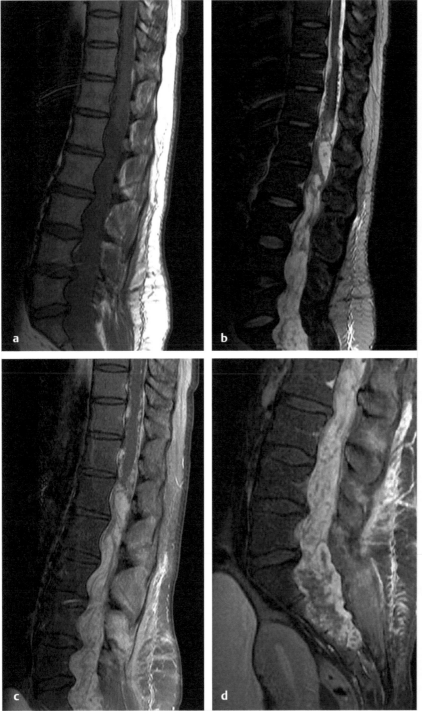

Fig. 7.17 Giant myxopapillary ependymomas in a patient who presented initially with subarachnoid hemorrhage. Sagittal T1 precontrast (**a**), T2 (**b**) and T1 postcontrast (**c, d**) magnetic resonance imaging (MRI) sequences demonstrate tumor extending from the conus into the sacral canal. There is heterogeneous T2 hyperintensity (**b**), and heterogeneous enhancement (**c, d**). Obliteration of the intradural space and scalloping and expansion of the spinal canal are seen, as is engorgement of the pial vasculature (**b**) due to tumor-related venous congestion.

subarachnoid nodular enhancement are considered diagnostic (▶ Fig. 7.19 and ▶ Fig. 7.20). Direct pial implants to the spinal cord incite intense reactive edema signal. The sensitivity of MRI in diagnosing leptomeningeal metastases is not especially high (30% false negative results), and thus a negative MRI does not exclude leptomeningeal disease.[33]

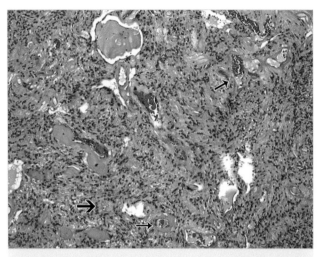

Fig. 7.18 Myxopapillary ependymoma. Tumor cells can be seen loosely arranged in perivascular pseudorosettes (*thick arrow*). Many thickened, hyalinized blood vessels are seen (*thin arrows*).

7.5.2 Leptomeningeal Metastases Histology

The sensitivity of CSF cytology in patients with leptomeningeal disease is reported to be 71% with a single sample, 86% after two samples, 90% after three samples, and 93% for more than three samples.[37] Flow cytometry may also be useful in patients with hematopoietic malignancies. The specific cytological features seen will vary according to the histology of the primary tumor.

7.6 Conclusion

IESTs are relatively rare lesions with a broad differential diagnosis. Radiographic evaluation is useful for patient discussion and preoperative planning, but the radiographic appearances of the various IESTs are not pathognomonic, and definitive diagnosis can only be made through tissue evaluation. Although often histologically benign, these tumors have the potential to cause considerable morbidity due to spinal cord or nerve root compression.

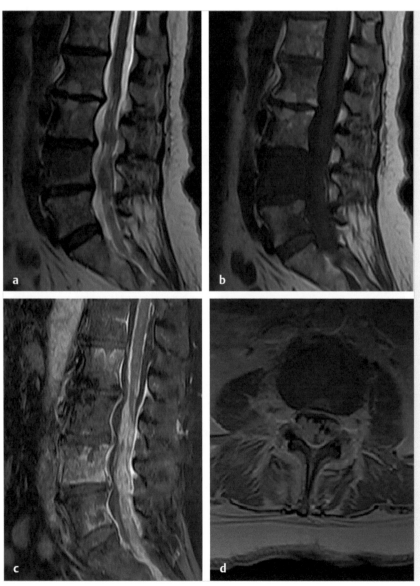

Fig. 7.19 Magnetic resonance imaging (MRI) of a patient with metastatic lung cancer to bone and leptomeninges. Sagittal T2 **(a)**, sagittal T1 precontrast **(b)**, sagittal T1 postcontrast **(c)**, and axial T1 postcontrast **(d)** images demonstrate typical clumping and nodularity of the roots of the cauda equina with extensive nerve root and pial enhancement at the distal spinal cord. Note heterogenous bone marrow replacement by tumor.

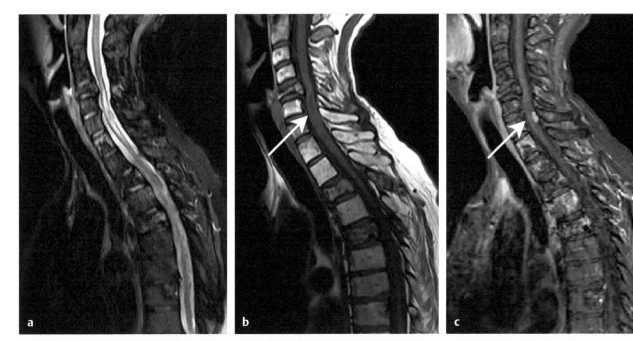

Fig. 7.20 Magnetic resonance imaging (MRI) of a patient with diffuse bone marrow replacement from metastatic breast cancer and a solitary dorsal pial-based metastasis at the C7 level. Sagittal T2 **(a)**, precontrast **(b)** and postcontrast **(c)** T1-weighted series demonstrate intense spinal cord edema related to the small, enhancing, noncompressive metastasis (*arrows*).

References

[1] Abul-Kasim K, Thurnher MM, McKeever P, Sundgren PC. Intradural spinal tumors: current classification and MRI features. Neuroradiology. 2008; 50(4): 301–314

[2] Arnautovic K, Arnautovic A. Extramedullary intradural spinal tumors: a review of modern diagnostic and treatment options and a report of a series. Bosn J Basic Med Sci. 2009; 9 Suppl 1:40–45

[3] Jeon JH, Hwang HS, Jeong JH, Park SH, Moon JG, Kim CH. Spinal schwannoma; analysis of 40 cases. J Korean Neurosurg Soc. 2008; 43(3):135–138

[4] Traul DE, Shaffrey ME, Schiff D. Part I: spinal-cord neoplasms-intradural neoplasms. Lancet Oncol. 2007; 8(1):35–45

[5] Louis DN, Ohgaki H, Wiestler OD, Cavenee WK, eds. WHO Classification of Tumours of the Central Nervous System. 4th ed. Lyon: International Agency for Research on Cancer (IARC); 2007

[6] Kornienko V, Pronin I, eds. Diagnostic Neuroradiology. Berlin: Springer-Verlag; 2009

[7] Van Goethem J, van den Hauwe L, Parizel P, eds. Spinal Imaging: Diagnostic Imaging of the Spine and Spinal Cord. Berlin: Springer-Verlag; 2007

[8] De Verdelhan O, Haegelen C, Carsin-Nicol B, et al. MR imaging features of spinal schwannomas and meningiomas. J Neuroradiol. 2005; 32(1):42–49

[9] Huang JH, Zhang J, Zager EL. Diagnosis and treatment options for nerve sheath tumors. Expert Rev Neurother. 2005; 5(4):515–523

[10] Cordera S, Bottacchi E, D'Alessandro G, Machado D, De Gonda F, Corso G. Epidemiology of primary intracranial tumours in NW Italy, a population based study: stable incidence in the last two decades. J Neurol. 2002; 249(3): 281–284

[11] Jääskeläinen J, Haltia M, Servo A. Atypical and anaplastic meningiomas: radiology, surgery, radiotherapy, and outcome. Surg Neurol. 1986; 25(3): 233–242

[12] Peker S, Cerçi A, Ozgen S, Isik N, Kalelioglu M, Pamir MN. Spinal meningiomas: evaluation of 41 patients. J Neurosurg Sci. 2005; 49(1):7–11

[13] Setzer M, Vatter H, Marquardt G, Seifert V, Vrionis FD. Management of spinal meningiomas: surgical results and a review of the literature. Neurosurg Focus. 2007; 23(4):E14

[14] Burger P, Scheithauer B, Vogel F. Surgical Pathology of the Nervous System and Its Coverings. 4th ed. Churchill Livingstone; 2002

[15] Wippold FJ II, Smirniotopoulos JG, Pilgram TK. Lesions of the cauda equina: a clinical and pathology review from the Armed Forces Institute of Pathology. Clin Neurol Neurosurg. 1997; 99(4):229–234

[16] Yang SY, Jin YJ, Park SH, Jahng TA, Kim HJ, Chung CK. Paragangliomas in the cauda equina region: clinicopathoradiologic findings in four cases. J Neurooncol. 2005; 72(1):49–55

[17] Sundgren P, Annertz M, Englund E, Strömblad LG, Holtås S. Paragangliomas of the spinal canal. Neuroradiology. 1999; 41(10):788–794

[18] Faro SH, Turtz AR, Koenigsberg RA, Mohamed FB, Chen CY, Stein H. Paraganglioma of the cauda equina with associated intramedullary cyst: MR findings. AJNR Am J Neuroradiol. 1997; 18(8):1588–1590

[19] Jeffs GJ, Lee GYF, Wong GT-H. Functioning paraganglioma of the thoracic spine: case report. Neurosurgery. 2003; 53(4):992–994, discussion 994–995

[20] Zileli M, Kalayci M, Başdemir G. Paraganglioma of the thoracic spine. J Clin Neurosci. 2008; 15(7):823–827

[21] Gelabert-González M. Paragangliomas of the lumbar region. Report of two cases and review of the literature. J Neurosurg Spine. 2005; 2(3):354–365

[22] Houten JK, Babu RP, Miller DC. Thoracic paraganglioma presenting with spinal cord compression and metastases. J Spinal Disord Tech. 2002; 15(4):319–323

[23] Conti P, Mouchaty H, Spacca B, Buccoliero AM, Conti R. Thoracic extradural paragangliomas: a case report and review of the literature. Spinal Cord. 2006; 44(2):120–125

[24] Telera S, Carosi M, Cerasoli V, et al. Hemothorax presenting as a primitive thoracic paraganglioma. Case illustration. J Neurosurg Spine. 2006; 4(6):515

[25] Słowiński J, Stomal M, Bierzyńska-Macyszyn G, Swider K. Paraganglioma of the lumbar spinal canal—case report. Folia Neuropathol. 2005; 43(2):119–122

[26] Pérez-López C, Sarmiento MA, Alvarez-Ruíz F, et al. [Paragangliomas of the cauda equina: report of two cases]. Neurocirugia (Astur). 2004; 15(6):565–570

[27] Fourney DR, Fuller GN, Gokaslan ZL. Intraspinal extradural myxopapillary ependymoma of the sacrum arising from the filum terminale externa. Case report. J Neurosurg. 2000; 93(2) Suppl:322–326

[28] Abdulaziz M, Mallory GW, Bydon M, et al. Outcomes following myxopapillary ependymoma resection: the importance of capsule integrity. Neurosurg Focus. 2015; 39(2):E8

[29] Sonneland PRL, Scheithauer BW, Onofrio BM. Myxopapillary ependymoma. A clinicopathologic and immunocytochemical study of 77 cases. Cancer. 1985; 56(4):883–893

[30] Warnick RE, Raisanen J, Adornato BT, et al. Intracranial myxopapillary ependymoma: case report. J Neurooncol. 1993; 15(3):251–256

[31] Lim SC, Jang SJ. Myxopapillary ependymoma of the fourth ventricle. Clin Neurol Neurosurg. 2006; 108(2):211–214

[32] Landriel F, Ajler P, Tedesco N, Bendersky D, Vecchi E. Multicentric extramedullary myxopapillary ependymomas: two case reports and literature review. Surg Neurol Int. 2012; 3:102

[33] Taillibert S, Chamberlain MC. Leptomeningeal metastasis. Handb Clin Neurol. 2018; 149:169–204

[34] Clarke JL. Leptomeningeal metastasis from systemic cancer. Continuum (Minneap Minn). 2012; 18(2):328:342

[35] Olson ME, Chernik NL, Posner JB. Infiltration of the leptomeninges by systemic cancer. A clinical and pathologic study. Arch Neurol. 1974; 30(2):122–137

[36] Boyle R, Thomas M, Adams JH. Diffuse involvement of the leptomeninges by tumour—a clinical and pathological study of 63 cases. Postgrad Med J. 1980; 56(653):149–158

[37] Glantz MJ, Cole BF, Glantz LK, et al. Cerebrospinal fluid cytology in patients with cancer: minimizing false-negative results. Cancer. 1998; 82(4):733–739

8 Treatment of Intradural Extramedullary Spinal Tumors

Ryan C. Hofler, Nicholas J. Szerlip, Anand V. Germanwala, and G. Alexander Jones

Summary

Intradural extramedullary spinal tumors represent about 80% of intradural spinal lesions in adults and 65% in children.[1,2] Numerous treatment strategies exist for the treatment of these lesions. Since most of these lesions are benign, surveillance with serial imaging and follow-up examinations may be a viable option depending on the presenting symptomatology.[3] However, if surgical resection is warranted, the goals of surgery include obtaining tissue for pathologic diagnosis and gross total resection of the lesion. Benign meningiomas, schwannomas, neurofibromas, and filum terminale ependymomas make up the vast majority of intradural extramedullary spinal tumors. Rare entities include lipomas, teratomas, inclusion cysts, melanocytic neoplasms, paragangliomas, and leptomeningeal carcinomatous spread. Most common tumors are well circumscribed, making them ideal targets for surgical resection.[1,3] In some cases, such as surgically inaccessible lesions, large lesions with subtotal resection, aggressive pathologies, or in patients who cannot tolerate surgery, radiation therapy may be an appropriate option.

Keywords: meningioma, schwannoma, neurofibroma, filum terminale ependymoma

8.1 Surveillance

Increased utilization of magnetic resonance imaging (MRI) of the spine has resulted in an increased rate of detection of incidental spinal cord lesions.[4,5] The overall risk of such surgery is relatively low; thus many of these lesions may be successfully and safely treated with surgical excision.[2] However, postoperative motor and sensory deficits may occur in up to 23% of cases, with permanent deficit in up to 8%.[6] Other complications such as cerebrospinal fluid (CSF) leak (with or without cauda equina entrapment) and progressive spinal deformity have been reported.[7,8,9] Risks of surgery must be weighed against a rather benign natural history. Growth rates in suspected benign intradural extramedullary spinal tumors are often low, with 33 to 44% of schwannomas showing a mean annual growth rate of 2.3 to 5.5%.[4,5] As a result, for patients with incidental or minimally symptomatic tumors, surveillance with serial imaging

and follow-up examinations have been advocated in order to avoid unnecessary surgery, while also allowing detection of tumor growth and development of new symptoms. Lesions that show no evidence of growth or localizing symptoms may be followed with interval surveillance. If symptoms develop or the lesion shows evidence of growth, surgical resection or other treatment options can be considered. Since surveillance is common, having a good understanding of the radiographic characteristics that define each tumor type is important.

8.2 Radiographic Characteristics

Meningioma: These are frequently found in the thoracic region where they are often located posterolaterally. Meningiomas occurring in the cervical region tend to be ventral, which can pose a significant surgical challenge. On MRI, they are well circumscribed with a broad dural attachment, and look similar to intracranial meningiomas. They are usually isointense to hypointense on T1 with avid homogenous enhancement with contrast.[10] A dural tail is often present (▶ Fig. 8.1 and ▶ Fig. 8.2). They can also be calcified which is important in surgical planning, so a computed tomography (CT) scan may be helpful in this regard.

Schwannoma: On MRI, schwannomas appear as mostly rounded lesions (▶ Fig. 8.3). They are isointense to hypointense on T1, and hyperintense on T2, often with mixed signal. Most schwannomas enhance avidly.[10] Larger lesions may protrude out of the neural foramen, forming a dumbbell-shaped mass that is characteristic for this histology. Bone remodeling, better visualized on CT, is classic for the benign nature of this mass and can be seen with widening of the neural exit foramen and thinning of the pedicle. Although they are often indistinguishable from neurofibromas, schwannomas are more frequently associated with hemorrhage, cyst formation, and fatty degeneration. These findings are rare in neurofibromas.

Neurofibroma: Radiographically, neurofibromas are not always distinguishable from schwannomas, but some features of their growth may set them apart. Schwannomas, as previously stated, are usually more round while neurofibromas are more fusiform (▶ Fig. 8.4). Instead of displacing the nerve root, these tumors tend to encase the root, making

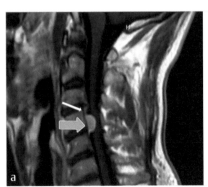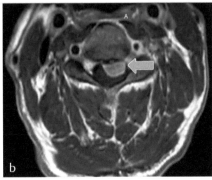

Fig. 8.1 Preoperative postcontrast sagittal **(a)** and axial **(b)** magnetic resonance (MR) images demonstrating a ventral dural based extramedullary mass at C4 (*blue arrow*). The lesion avidly enhances with contrast and has noted flattening along the dura and a dural tail (*white arrow*). This was noted to grow on surveillance imaging. These imaging characteristics are classic for spinal meningioma.

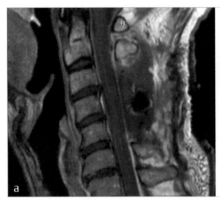
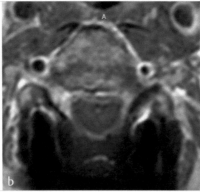

Fig. 8.2 Postoperative postcontrast sagittal (a) and axial (b) magnetic resonance (MR) images showing complete resection of lesion seen in ▶ Fig. 8.1 through a posterior approach. The dentate ligaments were cut to rotate the cervical cord for access. Final pathology was a meningioma.

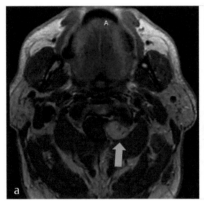
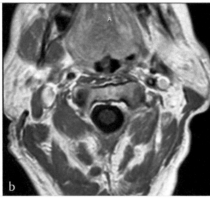

Fig. 8.3 (a) Preoperative postcontrast axial magnetic resonance imaging (MRI) showing an enhancing mass (*blue arrow*) enlarging and exiting the left C2 neural foramen in a patient presenting with neck pain and headaches. (b) Postoperative postcontrast axial MRI showing complete resection. Final pathology was a schwannoma.

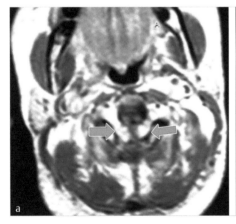
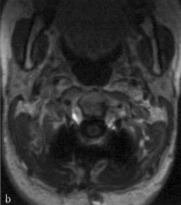

Fig. 8.4 (a) Preoperative postcontrast axial magnetic resonance imaging (MRI) showing bilateral enhancing dumbbell lesions (*blue arrows*) causing severe cord compression in a patient with neurofibromatosis type 1 presenting with quadriparesis. (b) Postoperative postcontrast axial MRI showing resection of neurofibromas within the spinal canal and spinal fixation.

complete resection with nerve sparing unlikely. They are usually hypointense on T1 and hyperintense on T2. Heterogeneous enhancement with areas of low signal is more characteristic of a neurofibroma rather than a schwannoma.[10] As with schwannomas, bone remodeling may be seen.

Filum terminale ependymoma: These lesions are usually hypointense on T1, but can be hyperintense due to a mucinous component that is sometimes present. They are typically hyperintense on T2, and can be prone to hemorrhage.[10] Enhancement is almost always seen (▶ Fig. 8.5 and ▶ Fig. 8.6). Myxopapillary ependymomas are the most common histological tumor type (▶ Fig. 8.7).

8.3 Operative Management

For lesions causing symptoms, including radiculopathy, myelopathy, weakness, or cauda equina syndrome, showing evidence of growth, or when tissue diagnosis is otherwise needed, surgical resection is warranted. The primary objectives for surgical resection of intradural extramedullary spinal tumors are gross total resection and preservation of neurologic function. Most lesions are accessible through a posterior approach. General anesthesia is normally utilized for these procedures. Due to the length of the surgery, mechanical venous thromboembolism prophylaxis and placement of a Foley catheter are considered.

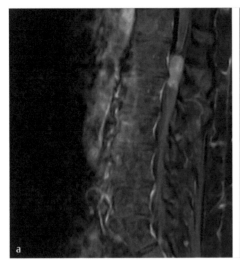
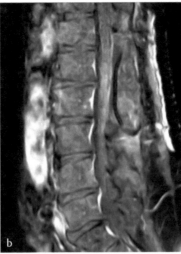

Fig. 8.5 **(a)** Preoperative postcontrast sagittal magnetic resonance imaging (MRI) in a patient presenting with leg pain and an enhancing L1/L2 mass. **(b)** Postoperative postcontrast sagittal MRI demonstrating a complete resection (and temporary surgical drain in the epidural space). Final pathology was a tancytic (variant of myxopapillary) ependymoma.

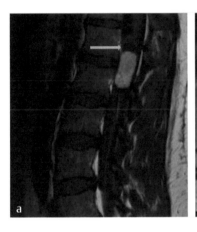
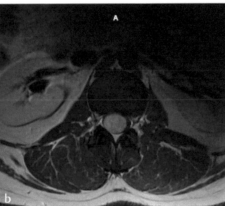

Fig. 8.6 Preoperative postcontrast sagittal **(a)** and axial **(b)** magnetic resonance (MR) images demonstrating avidly enhancing conus mass with capping (*blue arrow*) due to cerebrospinal fluid (CSF) obstruction. Final pathology was a myxopapillary ependymoma.

Intraoperative neuromonitoring, including somatosensory and/or motor evoked potentials, may be utilized; electromyography may be utilized to identify nerve roots, although care must be taken as false positives are common.[11] The patient is positioned in the prone position; for cervical, upper thoracic, or foramen magnum lesions, the head and neck may be immobilized in pins. Intraoperative ultrasound is useful to aid with tumor localization and to confirm adequate exposure prior to durotomy. Adequate exposure and sufficient dural opening are paramount for successful gross total resection; the amount of posterior and lateral bone removal depends on the location of the tumor (dorsal or ventral to the spinal cord). Competent dural closure, early mobilization, and rehabilitation are important for optimal outcomes.

Most nerve sheath tumors are positioned dorsal or dorsolateral to the spinal cord, which allows for excellent visualization through a laminectomy or hemilaminectomy approach.[12,13] Ventrally located tumors may require more complex surgical planning with inclusion of transpedicular, costotransvectomy, or lateral extracavitary approaches. In certain cases, ventral corpectomy may be considered, although this approach is technically difficult.[14] Ventral tumors of the foramen magnum may be approached through an extreme lateral approach.[15] Larger ventral tumors may be accessible through a midline posterior approach; lateral displacement of the spinal cord by the tumor itself can provide an excellent working corridor. In other cases, sectioning of dentate ligaments or noncritical dorsal nerve roots, with or without suture retraction, may be necessary in order to provide adequate ventral exposure. In the lumbar spine, lesions may be covered by the conus medullaris or nerve roots of the cauda equina, so careful dissection of these nerve roots from the tumor must be carried out.

Outcomes from surgical resection of intradural extramedullary spinal tumors are generally excellent. Mortality is rarely encountered and neurologic morbidity is typically less than 15%.[12,16] The most common surgical complications are related to CSF leakage and wound breakdown. CSF leakage is often adequately treated with lumbar drainage but may require exploration if persistent. New or worsened neurologic deficits are uncommon and typically improve postoperatively, although the degree of improvement depends on the patient's age and duration and severity of the deficit.

8.3.1 Meningioma

Meningiomas positioned dorsal and dorsolateral to the spinal cord can be gently delivered away from the spinal cord with use of careful traction on the dural margins. Excision of the origin on the dura is then carried out to complete removal. For ventral and lateral lesions, the arachnoid overlying the tumor is incised and dissection is carried out over the tumor surface (▶ Fig. 8.1 and ▶ Fig. 8.2). The exposed tumor surface may be cauterized to

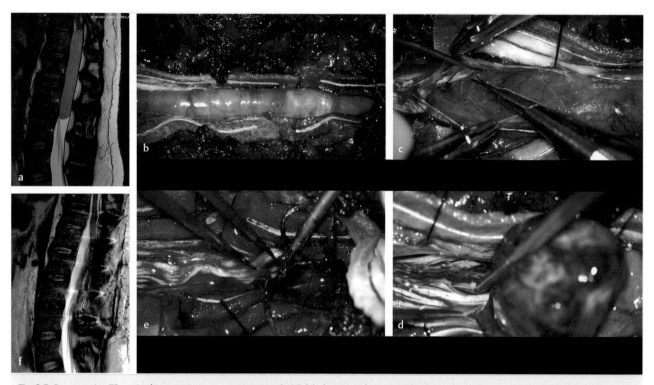

Fig. 8.7 Preoperative T2 sagittal magnetic resonance imaging (MRI) **(a)** showing a large intradural extramedullary mass extending from T12 to L2. Intraoperative photo showing **(b)** opened dura with a preserved arachnoid plane. The arachnoid plane is then opened sharply. The tumor has a purple salmon color, easily distinguishable from the spinal cord and nerves **(c)**. Dissecting the arachnoid plane is key to mobilizing these tumors and resecting them en bloc. A combination of blunt and sharp dissection is then used to roll the tumor out of the spinal canal **(d)**. The instrument denotes the attachment of the tumor to the nerve. In this case it was attached to the filum terminale, which was identified by its appearance and confirmed by its lack of electrical stimulation. Following resection of the tumor, careful coagulation of any bleeding is performed **(e)**. Postoperative T2 sagittal MRI **(f)** showing complete resection of the tumor. Final pathology was myxopapillary ependymoma.

reduce vascularity, blood loss and spillage, and tumor bulk. This may also cause the tumor capsule to contract, providing countertraction for further dissection. Central debulking of larger tumors can be performed to allow delivery of the segment opposing the spinal cord into the resection cavity. If resection of the dural attachment is not feasible, thorough cauterization of this portion of the dura is performed. Otherwise, the dural attachment is resected and dural closure is performed with a patch graft. Careful irrigation to remove blood products and debris prior to dural closure is essential to help prevent postoperative arachnoiditis.

After gross total resection of spinal meningiomas, recurrence rates are about 1% at 5 years and 6% at 14 years. With subtotal resection, recurrence rate rises to about 15%.[17,18] The recurrence rate for cases where the dural attachment was coagulated is reported to be similar to when it is resected.[18] Careful planning is necessary to optimize the degree of surgical resection. More difficult cases with en plaque lesions or extradural spread may be more prone to subtotal resection.

8.3.2 Schwannoma and Neurofibroma

As with other intradural extramedullary spinal tumors, the optimal approach to nerve sheath tumors depends on the anatomic position of the lesion. After achieving adequate exposure of the lesion, a plane is developed over its surface. A fenestrated layer of arachnoid, which separately ensheaths the dorsal and ventral nerve roots, typically overlies the surface of the lesion. This may be incised and reflected from the tumor surface to aid dissection.[19] Cauterization of the tumor capsule helps to reduce vascularity and shrink tumor bulk. In order to perform complete resection, sacrifice of the nerve fascicle proximal and distal to the tumor is often necessary. Much of the intradural nerve root can be preserved, however, as a result of the separation provided by the fenestrated arachnoid layer. Dumbbell-shaped lesions which extend through the root sleeve sometimes require sacrifice of the entire spinal nerve[19] (▶ Fig. 8.3 and ▶ Fig. 8.4). These lesions typically require complete facetectomy for adequate exposure; consideration should be given to instrumented fusion if this is done.

In patients without neurofibromatosis, complete resection of schwannomas and neurofibromas is typically curative.[12,20] In spite of this, tumors with large paraspinal portions present a particular challenge and are more prone to subtotal resection, leading to a tendency to recur. Deficits that result from the sacrifice of involved nerve roots are generally minor and usually well tolerated. Patients with neurofibromatosis have a higher propensity for recurrence and surgical intervention should be reserved for lesions that are clearly symptomatic or progressive.

8.3.3 Filum Terminale Ependymoma

Although filum terminale ependymomas, arising from neuro-ectodermal cells of the filum terminale, are histologically categorized as intramedullary tumors, the approach for surgical resection of these lesions is more similar to other extramedullary lesions[12,21] (▶ Fig. 8.5 and ▶ Fig. 8.6). Exposure of these tumors is carried out through standard laminectomies and dural opening over the involved levels. An arachnoid plane is developed over the tumor and the nerve roots are separated from the tumor surface. When possible, en bloc resection is performed in order to maximize the chances of gross total resection, and reduce risk of seeding due to tumor spillage (▶ Fig. 8.7 and ▶ Fig. 8.8). Larger tumors may densely associate with the nerve roots of the cauda equina, requiring careful piecemeal removal in an effort to avoid neural injury, often leading to subtotal resection.

Compared to meningiomas and nerve sheath tumors, resection of filum terminale ependymomas is associated with a higher rate of neurologic deterioration, especially when the lesion is closely associated with the conus medullaris or the nerve roots of the cauda equina.[21,22] Subtotally resected lesions have a

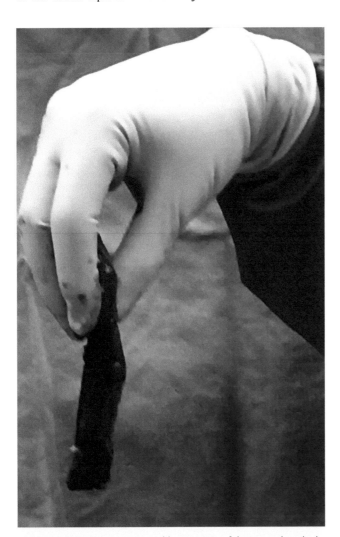

Fig. 8.8 Photo demonstrating en bloc resection of the tumor described in ▶ Fig. 8.7.

reported recurrence rate of up to 20%, compared to only rarely with complete resection. Similarly, survival after gross total resection approaches 100%, but drops to 69 and 62% at 5 and 10 years, respectively, for partially resected lesions.[12,22,23,24]

8.4 Radiation Therapy

Radiation therapy in the context of intradural extramedullary spinal tumors is primarily reserved for subtotally resected lesions that are clinically or histologically aggressive. In cases of tumor recurrence, the risks and benefits of reoperation and radiation therapy must be carefully weighed on a case-by-case basis. Many authors, however, advocate for reoperation prior to initiation of radiation therapy in these patients, provided a safe surgical corridor exists and the patient can tolerate surgery.[25,26] Radiation is, of course, not without risk, with some series reporting an approximately 3.5% risk of post-therapy neurologic decline.[27]

Although most authors would not typically recommend radiation therapy for most patients as a primary treatment option without surgery for benign intradural tumors, it may be a viable option in patients who are poor surgical candidates, or who harbor inoperable tumors. A number of series have evaluated the use of de novo radiation therapy for spinal meningiomas and nerve sheath tumors, which have demonstrated safety of the procedure for these patients, with myelopathy rates of about 0.4% post-treatment.[28,29] In addition, one series demonstrated an 85% pain improvement and 90% local control for patients undergoing stereotactic radiosurgery for spinal neoplasms including schwannoma, neurofibroma, meningioma, and metastasis.[28] Although strong evidence for efficacy is lacking for the use of radiation therapy for untreated benign intradural extramedullary spine tumors, it remains an option for select cases.

In patients with aggressive lesions such as filum terminale ependymomas, particularly when subtotally resected, recurrence tends to occur early. As such, adjuvant radiation therapy is an important consideration. In cases with substantive residual tumor or CSF dissemination, primary adjunctive radiation therapy should be pursued. However, in cases with near-total resection, careful surveillance with reoperation for repeat resection followed by radiation therapy remains the preferred option. It should be noted that while response of spinal ependymomas to radiation can be unpredictable, some patients can achieve lasting tumor control.[2]

8.5 Conclusion

The optimal treatment for intradural extramedullary spinal tumors must be determined on an individual basis, accounting for the size, location, and suspected histology of the tumor as well as age, medical condition, neurologic function, and preferences of the patient. In many cases, this involves surgical resection, with a goal of gross total resection without damage to surrounding neural structures. This can be achieved in many cases with minimal complications. When gross total resection is not possible without compromising neurologic function, subtotal resection followed by surveillance imaging or adjuvant radiation therapy are viable options depending on pathology. Careful case selection and preoperative surgical planning are paramount to treatment success and complication avoidance. Certain lesions will be best followed with serial imaging without operation; characteristics that favor surveillance include clearly benign radiographic appearance and lack of any neurological deficit.

References

[1] Abul-Kasim K, Thurnher MM, McKeever P, Sundgren PC. Intradural spinal tumors: current classification and MRI features. Neuroradiology. 2008; 50(4): 301–314

[2] Wein S, Gaillard F. Intradural spinal tumours and their mimics: a review of radiographic features. Postgrad Med J. 2013; 89(1054):457–469

[3] Chamberlain MC, Tredway TL. Adult primary intradural spinal cord tumors: a review. Curr Neurol Neurosci Rep. 2011; 11(3):320–328

[4] Lee CH, Chung CK, Hyun SJ, Kim CH, Kim KJ, Jahng TA. A longitudinal study to assess the volumetric growth rate of spinal intradural extramedullary tumour diagnosed with schwannoma by magnetic resonance imaging. Eur Spine J. 2015; 24(10):2126–2132

[5] Ozawa H, Onoda Y, Aizawa T, Nakamura T, Koakutsu T, Itoi E. Natural history of intradural-extramedullary spinal cord tumors. Acta Neurol Belg. 2012; 112 (3):265–270

[6] Nakamura M, Iwanami A, Tsuji O, et al. Long-term surgical outcomes of cervical dumbbell neurinomas. J Orthop Sci. 2013; 18(1):8–13

[7] Conti P, Pansini G, Mouchaty H, Capuano C, Conti R. Spinal neurinomas: retrospective analysis and long-term outcome of 179 consecutively operated cases and review of the literature. Surg Neurol. 2004; 61(1):34–43, discussion 44

[8] McGirt MJ, Garcés-Ambrossi GL, Parker SL, et al. Short-term progressive spinal deformity following laminoplasty versus laminectomy for resection of intradural spinal tumors: analysis of 238 patients. Neurosurgery. 2010; 66 (5):1005–1012

[9] Oterdoom DL, Groen RJ, Coppes MH. Cauda equina entrapment in a pseudomeningocele after lumbar schwannoma extirpation. Eur Spine J. 2010; 19 Suppl 2:S158–S161

[10] Ottenhausen M, Ntoulias G, Bodhinayake I, et al. Intradural spinal tumors in adults—update on management and outcome. Neurosurg Rev. 2019; 42(2): 371–388

[11] Malhotra NR, Shaffrey CI. Intraoperative electrophysiological monitoring in spine surgery. Spine. 2010; 35(25):2167–2179

[12] McCormick PC, Post KD, Stein BM. Intradural extramedullary tumors in adults. Neurosurg Clin N Am. 1990; 1(3):591–608

[13] Turel MK, D'Souza WP, Rajshekhar V. Hemilaminectomy approach for intradural extramedullary spinal tumors: an analysis of 164 patients. Neurosurg Focus. 2015; 39(2):E9

[14] O'Toole JE, McCormick PC. Midline ventral intradural schwannoma of the cervical spinal cord resected via anterior corpectomy with reconstruction: technical case report and review of the literature. Neurosurgery. 2003; 52(6): 1482–1485, discussion 1485–1486

[15] Sen CN, Sekhar LN. An extreme lateral approach to intradural lesions of the cervical spine and foramen magnum. Neurosurgery. 1990; 27(2):197–204

[16] Epstein FJ, Farmer JP. Pediatric spinal cord tumor surgery. Neurosurg Clin N Am. 1990; 1(3):569–590

[17] Levy WJ , Jr, Bay J, Dohn D. Spinal cord meningioma. J Neurosurg. 1982; 57 (6):804–812

[18] Solero CL, Fornari M, Giombini S, et al. Spinal meningiomas: review of 174 operated cases. Neurosurgery. 1989; 25(2):153–160

[19] McCormick PC. Anatomic principles of intradural spinal surgery. Clin Neurosurg. 1994; 41:204–223

[20] Schwade JG, Wara WM, Sheline GE, Sorgen S, Wilson CB. Management of primary spinal cord tumors. Int J Radiat Oncol Biol Phys. 1978; 4(5–6):389–393

[21] McCormick PC, Torres R, Post KD, Stein BM. Intramedullary ependymoma of the spinal cord. J Neurosurg. 1990; 72(4):523–532

[22] Sonneland PR, Scheithauer BW, Onofrio BM. Myxopapillary ependymoma. A clinicopathologic and immunocytochemical study of 77 cases. Cancer. 1985; 56(4):883–893

[23] Garrett PG, Simpson WJ. Ependymomas: results of radiation treatment. Int J Radiat Oncol Biol Phys. 1983; 9(8):1121–1124

[24] Whitaker SJ, Bessell EM, Ashley SE, Bloom HJ, Bell BA, Brada M. Postoperative radiotherapy in the management of spinal cord ependymoma. J Neurosurg. 1991; 74(5):720–728

[25] Cohen-Gadol AA, Zikel OM, Koch CA, Scheithauer BW, Krauss WE. Spinal meningiomas in patients younger than 50 years of age: a 21-year experience. J Neurosurg. 2003; 98(3) Suppl:258–263

[26] Roux FX, Nataf F, Pinaudeau M, Borne G, Devaux B, Meder JF. Intraspinal meningiomas: review of 54 cases with discussion of poor prognosis factors and modern therapeutic management. Surg Neurol. 1996; 46(5):458–463, discussion 463–464

[27] Engelhard HH, Villano JL, Porter KR, et al. Clinical presentation, histology, and treatment in 430 patients with primary tumors of the spinal cord, spinal meninges, or cauda equina. J Neurosurg Spine. 2010; 13(1):67–77

[28] Chang UK, Lee DH. Stereotactic radiosurgery for spinal neoplasms: current status and future perspective. J Neurosurg Sci. 2013; 57(2):87–101

[29] Monserrate A, Zussman B, Ozpinar A, Niranjan A, Flickinger JC, Gerszten PC. Stereotactic radiosurgery for intradural spine tumors using cone-beam CT image guidance. Neurosurg Focus. 2017; 42(1):E11

9 Minimally Invasive Approaches to Intradural Extramedullary Tumors

Owoicho Adogwa, Hani R. Malone, and John E. O'Toole

Summary

Minimally invasive approaches to intradural pathology, specifically intradural extramedullary tumors, have been shown to be safe and effective. In appropriately selected patients, minimally invasive surgical (MIS) techniques may potentially reduce complications, morbidity, and cost, compared to traditional open surgery. In this chapter, we will discuss the preoperative planning, technical details, and postoperative considerations related to the minimally invasive resection of intradural extramedullary tumors. Current evidence supporting the use of MIS techniques for intradural tumor surgery will also be discussed.

Keywords: minimally invasive spine surgery, intradural, intradural extramedullary, MIS, spinal tumor

9.1 Introduction

Intradural spinal tumors represent a relatively rare clinical entity with an annual incidence of approximately 1 in 10,000.[1] Intradural extramedullary (IDEM) tumors are more common than intramedullary tumors, representing 80% of all intradural tumors in adults and 65% of all intradural tumors in children; with the most common tumors being schwannomas, meningiomas, and neurofibromas.[2,3,4,5] Historically, and indeed currently, most intradural tumors are resected using a traditional midline incision, subperiosteal muscle dissection, and bilateral laminectomies. This dissection has been shown to cause denervation and devascularization of the paraspinal musculature, leading to significant loss of axial muscle strength.[6] By comparison, minimally invasive surgical (MIS) techniques utilize a tubular retractor system through a paramedian approach, sparing the midline ligaments, and minimizing damage to the paraspinal musculature.

The microsurgical resection of intradural spinal tumors can be one of the more technically challenging procedures in neurosurgery. Accordingly, some have avoided implementing MIS techniques due to the learning curve associated with performing this already difficult procedure through a tubular retractor system. Nevertheless, minimally invasive approaches to spinal tumors have evolved rapidly over the past 10 to 15 years, as more surgeons become efficient with MIS techniques and seek to avoid the morbidity associated with traditional open surgery.[7,8,9,10,11,12,13,14,15,16,17,18,19] This evolution was driven, in part, by the morbidity and significant complication rates associated with traditional surgical approaches to spinal tumors, particularly for metastatic disease.[20,21,22,23] There is a growing body of evidence demonstrating that minimally invasive approaches can be used to reduce the morbidity associated with the resection of intradural spinal tumors, without compromising the extent of resection or safety.[7,8,9,10,11,12,13,14,15,16,17,18,19]

In this chapter, we will discuss the technical details of using a minimally invasive approach for the resection of intradural spinal tumors, including: patient selection, surgical setup, MIS exposure, dural closure, and postoperative considerations. When properly performed, MIS techniques should aim to reduce operative time, blood loss, pain, postoperative immobilization, and length of hospital stay. These benefits should ultimately translate into faster recovery and cost reduction. The available evidence supporting these proposed benefits in IDEM tumor surgery will also be discussed.

9.2 Patient Selection: Indications, Advantages, and Disadvantages

The indications and limitations of minimally invasive spine surgery for degenerative disease continue to evolve, as advances in MIS instrumentation and surgical navigation expand spine surgeons' armamentarium. This evolution has led to corollary advances in MIS surgery for intradural spinal tumors.[7,8,9,10,11,12,13,14,15,16,17,18,19] Successful MIS resection of well-circumscribed intramedullary spinal tumors has been reported.[24,25] The ligation of spinal vascular malformations has also been shown to be safe and effective through a tubular retractor system.[26,27] However, minimally invasive approaches to intradural spinal pathology is most commonly used for IDEM spinal tumors, which will be the focus of this chapter.

There are a number of definitive advantages to traditional open surgical approaches to intradural tumors.[28] Midline approaches provide a wide exposure and large surgical corridor. This exposure may be necessary for large lesions that span multiple segments. Dural closure is also more facile when a large surgical corridor is created. However, this exposure comes at the cost of a larger excision with greater soft tissue destruction, blood loss, and recovery time.[8,9,10]

Open surgical approaches also sacrifice the support provided by posterior midline structures, specifically the interspinous ligaments. Compromise of this posterior tension band may predispose patients to segmental instability and/or postoperative kyphosis, necessitating instrumented fusion. The risk of postoperative kyphosis may be particularly significant following surgery for intradural tumors.[20,28,29] By comparison, MIS techniques generally utilize a unilateral paramedian approach that preserves the posterior tension band, mitigating the risk of postoperative instability and kyphosis.[20]

The fundamental advantages of minimally invasive spine surgery (reduced soft tissue destruction, blood loss, mobilization, and hospital stay) have been reproducible in series of patients with intradural tumors treated through an MIS approach.[7,8,9,10,11,12,13,14,15,16,17,18,19] There is also evidence that MIS approaches limit the risk of postoperative cerebrospinal fluid (CSF) leak following intended durotomies, which in turn reduces the risk of wound breakdown and postoperative infection.[10,11,30] This is most likely due to the relatively small amount of dead space that remains following removal of an MIS tubular retractor, compared to traditional midline approaches.

The appropriateness of an MIS approach to IDEM tumors is largely dictated by a preoperative assessment of the space required to remove the lesion. For example, tumors that lie ventral to the spinal cord are not amenable to an MIS approach. These lesions often require a larger dural opening to facilitate sectioning of the dentate ligaments and slight mobilization of the spinal cord. By comparison, dorsal and lateral intradural lesions are candidates for MIS surgery. Good visualization of these lesions can be achieved using a tubular retractor from a contralateral paramedian approach.[7] Size is not necessarily a counter indication, as rather large lesions (up to 4 cm) can be removed with the use of expandable retractors.[7] Nevertheless, MIS approaches should be limited to intradural lesions that are one or two levels in length.[19,20]

There is a learning curve associated with all minimally invasive techniques. This may be particularly true for intradural tumors and some repetition is necessary to become facile with dural closure in a limited corridor.[30] However, as minimally invasive surgery for degenerative spine pathology becomes more ubiquitous and is increasingly incorporated into residency training, more neurosurgeons are likely to consider MIS approaches to IDEM pathology.

9.3 Preoperative Assessment and Planning

The evaluation of any patient with a known or suspected spinal tumor begins with a detailed history and neurologic examination. Compared to patients with epidural disease or tumors of the vertebral column, those with intradural lesions are relatively less likely to present with severe radicular or axial back pain. However, these patients may develop neurological deficits from ongoing compression of the spinal cord or nerve roots.[31] Magnetic resonance imaging (MRI) is the primary imaging modality used to evaluate intradural spinal tumors.

T1-weighted sequences with gadolinium contrast are useful to define the extent and margins of intradural pathology. Although the degree of enhancement on postcontrast sequences may vary considerably for intramedullary pathology, commonly encountered IDEM lesions such as schwannomas, nerve sheath tumors, and meningiomas, tend to enhance avidly (▶ Fig. 9.1). T2-weighted sequences are useful for determining the nature and extent of cord deformation and/or nerve impingement, as well as cord edema and syrinx formation. For

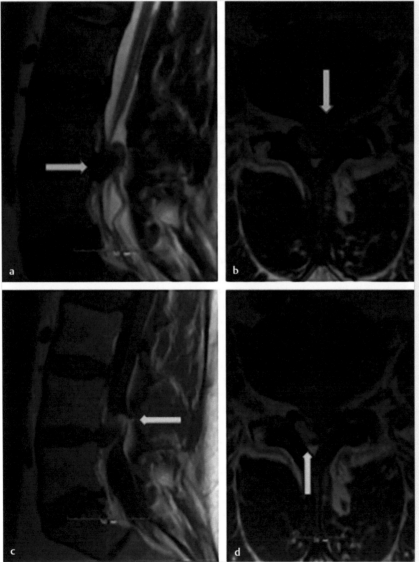

Fig. 9.1 Magnetic resonance imaging of a patient with a concurrent herniated lumbar disk and intradural extramedullary lesion. The hypointense herniated disk (*blue arrows*) on the left at L4–L5 can be well appreciated on T2-weighted sagittal (**a**) and axial (**b**) images. The intramedullary lesion enhances avidly (*green arrows*); seen here on sagittal (**c**) and axial (**d**) T1 postcontrast images.

patients with pacemakers, pain pumps, or other metallic foreign bodies precluding MRI, computed tomography (CT) myelography can be used as an alternative modality.

When reviewing imaging for intradural pathology, and considering a minimally invasive approach, special attention must be paid to the space required to remove the lesion. It is critical that the MIS retractor used allows for adequate visualization of the full length of the tumor. In ideal conditions, normal (nonpathologic) tissue rostral and caudal to the lesion should also be visualized to allow for accurate identification of tumor margins.[32] Inadequate visualization of IDEM tumors may lead to the piecemeal and subtotal resection of lesions that could otherwise be removed en bloc.[7,32] It is important to consider that adjustment of the tubular retractor system is limited after making a durotomy and any attempt to do so may introduce blood into the subarachnoid space and risk injury to exposed neural tissue. Some have advocated that the retractor used should be 5 to 10 mm larger than the planned length of the dural incision, in order to ensure enough length to reliably obtain a watertight dural closure.[7,32] It is also important to consider that the length of the durotomy should generally be 5 to 10 mm longer than the underlying intradural pathology to ensure adequate visualization.

When counseling patients with intradural pathology, expectations and operative goals must be frankly discussed prior to formulating a surgical plan. For intramedullary lesions, the nature of the pathology, and the presence or absence of a safe dissection plane, often limit extent of resection, making diagnosis the primary goal of surgery. Conversely, for IDEM tumors, surgical resection is often curative. Accordingly, careful surgical planning is critical to ensure maximal resection and definitive treatment when possible. Like all spinal tumor surgery, the primary goals for IDEM tumor surgery are pathologic diagnosis, symptomatic relief, tumor resection/source control, and decompression of the spinal cord and/or roots. The operating surgeon must be confident that these goals can be effectively addressed through an MIS approach before attempting a minimally invasive operation.

9.4 Surgical Technique

9.4.1 Positioning and Anesthesia

General anesthesia is recommended for all minimally invasive approaches to intradural pathology. We use intraoperative neurophysiologic monitoring with continuous somatosensory evoked potentials (SSEPs), electromyography (EMG), and when indicated, motor evoked potentials and/or a stimulation probe. Open communication between the anesthesia and neuromonitoring teams is critical to achieve the appropriate balance between muscle relaxation and accurate neurophysiologic recording. Prepositioning potentials may be necessary when intradural pathology has led to significant deformation of the spinal cord, but is generally not necessary.

Following the induction of anesthesia, the patient is placed in the prone position on a standard radiolucent spine table, such as a Jackson table (Mizuho OSI | Union City, CA). A Wilson frame (Mizuho OSI | Union City, CA) may be used to open the interlaminar space at lumbar levels, but at thoracic levels may limit anteroposterior (AP) fluoroscopy and complicate localization. In

the thoracic spine, we generally use a combination of standard radiolucent chest, hip, and thigh pads for this reason. With the patient positioned, fluoroscopy is used to identify the appropriate spinal level and mark the intended incision and site of dilation.

9.4.2 Exposure

We typically approach lateral IDEM tumors across the spinal canal from a contralateral approach. An approximately 3 cm paramedian skin incision is made several centimeters lateral to the midline. The position of the lesion in the spinal canal dictates the lateral extent of the incision, which can be measured on MRI preoperatively. An incision made too medial will prevent angulation of the tubular retractor and limit exposure of the midline and contralateral canal. Following skin incision, the opening is carried through the subcutaneous fat with monopolar cautery, achieving hemostasis and leaving the thoracolumbar fascia intact. We generally prefer to cut the fascia sharply prior to dilation, but others traverse the fascia upon dilation with K-wire and tubular dilators.

Dilation with the tubular retractor system then takes place in a stepwise fashion. We generally initiate dilation and localize with a K-wire, but some favor starting with the smallest dilator to mitigate the risk of passing the K-wire past the interlaminar space. The initial dilator should target the laminar/facet junction. Dilators of increasing caliber are then passed over each other using a circular motion to pass deep into the fascia. Lateral fluoroscopic guidance is used to ensure the correct depth at the level of the joint. Once the planned dilator width has been achieved and the depth of dilation measured, the corresponding tubular retractor can be placed and secured to the system's table-mounted articulating arm. Fluoroscopy should be used judiciously during minimally invasive surgery, given the cumulative risk of radiation exposure to the operating surgeon and ancillary staff. However, optimal retractor placement is paramount to success in MIS surgery for IDEM lesions and fluoroscopy should be used as needed until this can be confidently achieved.

The choice of tubular retractor should be based on the location and size of the IDEM tumor, with the retractor diameter ideally 5 to 10 mm larger than the length of the lesion. We have experience using fixed diameter tubes ranging from 18 to 26 mm for intradural pathology, which are significantly larger than the standard 18-mm diameter tubes commonly used for lumbar microdiskectomy. Expandable retractors can be used for larger lesions, which are capable of providing over 4 cm of longitudinal exposure. Once the retractor is secured in place, the microscope is brought into position focused to the depth of the operative site. We prefer a working distance of 350 mm, to allow for easy passing of instruments in and out of the tubular dilator without interference from the operative microscope.

At the depth of the tubular retractor, a soft tissue muscle plug is circumferentially sectioned and removed with monopolar cautery, exposing the underlying lamina and medial facet joint. Using a high-speed burr, a standard ipsilateral hemilaminectomy is performed, exposing the underlying ligamentum flavum, which is preserved. With the ligament serving as a protective barrier to the dura, the tubular retractor is then redirected medially. The high-speed burr can then be used to undercut the spinous process. The inner cortex of the contralateral lamina is then removed with a combination of drilling and the use of a Kerrison punch until the contralateral pedicle is visualized. This approach provides access to both the ipsilateral and contralateral sides of the spinal canal, while maintaining the integrity of the spinous process, interspinous ligaments, and posterior tension band.

Next, the ligamentum flavum, which has served as a barrier to the dura during drilling, can be efficiently removed. A straight curette can be used to separate the two bellies of the ligament in the midline, establishing an epidural plane. The ligament can then be freed from its rostral and caudal laminar attachments using a ball tip probe, an angled curette, and a Kerrison punch, exposing the underlying dura.

9.4.3 Tumor Resection

Prior to initiating the dural opening it is important to ensure that meticulous hemostasis is achieved to prevent blood running into the operative field and subarachnoid space. We use a long-handled no. 11 blade scalpel to initiate the durotomy in the midline, and then extend the opening rostrally and caudally using a nerve hook. The dural edges are then tacked up using 4–0 Nurolon or silk sutures.

Following the dural opening, tumor resection begins with careful dissection of the arachnoid layers overlying the mass and adjacent neural elements. At this stage in the operation, standard microsurgical techniques are used to remove the lesion. We most frequently utilize microscissors and Rhoton dissectors to create a plane around the mass. When addressing tumors in the thoracic and cervical spine, microdissection must free extramedullary tumors from the spinal cord and exiting nerve roots. In the lumbar spine, microsurgical technique must be similarly used to dissect the tumor free from the nerves of the cauda equina.

Once an IDEM tumor has been dissected from the adjunct neural tissue, the size and location of the mass dictate how it can be safely and efficiently resected. Large extramedullary lesions that deform the adjacent spinal cord, such as large thoracic meningiomas, generally have to be debulked prior to removal to avoid any additional physical stress to the spinal cord. In some cases, an ultrasonic aspirator with an MIS attachment can be used to perform debulking. Importantly, the ultrasonic aspirator must be used on low power settings to minimize the risk of collateral mechanical injury to the adjacent cord. Although piecemeal tumor removal is less efficient and may increase the likelihood of subtotal resection, it is occasionally necessary to avoid cord injury and neurologic deficit.

Conversely, schwannomas and other nerve sheath tumors at the level of the cauda equina can often be safely removed en bloc, without internal debulking.[31] For these lesions, microsurgical dissection is used to isolate the tumor and its associated afferent and efferent fascicles from all other roots in the thecal sac. Special care should be taken to ensure that no traversing roots are adherent to the ventral side of the mass, which may be originally difficult to identify. Once isolated, direct stimulation with a unipolar probe is applied to both the afferent and efferent nerve fascicles associated with the mass.

In the case of schwannoma, direct stimulation will produce a motor response in only rare cases. If a motor response is recorded, it is often because the nerve stimulated was not the nerve fascicle truly associated with the tumor, but rather a traversing nerve adherent to the mass. If there is no motor response, the afferent nerve is sectioned first and then the efferent nerve. This is to prevent rostral rebounding of the tumor mass above the dural opening from rostral nerve tension. Once the afferent and efferent roots are coagulated and sectioned, the mass can be removed en bloc. While performing microsurgery, surgeons accustomed to using the operating microscope may observe fewer differences than anticipated between MIS and open approaches, as the operation is reduced to a small corridor.

9.4.4 Dural Closure

Dural closure represents one of the more technically challenging components of minimally invasive surgery for intradural tumors. As with open surgery, a watertight dural closure is paramount to avoiding CSF leakage, pseudomeningocele formation, infection, and wound breakdown in the postoperative period. Prior to closing the dura, it is again critical to ensure that hemostasis is achieved, as the drainage of CSF during surgery precipitates bleeding from stretched epidural veins. Although a number of dural closure devices have been developed,[33] we prefer to repair the dura with a running stitch. With elongated instruments adapted for use through an MIS tubular retractor, dural closure can be performed in a manner similar to open techniques. We favor the strength of a 6.0 tapered Gor-Tex suture. Some advocate interrupted sutures or running interlocked suture lines, but we prefer a standard running suture. A Valsalva maneuver is performed at the end of the closure to evaluate for any defects in the suture line and to ensure a watertight closure. Hydrogel or fibrin-based dural sealants can be used as an adjunct to reinforce the suture line. At the conclusion of the case, the retractor system is removed slowly, taking care to identify and cauterize any sites of bleeding. The fascia and subcutaneous layers are closed with inverted 0 and 2.0 Vicryl sutures, respectively. We close the skin with a topical adhesive glue.

9.5 Postoperative Care and Concerns

CSF leakage is the primary postoperative concern specific to intradural spine tumor surgery. To reduce the amount of pressure on the healing durotomy closure, patients are kept flat on bed rest following surgery. Traditionally, open surgery postoperative protocols recommend that patients be kept flat and immobilized until postoperative day 2. Following minimally invasive surgery, this may not be necessary.[30] Compared to open intradural surgery, the minimal epidural dead space following MIS surgery reduces the risk of postoperative CSF leakage.[8,10,30] We routinely keep patients on bed rest the day of surgery, but mobilize them on postoperative day 1.

9.6 Discussion

Since first reported by Tredway et al in 2006, a growing body of evidence has demonstrated the safely and efficacy of minimally invasive surgery for IDEM spinal tumors.[7,8,9,10,11,12,13,14,15,16,17,18,19] Neurosurgeons who have become efficient using MIS retractors for degenerative disease may be well equipped to adapt MIS techniques for intradural tumors. However, success is contingent on an understanding of the proper indications and advantages/ disadvantages related to these techniques. MIS approaches work particularly well for well-circumscribed dorsal and lateral extra-medullary tumors. Lesions that lie ventral to the spinal cord or span more than two spinal segments are likely better approached with traditional open surgery.

In properly selected patients, minimally invasive surgery for IDEM tumors has been shown to offer a number of potential benefits over open surgery. These benefits are well summarized in a recent meta-analysis by Pham et al in which data for 114 patients was pooled from nine retrospective studies and analyzed.[8] Compared to open surgery, patients receiving MIS surgery for IDEM tumors experienced reduced CSF leakage, blood loss, length of hospital stay, and postoperative pain without an increased incidence of complications.[8]

The most common complication in this MIS meta-analysis was CSF leakage and/or pseudomeningocele formation, occurring in 5.3% of patients.[8,34] Yet compared to open surgery, MIS approaches are generally protective against CSF-related complications.[13,19,20] This is due to a reduction in tissue destruction and displacement that allows for re-expansion of the paraspinal musculature upon removal of the tubular retractors. This re-expansion obliterates much of the dead space that remains following open surgery and creates a physical barrier to CSF leakage. In a retrospective series directly comparing MIS to open surgery for IDEM tumors, Wong et al reported a significant difference in the number of postoperative CSF leaks between patients treated with MIS (1 patient, 3.7%) versus open approaches (3 patients, 16.7%).[10] In a study similarly comparing MIS to open surgery for IDEM lesions, Raygor et al report that 1 of 25 (4%) MIS patients had a CSF leak or pseudomeningocele, while 3 of 26 (11.5%) patients in the open cohort experienced CSF leaks.[11] In our own retrospective study of 23 consecutive patients with an MIS dural closure following intended durotomy, we did not experience any cases of CSF leakage or symptomatic pseudomeningocele.[30] All patients were allowed full activity less than 24 hours after surgery in this study, further suggesting that prolonged bed rest after successful primary dural closure appears unnecessary after MIS surgery.

Reports of MIS approaches to IDEM lesions have also consistently found reductions in blood loss (EBL) compared to open surgery. In the meta-analysis conducted by Pham et al, blood loss from MIS cohorts ranged from 134 to 153 mL, while EBL in open surgeries ranged from 320 to 558.8 mL.[10,11,35] In the comparative series by Wong et al, three open surgery patients required blood transfusions, but no MIS patients did.[10] Similarly, in the study by Raygor et al, three patients in the open group received a blood transfusion compared to one MIS patient.[11] This difference can be attributed to the decreased muscle cutting and soft tissue destruction caused by an MIS approach, as well as the tamponading effect of muscle re-expansion in the surgical cavity following retractor removal.

This reduction in dead space may also contribute to lower infection rates in MIS intradural surgery, as the volume of hematomas and seromas that may act as an infectious nidus is minimized. There is evidence suggesting that MIS surgery for degenerative spinal conditions may reduce postoperative wound infections by as much as 10-fold.[36] In their meta-analysis, Pham et al found evidence of postoperative infection in only 1 of the 114 patients analyzed (0.88%), a significantly lower rate compared to previous studies of open surgery for IDEM lesions.[8,37]

One of the primary reported benefits of minimally invasive surgery is reduced length of hospital stay (LOS), which often translates into cost reduction.[38] There is evidence that these benefits can be achieved when MIS techniques are applied to intradural spinal tumors. In a comparison between MIS and open surgery for IDEM tumors, Lu et al reported shorter hospital stays for patients in the MIS cohort (4.9 days vs. 8.2 days, $p = 0.003$).[35] Wong et al similarly found patients undergoing MIS resection to have a shorter LOS compared to patients receiving open surgery (3.9 vs. 6.1 days, $p < 0.01$).[10] However, Raygor et al found no significant difference between MIS and open groups (6.2 vs. 6.0 days, $p = 0.78$).[11] In our own cohort of patients with IDEM lesion, LOS and time spent in intensive care were both significantly reduced in the MIS cohort compared to patients receiving open surgery.[9] This shortened LOS and intensive care unit (ICU) time helped account for a nearly 30% reduction in cost in the MIS group.[9] As the emphasis on cost control in our healthcare systems continues to grow, the cost efficacy of MIS approaches to IDEM lesions may become increasingly important.

9.7 Conclusion

The use of minimally invasive retractor systems in the resection of intradural spinal tumors has been shown to be both safe and effective. There is increasing evidence from retrospective data that MIS techniques can be used to reduce the morbidity and cost of IDEM tumor resection, without compromising the extent of resection or safety. Due to the growth of minimally invasive spine surgery in residency training and an ever-increasing emphasis on cost effectiveness, more neurosurgeons are likely to adopt MIS techniques for IDEM pathology in the future.

References

[1] Kurland LT. The frequency of intracranial and intraspinal neoplasms in the resident population of Rochester, Minnesota. J Neurosurg. 1958; 15(6):627–641

[2] Abul-Kasim K, Thurnher MM, McKeever P, Sundgren PC. Intradural spinal tumors: current classification and MRI features. Neuroradiology. 2008; 50(4): 301–314

[3] Boström A, Kanther NC, Grote A, Boström J. Management and outcome in adult intramedullary spinal cord tumours: a 20-year single institution experience. BMC Res Notes. 2014; 7:908

[4] Brotchi J. Intramedullary astrocytomas surgery in adult patients: the rationale for cautious surgery. World Neurosurg. 2013; 80(5):e139–e140

[5] Chamberlain MC, Tredway TL. Adult primary intradural spinal cord tumors: a review. Curr Neurol Neurosci Rep. 2011; 11(3):320–328

[6] Sasaoka R, Nakamura H, Konishi S, et al. Objective assessment of reduced invasiveness in MED. Compared with conventional one-level laminotomy. Eur Spine J. 2006; 15(5):577–582

[7] Snyder L, Clark J, Nakaji P, Tumialán L. Minimally invasive surgical techniques for intradural extramedullary lesions of the thoracic spine. Barrow Quarterly. 2016; 26(1):20–25

[8] Pham M H, Chang K-E, Liu JC, Hsieh PC. Minimally invasive surgery for intradural extramedullary spinal tumors: a comprehensive review with illustrative clinical cases. World Spinal Column J. 2016; 7(2):84–96

[9] Fontes RB, Wewel JT, O'Toole JE. Perioperative cost analysis of minimally invasive vs open resection of intradural extramedullary spinal cord tumors. Neurosurgery. 2016; 78(4):531–539

[10] Wong AP, Lall RR, Dahdaleh NS, et al. Comparison of open and minimally invasive surgery for intradural-extramedullary spine tumors. Neurosurg Focus. 2015; 39(2):E11

[11] Raygor KP, Than KD, Chou D, Mummaneni PV. Comparison of minimally invasive transspinous and open approaches for thoracolumbar intradural-extramedullary spinal tumors. Neurosurg Focus. 2015; 39(2):E12

[12] Afathi M, Peltier E, Adetchessi T, Graillon T, Dufour H, Fuentes S. Minimally invasive transmuscular approach for the treatment of benign intradural extramedullary spinal cord tumours: technical note and results. Neurochirurgie. 2015; 61(5):333–338

[13] Nzokou A, Weil AG, Shedid D. Minimally invasive removal of thoracic and lumbar spinal tumors using a nonexpandable tubular retractor. J Neurosurg Spine. 2013; 19(6):708–715

[14] Gandhi RH, German JW. Minimally invasive approach for the treatment of intradural spinal pathology. Neurosurg Focus. 2013; 35(2):E5

[15] Lee B, Hsieh PC. Minimally invasive lumbar intradural extramedullary tumor resection. Neurosurg Focus. 2012; 33 Suppl 1:1

[16] Dahlberg D, Halvorsen CM, Lied B, Helseth E. Minimally invasive microsurgical resection of primary, intradural spinal tumours using a tubular retraction system. Br J Neurosurg. 2012; 26(4):472–475

[17] Mannion RJ, Nowitzke AM, Efendy J, Wood MJ. Safety and efficacy of intradural extramedullary spinal tumor removal using a minimally invasive approach. Neurosurgery. 2011; 68(1) Suppl Operative:208–216, discussion 216

[18] Dakwar E, Smith WD, Malone KT, Uribe JS. Minimally invasive lateral extracavitary resection of foraminal neurofibromas. J Clin Neurosci. 2011; 18 (11):1510–1512

[19] Tredway TL, Santiago P, Hrubes MR, Song JK, Christie SD, Fessler RG. Minimally invasive resection of intradural-extramedullary spinal neoplasms. Neurosurgery. 2006; 58(1) Suppl:ONS52–ONS58, discussion ONS52–ONS58

[20] O'Toole JE, Eichholz KM, Fessler RG. Minimally invasive approaches to vertebral column and spinal cord tumors. Neurosurg Clin N Am. 2006; 17(4): 491–506

[21] Klimo P , Jr, Kestle JR, Schmidt MH. Treatment of metastatic spinal epidural disease: a review of the literature. Neurosurg Focus. 2003; 15(5):E1

[22] Weigel B, Maghsudi M, Neumann C, Kretschmer R, Müller FJ, Nerlich M. Surgical management of symptomatic spinal metastases. Postoperative outcome and quality of life. Spine. 1999; 24(21):2240–2246

[23] Ghogawala Z, Mansfield FL, Borges LF. Spinal radiation before surgical decompression adversely affects outcomes of surgery for symptomatic metastatic spinal cord compression. Spine. 2001; 26(7):818–824

[24] Haji FA, Cenic A, Crevier L, Murty N, Reddy K. Minimally invasive approach for the resection of spinal neoplasm. Spine. 2011; 36(15):E1018–E1026

[25] Ogden AT, Fessler RG. Minimally invasive resection of intramedullary ependymoma: case report. Neurosurgery. 2009; 65(6):E1203–E1204, discussion E1204

[26] On Tsang AC, Hang Tse PY, Ting Ng GH, Kit Leung GK. Minimal access microsurgical ligation of spinal dural arteriovenous fistula with tubular retractor. Surg Neurol Int. 2015; 6:99

[27] Patel NP, Birch BD, Lyons MK, DeMent SE, Elbert GA. Minimally invasive intradural spinal dural arteriovenous fistula ligation. World Neurosurg. 2013; 80(6):e267–e270

[28] Fassett DR, Clark R, Brockmeyer DL, Schmidt MH. Cervical spine deformity associated with resection of spinal cord tumors. Neurosurg Focus. 2006; 20 (2):E2

[29] McGirt MJ, Chaichana KL, Atiba A, et al. Incidence of spinal deformity after resection of intramedullary spinal cord tumors in children who underwent laminectomy compared with laminoplasty. J Neurosurg Pediatr. 2008; 1(1): 57–62

[30] Tan LA, Takagi I, Straus D, O'Toole JE. Management of intended durotomy in minimally invasive intradural spine surgery: clinical article. J Neurosurg Spine. 2014; 21(2):279–285

[31] Tan LA, Kasliwal MK, Wewel J, Fontes RB, O'Toole JE. Minimally invasive surgery for synchronous, same-level lumbar intradural-extramedullary neoplasm and acute disc herniation. Neurosurg Focus. 2014; 37(2) Suppl 2: Video 16

[32] Tan LA, O'Toole JE. Tubular retractor selection in minimally invasive spinal tumor resection. J Neurosurg Spine. 2014; 20(5):596–597, author reply 597–598

[33] Park P, Leveque JC, La Marca F, Sullivan SE. Dural closure using the U-clip in minimally invasive spinal tumor resection. J Spinal Disord Tech. 2010; 23(7): 486–489

[34] Hoover JM, Clarke MJ, Wetjen NM, Mandrekar J, Puffer RC, Krauss WE. Complications necessitating a return to the operating room following intradural spine surgery. World Neurosurg. 2012; 78(3–4):344–347

[35] Lu DC, Chou D, Mummaneni PV. A comparison of mini-open and open approaches for resection of thoracolumbar intradural spinal tumors. J Neurosurg Spine. 2011; 14(6):758–764

[36] O'Toole JE, Eichholz KM, Fessler RG. Surgical site infection rates after minimally invasive spinal surgery. J Neurosurg Spine. 2009; 11(4):471–476

[37] Omeis IA, Dhir M, Sciubba DM, et al. Postoperative surgical site infections in patients undergoing spinal tumor surgery: incidence and risk factors. Spine. 2011; 36(17):1410–1419

[38] Wang MY, Lerner J, Lesko J, McGirt MJ. Acute hospital costs after minimally invasive versus open lumbar interbody fusion: data from a US national database with 6106 patients. J Spinal Disord Tech. 2012; 25(6):324–328

10 Intradural Extramedullary Spinal Cord Tumors: Current Research and Potential Therapeutics

James S. Ryoo, Abhinav K. Reddy, Nikki M. Barrington, and Ankit I. Mehta

Summary

Intradural extramedullary (IDEM) spinal cord tumors are rare, primary intraspinal neoplasms that may cause significant radicular pain, motor disturbances, and sensory loss. The majority of patients benefit from complete resection with decompression of the surrounding neural structures, and surgery remains an effective approach of treatment. However, treatment options are very limited in patients who are deemed to be poor surgical candidates. These patients may have systemic conditions such as neurofibromatosis, significant comorbidities, or unfavorable tumor locations or pathologies, all of which can reduce the odds of successful treatment. The following chapter highlights the most recent therapeutic developments for this small subpopulation of IDEM tumor patients. We mainly describe the most recent research in systemic therapies for neurofibromatosis patients, stereotactic radiosurgery, and robot-assisted surgery while providing future directions of investigation that may aid in expanding the applicability of such treatments.

Keywords: intradural extramedullary spinal tumors, neurofibromatosis, stereotactic radiosurgery, robotic surgery

10.1 Systemic Therapies for IDEM Spine Tumors in Neurofibromatosis

10.1.1 Introduction

Intradural extramedullary (IDEM) tumors associated with neurofibromatosis, such as spinal neurofibromas and spinal plexiform neurofibromas in neurofibromatosis type 1 (NF1) or spinal schwannomas and meningiomas in neurofibromatosis type 2 (NF2), pose a special difficulty in management due to the multiplicity of tumors and the associated extensive tumor load. Although surgery is indicated for patients with significant spinal cord compression causing sensorimotor dysfunction, those with-

out clinical deficits are usually managed conservatively through watchful waiting.[1] The timing of intervention is a difficult decision and, in many cases, surgical removal of every lesion is not possible. Consequently, advancements in systemic therapies are of great interest in order to provide a safe means of achieving volumetric control and symptom management. Recently, the increased understanding of the molecular pathways involved in NF1/2 has led to the development of several biologically targeted therapeutic agents, which are currently employed in clinical trials. Although most of the therapeutics that are discussed here were not initially designed to treat IDEM tumors specifically, targeting the common molecular pathways in NF1/2-related tumors may provide an effective method to reduce tumor burden for surgical resection, or even remove the necessity of surgical intervention altogether.

10.1.2 NF1: Genetic Pathophysiology

NF1 is an autosomal dominant disorder caused by mutations in the NF1 tumor suppressor gene, which encodes neurofibromin. The average global prevalence of NF1 is around 1 per 3,000, although estimates vary by country.[2] Neurofibromas arising from the nerve sheath of spinal nerve roots account for the large majority of spinal tumors seen in this condition, with studies reporting 13 to 40% of NF1 patients to have neurofibromas in the spine.[3,4]

NF1 results from a germline mutation in the NF1 gene encoding neurofibromin on chromosome 17q11.2.[5] The mutations causing loss of function of neurofibromin vary incredibly due to the large size of the gene and the relative lack of mutation hotspots. Most clinical manifestations of NF1 syndrome result from a haploinsufficiency of neurofibromin; however, the development of tumors requires biallelic loss of function of NF1, which is in line with Knudson's two-hit hypothesis of tumor suppressors.

Neurofibromin functions as a GTP-ase activating protein and plays a large role in the maintenance of Ras in its inactive state, Ras-GDP (▶ Fig. 10.1). In normal cells, Ras is a proto-oncogene

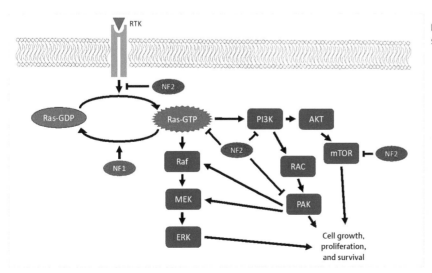

Fig. 10.1 Schematic representation of cell signaling pathways involved in NF1/2.

that regulates proliferation and growth and remains mainly in the inactive Ras-GDP conformation. The removal of neurofibromin results in the constitutive loading of the active Ras-GTP state and the consequent hyperactivation of downstream growth-promoting pathways such as RAF/MEK/ERK and PI3K/AKT/mTOR pathways.[6]

10.1.3 NF1: Therapeutic Advances

Targeted systemic therapy has a large role to play in NF1 patients with spinal tumors considering that many of these patients present with multiple neurofibromas or large, plexiform neurofibromas, which have been shown to be resistant to treatment with surgery or radiation.[7] The increasing understanding of tumorigenesis in NF1 through robust preclinical studies has allowed for the identification of several biologically targeted therapies, especially to treat plexiform neurofibromas.[8] To date, therapies have aimed to either affect the tumor microenvironment or target specific nodes in the Ras signaling pathway (▶ Table 10.1), both of which will be discussed in the following section.

The genetically altered microenvironment of neurofibromas has been shown to contribute to tumorigenicity through recruitment of inflammatory cells by surrounding NF1 haploinsufficient Schwann cells.[14,15,16] Mast cell infiltration in plexiform neurofibromas had been solely an observed phenomenon before the identification of a c-kit mediated mechanism of mast cell recruitment, which was found to be critical for tumor development.[17] This discovery prompted a phase 2 clinical trial with imitanib in which 26% of evaluable patients had a volumetric response, while 30% achieved symptomatic response after ≥ 6 months of treatment.[9] However, subsequent studies with agents targeting this mechanism have yet to yield such favorable results and warrants further trials.

The Ras signal transduction pathway has been regarded an ideal target for treatment since Ras-GTP amplification has been observed in NF1 tumors.[18] Farnesyl-transferase inhibitors, such as tipifarnib, were identified through preclinical studies to specifically block Ras signaling at its node of dysfunction by selectively inhibiting Ras farnesylation, which is a post-translational modification required for Ras activity.[19] A phase 2 trial with this agent, however, was not able to demonstrate a prolonged time-to-progression (TTP) compared to the placebo group.[11] Despite the lack of positive results, the study was instrumental in establishing a baseline average of 10.6-month TTP in plexiform neurofibromas through observation of the placebo group, thus providing a historical control group for future single-arm trials.

More recent studies have been focusing on antagonizing downstream targets in the Ras pathway such as mTOR and MEK. A clinical trial with sirolimus, an mTOR inhibitor, found an increase in the median TTP to 15.4 months, which was significantly longer than the median TTP of the placebo arm of the tipifarnib trial mentioned above.[12] Studies using MEK inhibitors have demonstrated superior outcomes compared to the modest results seen in the sirolimus trial. In a recent phase 1 trial with selumetinib, partial responses of ≥ 20% volume reduction were seen in 71% of study participants, with no disease progression seen in any of the patients.[13] The authors also observed that intermittent dosing of selumetinib was efficacious in a genetically engineered mouse model, opening the possibility of utilizing intermittent dosing in human patients to minimize toxicity.[13] A subsequent phase 2 trial (ClinicalTrials.gov number, NCT02407405) is currently being performed to observe the relationship between inhibition of phosphorylated extracellular-signal-regulated kinase (pERK), a downstream target of MEK, and volumetric tumor response.

10.1.4 NF2: Genetic Pathophysiology

NF2 is an autosomal dominant disorder caused by mutations in the NF2 gene, which encodes the tumor suppressor protein merlin. NF2 is rarer than NF1, with an estimated birth incidence of about 1 per 33,000~40,000[20,21] and, like NF1, has been shown to be associated with multiple nervous system tumors.[22] Spinal cord tumors have shown to arise in 60 to 90% of NF2 patients both as intramedullary and IDEM lesions, with no apparent predilection for cervical, thoracic, or lumbar regions.[23,24]

Patients with NF2 present with genetic alterations to the NF2 gene coding for the merlin (or schwannomin) protein, leading to loss of function or truncation of the tumor suppressor. Much like NF1, biallelic loss of function of the tumor suppressor is what drives the near complete incidence of tumorigenesis in these patients. Mutations in NF2 can occur through both autosomal dominant familial inheritance or through de novo mutations during development. Approximately half of all patients with NF2 have a familial inheritance, with over 90% of patients with a family history of individuals with NF2 having an inherited mutation in the gene. Tumors in these patients express a second hit either through loss of heterozygosity (LOH) of the gene or through a second mutational event. Studies of NF2 schwannomas suggest that LOH at the allele is the most common form of second hit in these patients.[25]

The ways in which alterations in NF2 (and subsequently merlin) lead to tumorigenesis through dysregulation of tumor suppressor properties is not entirely clear at this time. It is known that merlin is associated with regulation of the Ras/RAC pathways implicated in many other cancers through loss of inhibition of PI3K and PAK.[26] Merlin serves as a stabilizer of cadherin dependent cell–cell junctions and inhibits receptor tyrosine kinases at the cell membrane.[27] Thus, loss of merlin permits unchecked signaling of the ErbB/EGFR family RTKs[28] and other proliferation pathways such as Ras/RAC,[29] sharing many of the same targets identified for NF1 (▶ Fig. 10.1). Several therapeutic agents that target points along these pathways such as increased mTOR, EGFR/ErBb2, and MEK are currently under investigation (▶ Table 10.2), particularly in the treatment of vestibular schwannomas and NF2-related meningiomas.

10.1.5 NF2: Therapeutic Advances

The impact of NF2 protein on multiple intracellular signaling pathways has led to investigation of several molecular and cellular targets of therapy, some of which have progressed to clinical trials. Early molecular research has demonstrated that abnormal mTORC1/mTORC2 signaling was present in NF2-associated meningiomas and schwannomas,[40,41] which led to several clinical trials involving the use of everolimus, a rapamycin analog and mTORC1 inhibitor. However, results of these studies were not favorable, and no clinical or volumetric responses occurred from therapy with questionable stabilization

Table 10.1 Therapeutic advances in NF1

	Drug	Mechanism	Study type	Results	Age; n	Endpoint (clinical)	Reference
1	Imatinib (NCT01673009)	Antihistamine	Phase 2, open label	26% of evaluable patients with volumetric response 30% of patients with symptomatic improvement	3–65; 36	Volumetric response of ≥20% reduction	[9]
2	Imitanib (NCT01140360)	Antihistamine	Phase 2, open label	100% patients with stable disease progression, no patients with volumetric response	3–65; 12	Complete disappearance of tumor defined as full response, volumetric response of ≥30% reduction defined as partial response	None
3	Ketitofen fumarate	Antihistamine	Case study	Symptomatic improvement	30; 1	n/a	[10]
4	Tipifarnib (NCT00021541)	Farnesyl-transferase inhibitor	Phase 2, random-ized, cross-over, double-blinded, placebo-controlled	Tipifarnib did not significantly prolong TTP compared to placebo	3–25; 60	Time-to-progression (volumetric increase of ≥20% was defined as progression)	[11]
5	Sirolimus	mTOR inhibitor	Phase 2, 2 stratum	Estimated median TTP of subjects receiving sirolimus was 15.4 months	>3; 49	Time-to-progression (volumetric increase of ≥20% was defined as progression)	[12]
6	Selumetinib (NCT01362803)	MEK inhibitor	Phase 1, open label	Partial responses were obtained in 71% of patients No disease progression of tumor volume increase ≥20% has been observed to date	2–18; 24, on-going	Partial response defined as a volumetric decrease of ≥20% for at least 4 weeks	[13]
7	Selumetinib (NCT02407405)	MEK inhibitor	Phase 2, open label	None	>18; ongoing	Volumetric decrease of ≥20%	None
8	PD-0325901 (NCT02096471)	MEK inhibitor	Phase 2, open label	Partial responses were obtained in 42.1% of participants, the remainder had stable responses	≥16; 19	Partial response defined by a volumetric decrease of ≥20% Stable response defined by a volumetric increase <20% and decrease <20%	None
9	Trematinib (NCT02124772)	MEK inhibitor	Phase 1/2a, open label, 4 part	None	<18; ongoing	Safety assessment by means of adverse events, electrocardiogram, echocardiogram, changes in lab values, and changes in vital signs	None

Abbreviations: NF1, neurofibromatosis type 1; TTP, time-to-progression.

Table 10.2 Therapeutic advances in NF2

	Drug	Mechanism	Study type	Results	Age; n	Endpoint (clinical)	Reference
1	Everolimus (NCT01419639)	mTORC1 inhibitor	Phase 2, open label	No hearing or volumetric responses	>3; 9	VS: ≥15% volume reduction, objective hearing response	[30]
2	Everolimus (NCT01490476) (NCT01345136)	mTORC1 inhibitor	Phase 2, open label	No hearing or volumetric responses; stabilization/delay of tumor growth	≥15; 10	VS: radiographic tumor response (maximum tumor shrinkage), objective hearing response	[31,32]
3	Everolimus (NCT01880749)	mTORC1 inhibitor	Phase 0	Ongoing	≥18; ongoing	VS, MN: estimate proportions of tumors with complete inhibition of phospho-S6	None
4	Bevacizumab (NCT01207687)	VEGF inhibitor	Phase 2, open label	Durable hearing response in 36% of patients	≥12; 14	VS: hearing response measured by word recognition score	[33]
5	Bevacizumab (NCT01767792)	VEGF inhibitor	Phase 2, open label	Ongoing	≥6; ongoing	VS: determine the hearing response rate at 24 weeks after treatment	None
6	Lapatinib (NCT00973739)	EGFR/ErBb2 inhibitor	Phase 2, open label	Volumetric response in 23.5%, hearing response in 30.8% of patients	>3; 17	VS: volumetric response of ≥15% reduction; hearing response measured by word recognition score	[34]
7	Lapatinib (NCT00863122)	EGFR/ErBb2 inhibitor	Early Phase 1	None	≥18; 26	VS: assess steady-state lapatinib plasma concentrations at the time of surgical resection and minimum tumor concentration level of > 3 uM after oral dosing	None
8	Ataxinib (NCT02129647)	VEGFR2, PDGFR, c-kit inhibitor	Phase 2, open-label	None	≥18; ongoing	VS: volumetric response of ≥20% reduction; hearing response measured by increased speech discrimination score	None
9	AZD2014	mTORC1/mTORC2 inhibitor	Preclinical (in vitro)	AZD2014 leads to more profound suppression of primary human NF2-deficient meningioma cell proliferation when compared with rapamycin	n/a	n/a	[35]
10	Ponatinib	BCR-ABL/SRC inhibitor	Preclinical (in vitro)	Stimulated a robust G1 cell cycle arrest of merlin-deficient HSC in a dose-dependent manner	n/a	n/a	[36]
11	AR42 (NCT02282917)	HDAC	Early Phase 1	Ongoing	≥18; ongoing	Estimate the expression levels of phospho-Akt (p-AKT) and p16INKA after oral AR42	[37,38]
12	Nilotinib + selumetinib (AZD6244)	PDGFR/c-KIT inhibitor + MEK1/2 inhibitor	Preclinical (in vitro)	Nilotinib inhibited PDGF-DD mediated proliferation of NF2 schwannoma cells, while the addition of selumetinib increased this inhibitory effect	n/a	n/a	[39]

Abbreviations: EGFR, epithelial growth factor receptor; HSC, human schwan cells; MN, meningioma; NF2, neurofibromatosis type 2; PDGFR, platelet-derived growth factor receptor; VEGF, vascular endothelial growth factor; VEGFR2, vascular endothelial growth factor receptor 2; VS, vestibular schwannoma.

of tumor growth in some patients.[30,31] Nonetheless, the mTOR pathway is still under investigation as a recent preclinical study has demonstrated the superiority of AZD2014, a dual mTORC1/2 inhibitor, over rapamycin in suppressing proliferation of NF2-deficient meningioma cells.[35]

Antagonists of the Her1–2 members of the ERbB family of tyrosine receptor kinases (i.e., lapatinib) have demonstrated marginally better results on clinical trials, which were based on particularly encouraging results from in vivo mice models of vestibular schwannoma.[42] A phase 2 trial of lapatinib in 17 patients with NF2-related progressive vestibular schwannomas showed a ≥15% decrease in volume in 4 patients (23.5%) and 70.6% volumetric progression-free survival with minimal toxicity.[34] However, the authors did not observe volumetric responses in meningiomas and questioned the applicability of lapatinib in other NF2-related tumors. In contrast, a more recent retrospective study of patients with NF2-related vestibular schwannomas treated on a phase 2 clinical trial with lapatinib demonstrated modest growth-inhibitory effects on coincidental meningiomas.[43] Such discrepant results highlight the need for further prospective studies of lapatinib treatment for NF2 patients with meningiomas, considering the positive results seen in the treatment of NF2 vestibular schwannomas.

Bevacizumab, an antivascular endothelial growth factor (anti-VEGF) monoclonal antibody, has demonstrated the most promising results in tumor volume reduction and stabilization. A retrospective review of 31 NF2 patients with progressive vestibular schwannoma treated with bevacizumab reported 61% of patients with stable or improved hearing and 54% of patients with stable or decreased tumor size after 3 years of treatment.[44] Another review observed that 29% of meningiomas in the same patient cohort also had volumetric responses to bevacizumab treatment; however, tumor shrinkage was not durable, with median duration of response at 3.7 months and median time to progression at 15 months.[45] The relatively positive results in these studies have led to two prospective phase 2 clinical trials (ClinicalTrials.gov number NCT01207687, NCT01767792) assessing hearing responses rates in vestibular schwannoma patients. In addition, the potential of combination therapy with bevacizumab and lapatinib has been suggested,[34] considering preclinical models which show a functional link between the EGFR/ErbB2 signaling pathway and VEGF-dependent angiogenesis.[46]

10.2 Stereotactic Radiosurgery

10.2.1 Introduction

Stereotactic radiosurgery (SRS) is known to be an effective method of managing a variety of intracranial tumors. Once limited by the lack of fixation devices to the spine, SRS is increasingly being used to treat spinal lesions due to advancements in image-guidance technology.[47,48,49] Most studies of SRS in managing spinal tumors have been limited to vertebral and metastatic lesions[49,50,51,52,53]; however, SRS may have a role in treating primary intradural tumors as well. Although microsurgical resection remains the primary treatment modality of benign, IDEM tumors,[54,55,56,57] SRS may prove to be an effective option in patients who are poor surgical candidates due to comorbidities, multiplicity of tumors, or tumor recurrence

associated with pathology. The following section reviews the current literature on SRS in the management of benign IDEM spine tumors and future directions of research that may help in establishing SRS as a safe and efficacious treatment option.

10.2.2 Recent Research of SRS Use in IDEM Tumors

The first documented use of SRS in treatment of IDEM tumors was by Ryu et al in their study of 16 spinal lesions, which included 2 schwannomas and 1 meningioma. The study demonstrated the possibility of SRS as an option for treating a variety of primary spine tumors.[49] Another small study of 22 spinal tumors, which included 2 neurofibromas and 1 meningioma, treated with SRS reported favorable results as well and provided additional evidence on the feasibility of using SRS to treat IDEM tumors.[50]

A prospective study by Dodd et al described outcomes in the primary management of 55 IDEM spinal tumor, including 9 neurofibromas, 30 schwannomas, and 16 meningiomas, with CyberKnife radiosurgery at Stanford University Medical Center from 1999 to 2005.[58] Treatment doses of 1,600 to 3,000 cGy were delivered in 1 to 5 fractions to tumor volumes of 0.136 to 24.6 cm³. After more than 24 months of follow-up, 28 of the 55 lesions were either stable in size (61%) or smaller (39%), indicating that radiosurgery may not be effective in reversing the mass effect produced by these tumors. As such, two patients without reduction in tumor size had to receive further surgical resection due to progression of myelopathy. In addition, three tumors were enlarged, although by less than 10%, despite SRS. Only a single patient experienced radiation-induced myelopathy 8 months after treatment. Notably, a majority of patients (70% of meningiomas, 50% of schwannomas) reported significant pain relief, which was interestingly not correlative with total dosage, fractionation number, or reduction in tumor size. Despite favorable results reported in this study, the authors noted that longer follow-up was needed to determine the long-term efficacy in treating IDEM tumors due to their slow-growing nature.

A more recent study by Sachdev et al from the same institution described the outcomes of 103 IDEM tumors (24 neurofibromas, 47 schwannomas, and 32 meningiomas) after SRS during 1999 to 2008.[59] Total treatment dose ranging from 1,400 to 3,000 cGy were delivered in 1 to 5 fractions to tumor volumes ranging from 0.049 to 54.52 cm³. All tumors except for a single schwannoma demonstrated radiographic control after a mean of 33 months of follow-up. At latest follow-up, 91, 67, and 86% of meningiomas, neurofibromas, and schwannomas, respectively, showed improvement or long-term stability of clinical symptoms. A single patient with a C7–T2 recurrent meningioma developed transient radiation myelitis 9 months after treatment. However, the patient became neurologically stable after treatment with corticosteroids, and showed continued radiographic control until last follow-up (▶ Fig. 10.2).

Another study by Gerszten et al prospectively evaluated the efficacy of radiosurgery in 73 IDEM tumors, including 25 neurofibromas, 35 schwannomas, and 13 meningiomas, between 2001 and 2006 at the University of Pittsburgh Medical Center.[60] Single fraction doses (except for a single patient who underwent 3 fractions of treatment) of 1,500 to 2,500 cGy were delivered to tumors ranging from 0.3 to 93.4 cm³ in size.

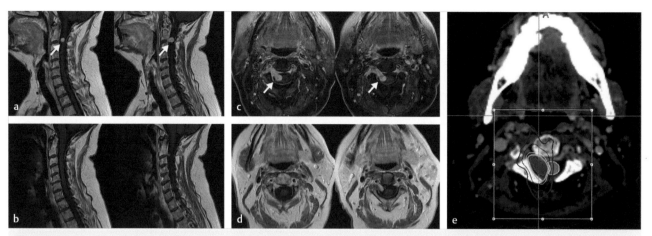

Fig. 10.2 Temporal response to radiosurgery shown in a 57-year-old patient with a C2 to C3 neurofibroma treated with 20 Gy in 2 fractions. **(a)** Sequential pretreatment postcontrast sagittal magnetic resonance imaging (MRI) images with the tumor highlighted by *arrows*. **(b)** 3 years posttreatment. **(c)** Sequential pretreatment postcontrast axial MRI images with the tumor highlighted by *arrows*. **(d)** 3 years posttreatment. **(e)** Treatment planning view, with tumor outlined in *red* and the spinal cord (identified as a critical structure) outlined in *blue*. (Reproduced with permission from Sachdev et al.[59])

Radiographic tumor control was achieved in all patients, and pain improvement was seen in 73% of cases with previous reports of pain. Three patients experienced radiation-related complications with symptoms of Brown–Sequard syndrome 5 to 13 months after treatment. In contrast to the study performed by Dodd et al, SRS was not used as the primary treatment for this patient cohort. SRS was the primary treatment modality in only 14 cases, while it was used as part of a multimodal treatment plan for the remaining tumors.

10.2.3 Future Directions

All of the aforementioned prospective studies described cases of radiation-induced myelopathy as a complication of SRS for IDEM tumors. The main factors associated with a risk of radiation-induced myelopathy are total dose and fraction sizes of radiation, length of spinal cord treated, and duration of treatment.[61,62,63] However, it is unclear which factors played a role in the development of myelopathy in these studies. For example, the cases of radiation-induced myelopathy observed in these studies were not significant outliers in terms of radiation dosage or tumor volume. Although animal studies have demonstrated a correlation between radiation dose and degree of radiation myelopathy,[64] such a relationship has not been apparent in actual clinical practice.[65] With insufficient data to establish a relationship between radiation dose and injury to the spinal cord, determining therapeutic ranges of radiation treatment in IDEM spine tumors remains an obstacle.

The prevention of radiation-induced injury may also be hindered by difficulties in precisely targeting tumor tissue within the spinal cord. Although utilization of high-resolution imaging has allowed us to accurately delineate tumor tissue in relation to the surrounding normal structures, static MRI images are insufficient to accurately account for oscillations of the spinal cord due to respiration or CSF pulsations. Such oscillatory movement is enhanced with compression of the spinal cord, resulting in increased movement at the site of the tumor.[66] The implications of such oscillatory movements cannot be overlooked especially considering the delivery of high-dose radiation to the sensitive

spinal cord. Dynamic MRI or CT myelograms can provide a breakthrough to cyclic radiation dosage that has the potential to improve precision and reduce radiation-induced injury.

The results of these studies also suggest that IDEM tumors with a concurrent diagnosis of NF1 may not respond to radiation in the same way as other sporadic IDEM tumors. Dodd et al noted that patients with NF1 were the least likely to report improvement in clinical symptoms such as pain, sensory loss, or weakness despite radiographic response to radiation.[58] Similarly, in the study by Gerszten et al, all three neurofibroma patients with a diagnosis of NF1 reported no improvement in pretreatment pain symptoms.[60] SRS treatment in NF1 patients may be complicated by the fact that these patients usually present with numerous spine lesions, which makes it difficult to target the tumor that is responsible for the patient's clinical symptoms. The persistence of pain may also be due to the infiltrative nature of neurofibromas, which are the primary spinal nerve root tumors seen in NF1 patients.[67] Comparable results in terms of pain are seen with surgical resection of neurofibromas as well,[68] suggesting that tumor pathology may contribute to the observed poor results. As such, Sachdev et al showed that neurofibromas, 87% of which had underlying NF1, were the most symptomatic and showed the poorest radiographic and clinical response to SRS among the treated lesions.[59] The poor response to SRS seen in neurofibromas in NF1 suggest that this treatment modality may not be the best option in these patients.

10.3 Robot-Assisted Surgery

10.3.1 Introduction

Among the most recent technological developments in medicine, robot-assisted surgical devices have shown remarkable value, especially in the fields of surgical oncology, urology, general surgery, and gynecology.[69,70,71] Robotics in spine surgery is less advanced and is mainly used in aiding accurate pedicle screw placement. Several successful cases have been reported in tumor resections as well, broaching the possibility of using robotic surgery in treating IDEM tumors. Although robot-assisted surgery provides several benefits such as improved accuracy, decreased radiation exposure, reduced length of stay, and reduced postoperative complications, it is not without its drawbacks, and several obstacles must be addressed to fully exploit its advantages for treating IDEM tumors.

10.3.2 Progress in Robot-Assisted Spine Tumor Surgery

To date, there have been very few studies evaluating robot-assisted surgery in spinal oncology. Case studies published in the literature demonstrate feasibility of robotics in spinal tumor resection in various locations. For example, the da Vinci system has been used in resecting paravertebral masses with an anterior approach through the thoracic cavity or abdomen. One study reported two cases of paravertebral spinal schwannomas, one in the superior sulcus and one in the inferior sulcus of the thoracic cavity, which are regions where standard surgical approaches could be challenging.[72] Complete resections were achieved with no postoperative complications for either patient.[72] Another paraspinal schwannoma at the L4–L5 level was able to be resected with a robotic transperitoneal approach, resulting in minimal bleeding and no damage to the surrounding structures.[73]

The advantages of the da Vinci system were also highlighted in cases of large presacral tumors, in which a conventional open approach is complicated by a limited surgical field despite using wide incisions and extensive retraction of the surrounding organs. The use of the da Vinci system in such situations allows for superior visualization and dissection of the tumor within a limited surgical corridor with minimal tissue injury, which in turn allows for faster recovery. One study reported nine patients with presacral tumors greater than 10 cm in diameter, all treated with robot-assisted resection resulting in shorter operation times, shorter hospital stays, and markedly less bleeding compared to open approaches.[74] A similar series of seven patients with presacral tumors underwent transperitoneal excision following the da Vinci system, all of which were resected successfully with decreased blood loss compared to an open approach.[75]

Robot-assisted surgery may also play a large role in the excision of primary and metastatic tumors in the vertebral columns. En bloc resections of bony tumors are challenging due to difficulties in determining intraoperative tumor resection margins within the complex anatomy of the spine. Bederman et al demonstrated the use of robotic guidance in a case of en bloc resection of primary sacral osteosarcoma.[76] In this case, a robot synchronized with preoperative images defining tumor margins was employed to drill pilot holes along the planned resection margins. The authors were able to achieve negative tumor margins and improve patient outcomes through such robotic guidance. As radiographic imaging systems become more developed, it is not too difficult to envision the use of robotic systems to intraoperatively help define predetermined borders of resection, maximizing tumor extirpation while limiting damage to critical surrounding tissues.

Despite the range of robotic advances seen in spinal oncology, there are no publications in the literature describing the use of robotic surgery for the treatment of intradural spine tumors at this time. However, the potential of robot-assisted guidance for resection margins demonstrated by Bederman et al cannot be overlooked and may play a large role in intradural tumor surgery, especially given that these tumors are often surrounded by critical neural elements. One can imagine a robotic microinstrument resection for an upper thoracic meningioma that is anterior to the spinal cord with optimum visualization. Further research in this field will be required to possibly treat patients who would not have been good candidates for surgery in the past.

10.3.3 Future Directions

Although the implications of robotic spine surgery are exciting, there are several drawbacks that must be addressed to standardize its use while improving patient outcomes. The most obvious disadvantage of robot-assisted surgery is the initial cost and continued burden of maintenance. A system costs upwards of $850,000 and annual expenses of disposable elements are estimated to be around $2,000.[77] Additionally, many cases of robotic spine surgeries are noted to have longer operation times, mostly due to inexperience in using the system and prolonged time needed for device setup.[77,78] Gaining full familiarity using the system is associated with a steep learning curve, taking more than 30 cases for even experienced surgeons.[79]

One of the largest barriers to the routine utilization of robotic assistance in IDEM tumors is the limitations in haptic feedback technology. Although high-definition endoscope optics can provide comparable or, in some cases, perhaps even superior means of visual feedback compared to open resection, other sensory cues such as tactile and proprioceptive stimuli are currently very lacking. The margin of error resulting from this deficiency may be tolerable in other surgical fields; however, such feedback is absolutely necessary when manipulating central nervous system tissues in order to minimize potentially irreversible injury. Future research to develop more realistic, responsive haptic feedback systems is crucial for the routine implementation of robotics in IDEM treatment.

Robot-assisted surgery of IDEM tumors is also deterred by the fact that most current robotic systems are designed to focus on a single type of surgery. As a result, resection of IDEM tumors, which comprises both bony and soft tissue stages within one surgery, is impossible to perform with one robotic system. A cadaveric study experimented the possibility of performing a conventional open laminectomy followed by intradural surgery using the da Vinci system to separate cauda equina nerve roots from the filum terminale.[80] Although such an approach may help with small aspects of surgery such as physiologic tremor reduction, it would fail to capitalize on the minimally invasive approach of robotic surgery while sacrificing real-time, tactile feedback. Development of an "all-in-one" system with the ability to provide both sufficient force for bone remodeling and sensitive feedback for soft tissue manipulation may be warranted.

An interesting aspect of robot-assisted surgery lies in the interchangeable arms that may be designed to perform specific functions needed by the surgeon. In the context of IDEM tumor treatment, robotic arms containing special sensors that can detect and delineate different types of tissues in the intraoperative setting may allow for more accurate and efficient surgeries. For example, fluorescent probe arms may be used to detect residual tumor in real-time following intravenous injection of fluorescent agents, thus allowing constant intraoperative feedback for identifying tumor margins. Even more creative modalities of feedback integrated into these robotic arms may be beneficial in ensuring the efficacy and safety of robotic-assisted intradural tumor surgeries.

10.4 Conclusion

Intradural extramedullary (IDEM) tumors are generally treated with surgical resection and decompression of the surrounding neural structures; however, the presence of systemic disease (i.e., neurofibromatosis), severe comorbidities, and the challenging anatomical location of the tumor may make such a task difficult to achieve. A gamut of systemic chemotherapies are being studied and developed for use in patients with IDEM tumors associated with NF1 and NF2. These systemic therapeutics have shown to decrease total tumor burden and relieve the patient of other symptomatology secondary to neurofibromatosis. Stereotactic radiosurgery has been shown to be efficacious in treating IDEM tumors, either as a primary treatment course or as part of a multimodal treatment plan, though the select patient populations in which its benefit is greatest remains to be elucidated. Robotic surgery for IDEM tumors has shown to result in improved visualization and accuracy of resection, reduced length-of-stay, and decreased postoperative complications. However, several obstacles such as cost, limited haptic feedback, and lack of flexibility in manipulating both bony and soft tissue structures remain before implementation in routine practice is achieved.

References

[1] Asthagiri AR, Parry DM, Butman JA, et al. Neurofibromatosis type 2. Lancet. 2009; 373(9679):1974–1986

[2] Uusitalo E, Leppävirta J, Koffert A, et al. Incidence and mortality of neurofibromatosis: a total population study in Finland. J Invest Dermatol. 2015; 135(3):904–906

[3] Khong P-L, Goh WHS, Wong VCN, Fung C-W, Ooi G-C. MR imaging of spinal tumors in children with neurofibromatosis 1. AJR Am J Roentgenol. 2003; 180(2):413–417

[4] Thakkar SD, Feigen U, Mautner VF. Spinal tumours in neurofibromatosis type 1: an MRI study of frequency, multiplicity and variety. Neuroradiology. 1999; 41(9):625–629

[5] Martin GA, Viskochil D, Bollag G, et al. The GAP-related domain of the neurofibromatosis type 1 gene product interacts with ras p21. Cell. 1990; 63 (4):843–849

[6] Weiss B, Bollag G, Shannon K. Hyperactive Ras as a therapeutic target in neurofibromatosis type 1. Am J Med Genet. 1999; 89(1):14–22

[7] Gottfried ON, Viskochil DH, Couldwell WT. Neurofibromatosis Type 1 and tumorigenesis: molecular mechanisms and therapeutic implications. Neurosurg Focus. 2010; 28(1):E8

[8] Gutmann DH, Blakeley JO, Korf BR, Packer RJ. Optimizing biologically targeted clinical trials for neurofibromatosis. Expert Opin Investig Drugs. 2013; 22(4): 443–462

[9] Robertson KA, Nalepa G, Yang F-C, et al. Imatinib mesylate for plexiform neurofibromas in patients with neurofibromatosis type 1: a phase 2 trial. Lancet Oncol. 2012; 13(12):1218–1224

[10] Riccardi VM. Ketotifen suppression of NF1 neurofibroma growth over 30 years. Am J Med Genet A. 2015; 167(7):1570–1577

[11] Widemann BC, Dombi E, Gillespie A, et al. Phase 2 randomized, flexible crossover, double-blinded, placebo-controlled trial of the farnesyltransferase inhibitor tipifarnib in children and young adults with neurofibromatosis type 1 and progressive plexiform neurofibromas. Neuro-oncol. 2014; 16(5):707–718

[12] Weiss B, Widemann BC, Wolters P, et al. Sirolimus for progressive neurofibromatosis type 1-associated plexiform neurofibromas: a neurofibromatosis Clinical Trials Consortium phase II study. Neuro-oncol. 2015; 17(4):596–603

[13] Dombi E, Baldwin A, Marcus LJ, et al. Activity of selumetinib in neurofibromatosis type 1-related plexiform neurofibromas. N Engl J Med. 2016; 375(26):2550–2560

[14] Yang F-C, Chen S, Clegg T, et al. Nf1 +/- mast cells induce neurofibroma like phenotypes through secreted TGF-beta signaling. Hum Mol Genet. 2006; 15 (16):2421–2437

[15] Zhu Y, Ghosh P, Charnay P, Burns DK, Parada LF. Neurofibromas in NF1: Schwann cell origin and role of tumor environment. Science. 2002; 296 (5569):920–922

[16] Yang F-C, Ingram DA, Chen S, et al. Neurofibromin-deficient Schwann cells secrete a potent migratory stimulus for Nf1 +/- mast cells. J Clin Invest. 2003; 112(12):1851–1861

[17] Yang F-C, Ingram DA, Chen S, et al. Nf1-dependent tumors require a microenvironment containing Nf1 +/- and c-kit-dependent bone marrow. Cell. 2008; 135(3):437–448

[18] Guha A, Lau N, Huvar I, et al. Ras-GTP levels are elevated in human NF1 peripheral nerve tumors. Oncogene. 1996; 12(3):507–513

[19] Crul M, de Klerk GJ, Beijnen JH, Schellens JH. Ras biochemistry and farnesyl transferase inhibitors: a literature survey. Anticancer Drugs. 2001; 12(3): 163–184

[20] Evans DG, Howard E, Giblin C, et al. Birth incidence and prevalence of tumor-prone syndromes: estimates from a UK family genetic register service. Am J Med Genet A. 2010; 152A(2):327–332

[21] Evans DG, Huson SM, Donnai D, et al. A genetic study of type 2 neurofibromatosis in the United Kingdom. I. Prevalence, mutation rate, fitness, and confirmation of maternal transmission effect on severity. J Med Genet. 1992; 29(12):841–846

[22] Evans DGR, Moran A, King A, Saeed S, Gurusinghe N, Ramsden R. Incidence of vestibular schwannoma and neurofibromatosis 2 in the North West of England over a 10-year period: higher incidence than previously thought. Otol Neurotol. 2005; 26(1):93–97

[23] Mautner VF, Tatagiba M, Lindenau M, et al. Spinal tumors in patients with neurofibromatosis type 2: MR imaging study of frequency, multiplicity, and variety. AJR Am J Roentgenol. 1995; 165(4):951–955

[24] Patronas NJ, Courcoutsakis N, Bromley CM, Katzman GL, MacCollin M, Parry DM. Intramedullary and spinal canal tumors in patients with neurofibromatosis 2: MR imaging findings and correlation with genotype. Radiology. 2001; 218(2):434–442

[25] Hadfield KD, Smith MJ, Urquhart JE, et al. Rates of loss of heterozygosity and mitotic recombination in NF2 schwannomas, sporadic vestibular schwannomas and schwannomatosis schwannomas. Oncogene. 2010; 29(47):6216–6221

[26] Yohay KH. The genetic and molecular pathogenesis of NF1 and NF2. Semin Pediatr Neurol. 2006; 13(1):21–26

[27] Qian X, Karpova T, Sheppard AM, McNally J, Lowy DR. E-cadherin-mediated adhesion inhibits ligand-dependent activation of diverse receptor tyrosine kinases. EMBO J. 2004; 23(8):1739–1748

[28] Curto M, Cole BK, Lallemand D, Liu C-H, McClatchey AI. Contact-dependent inhibition of EGFR signaling by Nf2/Merlin. J Cell Biol. 2007; 177(5):893–903

[29] Morrison H, Sperka T, Manent J, Giovannini M, Ponta H, Herrlich P. Merlin/neurofibromatosis type 2 suppresses growth by inhibiting the activation of Ras and Rac. Cancer Res. 2007; 67(2):520–527

[30] Karajannis MA, Legault G, Hagiwara M, et al. Phase II study of everolimus in children and adults with neurofibromatosis type 2 and progressive vestibular schwannomas. Neuro-oncol. 2014; 16(2):292–297

[31] Goutagny S, Raymond E, Esposito-Farese M, et al. Phase II study of mTORC1 inhibition by everolimus in neurofibromatosis type 2 patients with growing vestibular schwannomas. J Neurooncol. 2015; 122(2):313–320

[32] Goutagny S, Giovannini M, Kalamarides M. A 4-year phase II study of everolimus in NF2 patients with growing vestibular schwannomas. J Neurooncol. 2017; 133(2):443–445

[33] Blakeley JO, Ye X, Duda DG, et al. Efficacy and biomarker study of bevacizumab for hearing loss resulting from neurofibromatosis type 2-associated vestibular schwannomas. J Clin Oncol. 2016; 34(14):1669–1675

[34] Karajannis MA, Legault G, Hagiwara M, et al. Phase II trial of lapatinib in adult and pediatric patients with neurofibromatosis type 2 and progressive vestibular schwannomas. Neuro-oncol. 2012; 14(9):1163–1170

[35] Beauchamp RL, James MF, DeSouza PA, et al. A high-throughput kinome screen reveals serum/glucocorticoid-regulated kinase 1 as a therapeutic target for NF2-deficient meningiomas. Oncotarget. 2015; 6(19):16981–16997

[36] Petrilli AM, Garcia J, Bott M, et al. Ponatinib promotes a G1 cell-cycle arrest of merlin/NF2-deficient human schwann cells. Oncotarget. 2017; 8(19):31666–31681

[37] Bush ML, Oblinger J, Brendel V, et al. AR42, a novel histone deacetylase inhibitor, as a potential therapy for vestibular schwannomas and meningiomas. Neuro-oncol. 2011; 13(9):983–999

[38] Cheng H, Xie Z, Jones WP, et al. Preclinical pharmacokinetics study of R- and S-enantiomers of the histone deacetylase inhibitor, AR-42 (NSC 731438), in rodents. AAPS J. 2016; 18(3):737–745

[39] Ammoun S, Schmid MC, Triner J, Manley P, Hanemann CO. Nilotinib alone or in combination with selumetinib is a drug candidate for neurofibromatosis type 2. Neuro-oncol. 2011; 13(7):759–766

[40] James MF, Han S, Polizzano C, et al. NF2/merlin is a novel negative regulator of mTOR complex 1, and activation of mTORC1 is associated with meningioma and schwannoma growth. Mol Cell Biol. 2009; 29(15):4250–4261

[41] James MF, Stivison E, Beauchamp R, et al. Regulation of mTOR complex 2 signaling in neurofibromatosis 2-deficient target cell types. Mol Cancer Res. 2012; 10(5):649–659

[42] Clark JJ, Provenzano M, Diggelmann HR, Xu N, Hansen SS, Hansen MR. The ErbB inhibitors trastuzumab and erlotinib inhibit growth of vestibular schwannoma xenografts in nude mice: a preliminary study. Otol Neurotol. 2008; 29(6):846–853

[43] Osorio DS, Hu J, Mitchell C, et al. Effect of lapatinib on meningioma growth in adults with neurofibromatosis type 2. J Neurooncol. 2018; 139(3):749–755

[44] Plotkin SR, Merker VL, Halpin C, et al. Bevacizumab for progressive vestibular schwannoma in neurofibromatosis type 2: a retrospective review of 31 patients. Otol Neurotol. 2012; 33(6):1046–1052

[45] Nunes FP, Merker VL, Jennings D, et al. Bevacizumab treatment for meningiomas in NF2: a retrospective analysis of 15 patients. PLoS One. 2013; 8(3):e59941

[46] Tortora G, Ciardiello F, Gasparini G. Combined targeting of EGFR-dependent and VEGF-dependent pathways: rationale, preclinical studies and clinical applications. Nat Clin Pract Oncol. 2008; 5(9):521–530

[47] Hsu W, Nguyen T, Kleinberg L, et al. Stereotactic radiosurgery for spine tumors: review of current literature. Stereotact Funct Neurosurg. 2010; 88 (5):315–321

[48] Yin F-F, Ryu S, Ajlouni M, et al. Image-guided procedures for intensity-modulated spinal radiosurgery. Technical note. J Neurosurg. 2004; 101(3) Suppl 3:419–424

[49] Ryu SI, Chang SD, Kim DH, et al. Image-guided hypo-fractionated stereotactic radiosurgery to spinal lesions. Neurosurgery. 2001; 49(4):838–846

[50] De Salles AAF, Pedroso AG, Medin P, et al. Spinal lesions treated with Novalis shaped beam intensity-modulated radiosurgery and stereotactic radiotherapy. J Neurosurg. 2004; 101(3) Suppl 3:435–440

[51] Gerszten PC, Burton SA, Ozhasoglu C, Welch WC. Radiosurgery for spinal metastases: clinical experience in 500 cases from a single institution. Spine. 2007; 32(2):193–199

[52] Rock JP, Ryu S, Yin F-F. Novalis radiosurgery for metastatic spine tumors. Neurosurg Clin N Am. 2004; 15(4):503–509

[53] Degen JW, Gagnon GJ, Voyadzis J-M, et al. CyberKnife stereotactic radiosurgical treatment of spinal tumors for pain control and quality of life. J Neurosurg Spine. 2005; 2(5):540–549

[54] Parsa AT, Lee J, Parney IF, Weinstein P, McCormick PC, Ames C. Spinal cord and intradural-extraparenchymal spinal tumors: current best care practices and strategies. J Neurooncol. 2004; 69(1–3):291–318

[55] Zuckerman SL, Chotai S, Devin CJ, et al. Surgical resection of intradural extramedullary spinal tumors: patient reported outcomes and minimum clinically important difference. Spine. 2016; 41(24):1925–1932

[56] Conti P, Pansini G, Mouchaty H, Capuano C, Conti R. Spinal neurinomas: retrospective analysis and long-term outcome of 179 consecutively operated cases and review of the literature. Surg Neurol. 2004; 61(1):34–43, discussion 44

[57] Cohen-Gadol AA, Zikel OM, Koch CA, Scheithauer BW, Krauss WE. Spinal meningiomas in patients younger than 50 years of age: a 21-year experience. J Neurosurg. 2003; 98(3) Suppl:258–263

[58] Dodd RL, Ryu M-R, Kamnerdsupaphon P, Gibbs IC, Chang SD , Jr, Adler JR , Jr. CyberKnife radiosurgery for benign intradural extramedullary spinal tumors. Neurosurgery. 2006; 58(4):674–685, discussion 674–685

[59] Sachdev S, Dodd RL, Chang SD, et al. Stereotactic radiosurgery yields long-term control for benign intradural, extramedullary spinal tumors. Neurosurgery. 2011; 69(3):533–539, discussion 539

[60] Gerszten PC, Burton SA, Ozhasoglu C, McCue KJ, Quinn AE. Radiosurgery for benign intradural spinal tumors. Neurosurgery. 2008; 62(4):887–895, discussion 895–896

[61] Schultheiss TE, Kun LE, Ang KK, Stephens LC. Radiation response of the central nervous system. Int J Radiat Oncol Biol Phys. 1995; 31(5):1093–1112

[62] Isaacson SR. Radiation therapy and the management of intramedullary spinal cord tumors. J Neurooncol. 2000; 47(3):231–238

[63] Rampling R, Symonds P. Radiation myelopathy. Curr Opin Neurol. 1998; 11 (6):627–632

[64] Hopewell JW, Morris AD, Dixon-Brown A. The influence of field size on the late tolerance of the rat spinal cord to single doses of X rays. Br J Radiol. 1987; 60(719):1099–1108

[65] Gibbs IC, Patil C, Gerszten PC, Adler JR , Jr, Burton SA. Delayed radiation-induced myelopathy after spinal radiosurgery. Neurosurgery. 2009; 64(2) Suppl:A67–A72

[66] Jokich PM, Rubin JM, Dohrmann GJ. Intraoperative ultrasonic evaluation of spinal cord motion. J Neurosurg. 1984; 60(4):707–711

[67] Halliday AL, Sobel RA, Martuza RL. Benign spinal nerve sheath tumors: their occurrence sporadically and in neurofibromatosis types 1 and 2. J Neurosurg. 1991; 74(2):248–253

[68] Seppälä MT, Haltia MJ, Sankila RJ, Jääskeläinen JE, Heiskanen O. Long-term outcome after removal of spinal neurofibroma. J Neurosurg. 1995; 82(4):572–577

[69] Zou H, Luo L, Xue H, et al. Preliminary experience in laparoscopic resection of hepatic hydatidectocyst with the Da Vinci Surgical System (DVSS): a case report. BMC Surg. 2017; 17(1):98

[70] Novara G, La Falce S, Kungulli A, Gandaglia G, Ficarra V, Mottrie A. Robot-assisted partial nephrectomy. Int J Surg. 2016; 36(Pt C):554–559

[71] Sinno AK, Fader AN. Robotic-assisted surgery in gynecologic oncology. Fertil Steril. 2014; 102(4):922–932

[72] Pacchiarotti G, Wang MY, Kolcun JPG, et al. Robotic paravertebral schwannoma resection at extreme locations of the thoracic cavity. Neurosurg Focus. 2017; 42(5):E17

[73] Yang MS, Kim KN, Yoon DH, Pennant W, Ha Y. Robot-assisted resection of paraspinal schwannoma. J Korean Med Sci. 2011; 26(1):150–153

[74] Oh JK, Yang MS, Yoon DH, et al. Robotic resection of huge presacral tumors: case series and comparison with an open resection. J Spinal Disord Tech. 2014; 27(4):E151–E154

[75] Yin J, Wu H, Tu J, et al. Robot-assisted sacral tumor resection: a preliminary study. BMC Musculoskelet Disord. 2018; 19(1):186

[76] Bederman SS, Lopez G, Ji T, Hoang BH. Robotic guidance for en bloc sacrectomy: a case report. Spine. 2014; 39(23):E1398–E1401

[77] Ghasem A, Sharma A, Greif DN, Alam M, Maaieh MA. The arrival of robotics in spine surgery: a review of the literature. Spine. 2018; 43(23): 1670–1677

[78] Yu L, Chen X, Margalit A, Peng H, Qiu G, Qian W. Robot-assisted vs freehand pedicle screw fixation in spine surgery—a systematic review and a meta-analysis of comparative studies. Int J Med Robot. 2018; 14(3): e1892

[79] Hu X, Lieberman IH. What is the learning curve for robotic-assisted pedicle screw placement in spine surgery? Clin Orthop Relat Res. 2014; 472(6): 1839–1844

[80] Karas CS, Chiocca EA. Neurosurgical robotics: a review of brain and spine applications. J Robot Surg. 2007; 1(1):39–43

Section III

Peripheral Nerve Tumors

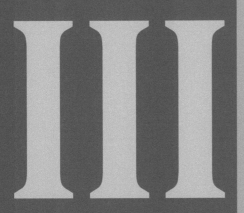

11 Peripheral Nerve Tumor: Histopathology and Radiology

Luis Manon, David Nai, Akua Graf, Amanda Allen, Christopher Florido, Young Jun Lee, and Tibor Valyi-Nagy

Summary

This chapter will review the histologic and radiographic findings associated with tumors of peripheral nerves with a focus on nerve sheath tumors including neurofibroma, schwannoma, perineurioma, and malignant peripheral nerve sheath tumor. Partially overlapping morphologic features and an association of several of these tumors with genetic disorders can make the diagnosis of these neoplasms difficult.

Keywords: peripheral nerve sheath tumor, histology, radiology, schwannoma, neurofibroma, perineurioma, hybrid nerve sheath tumor, malignant peripheral nerve sheath tumor

11.1 Neurofibroma

Neurofibroma is a common benign nerve sheath tumor that is composed of neoplastic Schwann cells and a variety of nonneoplastic cells including fibroblasts, perineurial-like cells, and mast cells and typically also residual axons.[1,2,3,4] A vast majority of neurofibromas are solitary lesions in patients without a clinical syndrome, while patients with neurofibromatosis type 1 (NF1) typically have multiple lesions. Neurofibroma can present as localized cutaneous neurofibroma, as a deeper circumscribed mass of peripheral nerve called localized intraneural neurofibroma, as plexiform neurofibroma with involvement of multiple nerve fascicles, as diffuse cutaneous neurofibroma, and as massive involvement of soft tissue in a body region.

Sporadic neurofibromas in individuals without NF1 are thought to be caused by somatic biallelic inactivation of neurofibromin. Neurofibromin is a product of the NF1 gene located at 17q11.2. Neurofibromin is a tumor suppressor protein—a negative regulator of Ras signaling related to cell survival and proliferation. Loss of neurofibromin increases Ras signaling with the potential of promotion of cell growth and proliferation. NF1 is an autosomal dominant syndrome associated with a germ-line inactivation of neurofibromin. In NF1, neurofibromas develop following somatic loss of the remaining wildtype NF1 allele.[1,2,3,4,5,6]

11.1.1 Pathologic/Anatomic Variants of Neurofibroma

Localized Cutaneous Neurofibroma

This most common form of neurofibroma presents as a painless, soft, up to 2 cm skin or subcutaneous nodule. Most are solitary and sporadic and present in young adults. In NF1 patients, they are typically multiple and increase in size and number after puberty.

Localized Intraneuronal Neurofibroma

These are neurofibromas confined to a single fascicle or nerve and much less common than localized cutaneous neurofibroma. They may appear at any point along a nerve, from the spinal root to the distal branches, but most affect large nerves of the cervical, brachial, or lumbosacral plexuses. Multiple tumors are usually associated with NF1. The perineurium and epineurium of the involved nerve form a thin sheath. Their gross appearance is gray to gray-tan, translucent, fusiform, and well circumscribed. Cut sections show the nerves from which the tumor originated, buried within the tumor.

Plexiform Neurofibroma

The plexiform neurofibroma variant involves and expands multiple nerve fascicles and is almost exclusively associated with NF1. It is more likely than other variants to undergo malignant transformation with a lifetime risk of progression to malignant peripheral nerve sheath tumors (MPNSTs) of approximately 10%.[7] It tends to occur in larger nerves and may grow in multiple branches of the same nerve. It may take the shape of multiple fusiform masses in an arbor-like pattern or that of a "bag of worms." Smooth-contoured, elongated ovoid structures—distorted nerve fascicles—may be involved. Tumor cells insinuate between the nerve fibers, distending the perineurial membrane. The tumor may invade through the epineurium and into the surrounding soft tissues; there can be microscopic involvement of organs and viscera.

Massive Soft Tissue Neurofibroma

All patients with this variant of neurofibroma have NF1. As the name suggests, it causes massive enlargement of the involved body region. The tumor can cause localized gigantism, producing distortion of a body part. The tumor often infiltrates deeper tissue, and the overlying skin may be pigmented.

Diffuse Cutaneous Neurofibroma

This uncommon tumor is ill-defined and features plaque-like cutaneous and subcutaneous lesions typically involving the head or neck region of children and young adults and is associated with NF1 in only a minority of cases. These tumors permeate the dermis, entrap cutaneous adnexa, and spread along subcutaneous adipose tissue and connective tissue septa.

11.1.2 Microscopic Pathology of Neurofibroma

Neurofibroma is composed of neoplastic Schwann cells and a variety of non-neoplastic cells including fibroblasts, perineurial-like cells, and mast cells, and typically also contains residual axons (▶ Fig. 11.1). Most neurofibromas are hypocellular and composed of widely spaced cells with ovoid, elongated nuclei that are often curved. They have scant cytoplasm embedded in gelatinous matrix. Mucopolysaccharide matrix appears watery blue on hematoxylin and eosin stained sections and positive on Alcian blue; it is weakly PAS-reactive. Nuclei are one-third to half the size of those of schwannoma cells. Compact "shredded carrots" bundles of collagen are present. Degenerative atypia is the most common benign atypical change and nuclear atypia alone is generally insignificant.[1,2,3,4,5,6]

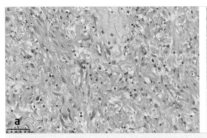 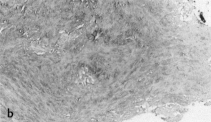 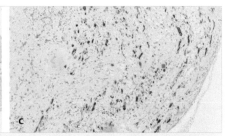

Fig. 11.1 Neurofibroma. (a) Hematoxylin and eosin (H&E) stained sections show spindle cell neoplasm with elongated nuclei in a collagenous matrix. (b) Many tumor cells are positive for S-100 (*brown staining*) by immunohistochemistry. (c) *Brown staining* highlights axons within neurofibroma (immunostaining for neurofilament).

There are enlarged nuclei, dense smudgy chromatin, inconspicuous nucleoli, and cytoplasmic nuclear pseudoinclusions. There is no significant MIB-1 labeling or mitotic activity.

Atypical neurofibroma is a variant that is difficult to distinguish from low-grade MPNST due to the presence of worrisome histologic features such as high cellularity, scattered mitotic activity, monomorphic cytology, and/or fascicular growth in addition to cytologic atypia.[1,2,5,6,8,9] Atypical neurofibromas may exhibit CDKN2A inactivation with loss of p16 expression.[9] In the context of NF1, the term atypical neurofibromatous neoplasm of uncertain biologic potential (ANNUBP) has recently been proposed for lesions with at least two features from a list that includes atypia, loss of neurofibroma architecture, high cellularity, and/or mitotic activity >1/50 but <3/10 high power fields.[5] This diagnosis should prompt additional sampling, clinical correlation, and possibly, expert pathology consultation to rule in or exclude MPNST.[5,6]

Neurofibromas stain for S-100, although staining typically does not involve all tumor cells. A similar pattern is seen with SOX-10. Only a limited number of EMA-positive cells are typically detected highlighting perineurial-like cells. Immunohistochemical analysis of neurofibromas does not show loss of H3K27me3 staining or increased p53 staining, which are features of MPNST.

11.1.3 Radiologic Features of Neurofibroma

On magnetic resonance imaging (MRI), intraneural neurofibromas appear elongated with a signal intensity similar to that of muscle on T1 sequences. There is high signal intensity on T2-weighted images and usually there is heterogeneous enhancement (▶ Fig. 11.2 and ▶ Fig. 11.3). On T2, central hypodense area, target sign is characteristic but not specific.[10,11,12,13] On computed tomography (CT) neurofibroma is hypodense and sometimes there is central hyperdensity. Plexiform neurofibromas appear as multilobulated masses extending along nerves.

Fluorodeoxyglucose (FDG)-positron emission tomography (PET) may be useful in distinguishing MPNSTs from benign peripheral nerve sheath tumors based on a tumor's metabolic activity, with malignant tumors demonstrating moderate to high FDG accumulation.[13,14,15,16,17]

11.2 Schwannoma

Schwannomas are benign peripheral nervous system tumors composed entirely of Schwann cells.[1,2,3,4] There are three major

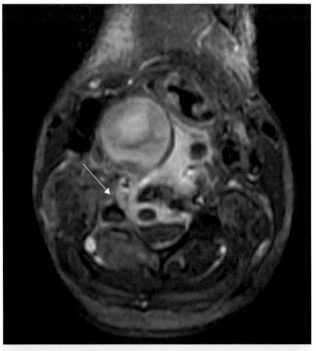

Fig. 11.2 Neurofibroma. Axial T1weighted postcontrast image of the upper cervical spine shows a peripheral enhancing extramedullary intradural mass displacing the spinal cord posteriorly and widening the left neural foramen (*arrow*).

forms: conventional schwannomas, cellular schwannomas, and plexiform schwannomas. Melanotic schwannomas are increasingly considered a unique entity rather than a variant of schwannoma.

The vast majority of schwannomas are single sporadic lesions affecting patients without a clinical syndrome. These lesions are thought to be caused by biallelic loss of function mutations affecting the NF2 gene located on 22q12.2 and encoding the protein merlin (also called schwannomin or neurofibromin 2). About 10% of schwannomas are associated with neurofibromatosis type 2 (NF2) or with schwannomatosis. NF2 is an autosomal dominant disorder associated with inactivating germline mutations of NF2.[1,18] Bilateral vestibular schwannomas are pathognomonic for NF2, and in addition to other tumors patients also present with schwannomas of other cranial, spinal, peripheral and cutaneous nerves. Schwannomatosis is characterized by multiple schwannomas and are associated SMARCB1 or LZTR1 on 22q mutations and inactivation of the NF2 gene in tumors but not in the germline.[1,2,4]

11.2.1 Conventional Schwannoma

Conventional, nonmelanotic schwannomas are benign typically encapsulated tumors with a peak incidence in the fourth to sixth decades of life with no gender prevalence. The gross appearance is smooth or lobulated, tan in color with gray and white patches. Schwannomas most commonly affect peripheral nerves of the skin and subcutaneous tissue. Peripheral nerve schwannomas often involve the head and neck region and flexor surfaces of the elbow, wrist, or knee. In the spine, most schwannomas affect sensory nerve roots. Intracranial schwannomas most commonly involve the eighth cranial nerve. Bilateral vestibular schwannomas are pathognomonic for NF2. Rarely schwannomas occur viscerally. Gross examination often shows globular tumor with hemorrhagic and cystic cut surfaces upon sectioning.

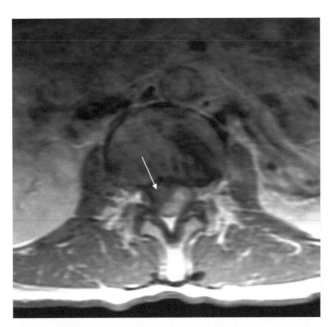

Fig. 11.3 Neurofibroma. Axial T2-weighted image of the lumbar spine demonstrates extramedullary intradural mass (*arrow*) displacing the conus medullaris to the left.

11.2.2 Microscopic Pathology of Conventional Schwannoma

Characteristic histopathologic findings associated with conventional schwannoma include detection of a spindle cell neoplasm with more cellular, denser and less cellular, looser tumor areas called Antoni A and B areas, respectively (▶ Fig. 11.4). A fibrous capsule, nuclear palisading (Verocay bodies), hyalinized blood vessels, cystic change, focal chronic inflammation, and remote hemorrhage are commonly found. Detection of degenerative nuclear atypia (ancient change) and scattered mitotic activity are consistent with the diagnosis of benign WHO grade I schwannoma. Nerve fibers, if detected, are adjacent to or at the periphery of the lesion.

Tumor cells are uniformly positive for S-100 by immunohistochemistry, are also positive for SOX10, and may focally express glial fibrillary acidic protein (GFAP). There is extensive membrane staining for collagen IV and ultrastructural studies show continuous basal lamina surrounding Schwann cells. Neurofilament immunostaining is typically negative within the tumor. Malignant transformation of conventional schwannoma is extremely rare.[1,2,3,4]

11.2.3 Cellular Schwannoma

This variant is highly cellular, and by definition is composed exclusively or predominantly of tumor areas with Antoni A histology. Cellular schwannoma demonstrates a female predominance and most common locations include the posterior mediastinum and pelvis. Mitotic activity may be prominent and can reach 10 mitoses per 10 high power microscopic fields. High cellularity and mitotic activity often raise the differential diagnostic concern of MPNST. Histopathologic and immunohistochemical findings that favor the diagnosis of cellular schwannoma include the detection of a peritumoral capsule, focal chronic inflammation, extensive expression of S-100 and SOX10, and retained H3K27me3 staining.[1,4,19] Cellular schwannomas are benign neoplasms and malignant transformation is extremely rare. However, recurrences are more common for cellular schwannomas of the intracranial, spinal, and sacral regions.[1,20]

11.2.4 Plexiform Schwannoma

This variant demonstrates a plexiform or multinodular growth pattern and may feature either conventional or cellular schwannoma histology.[1,2,3,4] Most of them involve the skin or subcutaneous tissues and are important to differentiate from plexiform

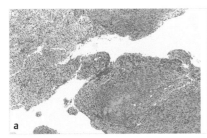

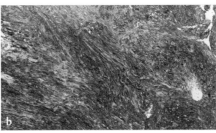

Fig. 11.4 Schwannoma. (a) Hematoxylin and eosin (H&E) stained section shows spindle cell neoplasm with more cellular and less cellular (Antoni A and Antoni B) areas. (b) Tumor cells are positive for S-100 (*brown staining*) by immunohistochemistry.

neurofibromas, as plexiform schwannomas do not have an increased potential for malignant transformation. There is an association of plexiform schwannoma with NF2 and schwannomatosis (5% each).[21]

11.2.5 Melanotic Schwannoma

Melanotic schwannoma is a tumor of melanin-producing Schwann cells that contain melanosomes and are increasingly considered a unique entity rather than a variant of schwannoma.[2,4,22] Melanotic schwannomas are rare and have a predilection for posterior spinal nerves and paraspinal ganglia. Melanotic schwannomas are immunoreactive for S-100, as well as melanoma immunohistochemical markers like HMB45 and melan-A. Some melanotic schwannomas contain laminated calcifications called psammoma bodies. Psammomatous melanotic schwannomas are often associated with Carney complex, an autosomal dominant disorder associated with lentiginous facial pigmentation; cutaneous, soft tissue, and cardiac myxomas; and endocrine dysregulation. Half of those with Carney complex have mutated PRKAR1A tumor suppressor gene. Loss of PRKAR1A protein staining can be detected by immunostaining in melanotic schwannomas not associated with Carney complex.[22] Unlike conventional schwannomas, a significant portion of melanotic schwannomas follow a malignant course.[1,22]

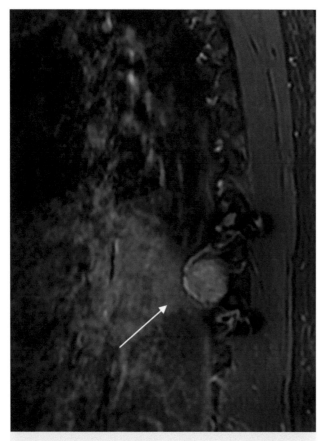

Fig. 11.5 Schwannoma. Sagittal T1-weighted postcontrast image shows a paraspinal mass with heterogeneous areas of enhancement (*arrow*).

11.2.6 Radiologic Features of Schwannoma

Conventional schwannomas appear as sharply circumscribed often globoid masses on radiographs with the origin of the tumor from a nerve often demonstrable. On MRI they are hypointense or isointense on T1 but are T2-bright and frequently show a low-intensity rim consistent with a capsule and cystic degeneration (▶ Fig. 11.5 and ▶ Fig. 11.6). A target sign is more common in neurofibroma than in schwannoma.

11.3 Perineurioma

Perineuriomas are rare tumors composed entirely of perineurial cells.[1,2,3,4] Intraneural perineuriomas are benign neoplasms and are located within the endoneurium of peripheral nerves. Soft tissue perineuriomas are typically not associated with nerve and are also benign, although rare malignant forms, perineurial MPNST, also exist. Molecular studies in perineuriomas demonstrate monosomy of chromosome 22. There is no association with NF1 or NF2.

Once termed "localized hypertrophic neuropathy," intraneural perineuriomas typically present as cylindrical enlargement of a peripheral nerve on an extremity during adolescence or early adulthood without gender predilection. Microscopically, perineurial cells are seen encircling individual nerve fibers or forming whorls without a central nerve fiber. There is no significant nuclear atypia or mitotic activity. The term pseudo-onion bulbing was adapted from the similarity between intraneural perineurioma and hypertrophic neuropathies. Immunohistochemically, there is membranous and widespread reactivity of the perineurial cells with EMA. There is no S-100 staining on the layers of perineurial cells encircling the nerve fiber (pseudo-onion bulbing). S-100 and neurofilament immunostains highlight enwrapped nerve fibers. Intraneural perineuriomas are benign but typically lead to loss of nerve function.

Soft tissue perineuriomas typically affect adults and are located in deep soft tissue without grossly apparent association with nerve. A small set of cases have been reported in the

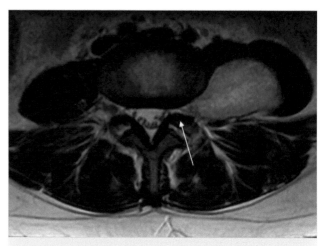

Fig. 11.6 Schwannoma. Axial T2-weighted image of the lumbar spine shows an expansile heterogeneous T2 high signal intensity mass in the left neural foramen (*arrow*).

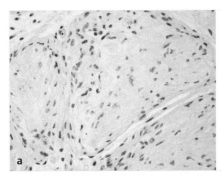 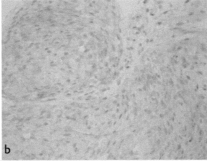 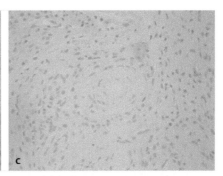

Fig. 11.7 (a) Soft tissue perineurioma. Upper panel: Hematoxylin and eosin (H&E) stained sections show spindle cell neoplasm with tumor cells forming storiform patterns. (b) Tumor cells are positive for EMA. (c) Tumor cells are negative for S-100.

intestine and have been termed as intestinal perineuriomas. Microscopically, tumor cells in soft tissue perineuriomas form storiform, fascicular, or bundled patterns. Individual cells may appear spindled. Tumor cells are positive for EMA and negative for S-100 (▶ Fig. 11.7). Mitosis and necrosis are generally absent. Reticular variants have a lace and net-like architecture with anastomosing cords of fusiform cells. The cells of a sclerosing variant of soft tissue perineurioma are often epithelioid and are embedded in a dense collagenous matrix. Soft tissue perineuriomas are benign although rare malignant forms, perineurial MPNSTs, also exist. These are characterized by hypercellularity and brisk mitotic activity and sometimes also necrosis.

11.4 Hybrid Nerve Sheath Tumors

Hybrid nerve sheath tumors are benign neoplasms demonstrating combined features of more than one benign peripheral nerve sheath tumor. Two notable more common types include schwannoma–perineurioma and neurofibroma–schwannoma.[1,2,4]

Hybrid schwannoma–perineurioma typically occurs sporadically. These lesions are usually circumscribed but not encapsulated. Microscopic examination shows benign spindle cell tumor with perineurioma-like architecture. Immunostaining have alternating staining patterns with S-100 and EMA-positive cells, Schwann cells, and perineurial cells, respectively.

Hybrid neurofibroma–schwannoma is a common tumor in schwannomatosis and also occurs in NF2 and NF1 patients. The schwannoma component in these tumors typically presents as cellular Antoni A areas with Verocay bodies in a background of neurofibroma.

11.5 Nerve Sheath Myxoma, Neurothekeoma, Ganglioneuroma, and Granular Cell Tumor

Benign neurogenic tumors also include nerve sheath myxoma, neurothekeoma, ganglioneuroma, and benign granular cell tumor[1,2,3,4]; however, a detailed discussion of these entities is beyond the scope of this chapter.

Nerve sheath myxoma is a benign, usually cutaneous, spindle cell neoplasm that features Schwann cell differentiation and most often affects the head and neck region of young adults. Tumors are solitary, firm, and circumscribed and are typically

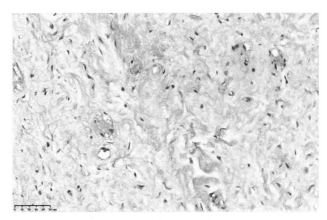

Fig. 11.8 Ganglioneuroma. Hematoxylin and eosin (H&E) stained section shows ganglioneuroma composed of ganglion cells, satellite cells, axons, and Schwann cells.

smaller than 3 cm. It is composed of lobules of S-100-positive spindle cells in a mucin-rich matrix; there is no tumor capsule.

Neurothekeoma is a benign cutaneous tumor that primarily affects the face, arm, and shoulders of children and young adults. Tumors are solitary, firm, and circumscribed and are typically smaller than 3 cm. It is composed of epithelioid or spindled cells in a myxoid stroma. Tumor cells are negative for S-100 by immunostaining.

Ganglioneuromas are benign neoplasms composed of ganglion cells, satellite cells, unmyelinated axons, and Schwann cells (▶ Fig. 11.8). Most are less than 15 cm, solitary, circumscribed, and thinly encapsulated masses located in the mediastinum, retroperitoneum, and pelvis of children under 10 years of age. Visceral involvement may be diffuse and associated with MEN-IIb. Gastrointestinal polypoid ganglioneuromas also occur in patients with Cowden syndrome, juvenile polyposis, tuberous sclerosis, and NF1.[2] Microscopic examination of ganglioneuroma reveals well differentiated but sometimes multinucleated ganglion cells that are clustered or scattered and have satellite cells fewer than ganglion cells in normal ganglia (▶ Fig. 11.8). Axonal processes in the background are unmyelinated. Progression to MPNST is rare.

Granular cell tumors feature tumor cells with characteristic granular cytoplasm due to abundant cytoplasmic lysosomes and are thought to be nerve sheath derived lesions. Most granular cell tumors are benign neoplasms and present as solitary, less than 3 cm nodules involving skin, subcutaneous tissue, tongue, or rarely viscera. Tumor cells are positive for S-100, SOX10, PAS, and CD68. Malignant granular cell tumors are extremely rare and either qualify as a malignancy because of malignant histologic features or because of clinically malignant behavior in spite of benign histology.[23] The histologic diagnosis of malignant granular cell tumor requires the detection of three features from a list consisting of marked cellularity, cellular pleomorphism, high nucleus to cytoplasm ratio, prominent nucleoli, brisk mitotic activity, presence of spindle cells, and necrosis.[2,23]

11.6 Malignant Peripheral Nerve Sheath Tumor

MPNSTs are malignant neoplasms demonstrating evidence of Schwann cell or perineurial cell differentiation.[1,2,4,24] These neoplasms may arise in the peripheral nerve or in the extraneural soft tissue. A slight majority of MPNSTs are NF1 associated and develop as malignant progression of a plexiform or intraneural neurofibroma in patients with a median age at presentation of 26 years.[24] Sporadic MPNSTs typically arise from large peripheral nerves without a benign precursor affecting patients with a median age of 62 years.[24] About 10 to 20% of MPNSTs develop in the site of previous irradiation. MPNSTs associated with NF1 as well as sporadic cases share highly recurrent inactivation of NF1, CDKN2A, and the polycomb repressor complex components EED and SUZ12.

The gross presentation of MPNSTs involving a nerve is often fusiform, while those grossly not associated with a nerve are often globular. At diagnosis, MPNSTs are often larger than 5 cm. The cut surfaces of MPNSTs may show obvious necrosis and hemorrhage.

The histopathologic presentation of MPNST is highly varied. Most MPNSTs are high-grade hypercellular neoplasms, and contain tightly packed spindle cells with enlarged hyperchromatic nuclei and variable amount of cytoplasm growing in a herringbone or fasciculated pattern (▶ Fig. 11.9). Most demonstrate more than 10 mitoses per 10 high power microscopic fields and necrosis or more than 20 mitoses per 10 high power microscopic fields and no necrosis. The cells are interspersed with faint collagen fibers. The nuclei are at least three times the size of the nuclei in neurofibroma. Cellular pleomorphism may be seen, usually in the form of scattered tumor giant cells. About 15% of MPNSTs are low grade and feature lower cellularity and mitotic activity and a lack of necrosis. As discussed in the neurofibroma segment above, atypical neurofibroma is a neurofibroma variant that is difficult to distinguish from low-grade MPNST.[1,2,5,6,8,9] In the context of NF1, the term atypical neurofibromatous neoplasm of uncertain biologic potential (ANNUBP) has recently been proposed for lesions with at least two features from a list that includes atypia, loss of neurofibroma architecture, high cellularity, and/or mitotic activity > 1/50 but < 3/10 high power fields.[5,6] This diagnosis should prompt additional sampling, clinical correlation, and possibly, expert pathology consultation to rule in or exclude low-grade MPNST.[5,6]

Immunohistochemical studies are important for the diagnosis of MPNST. Although widespread S-100 expression can

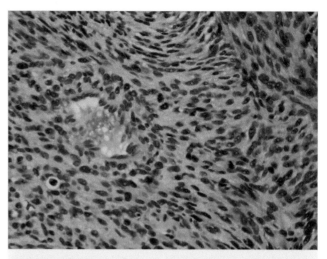

Fig. 11.9 Malignant peripheral nerve sheath tumor. Hematoxylin and eosin (H&E) stained section shows high-grade hypercellular spindle cell neoplasm with enlarged hyperchromatic nuclei and prominent mitotic activity.

be seen in low-grade MPNSTs, S-100 expression in the much more common high-grade MPNSTs is often only focal and is not detectable in a significant minority of cases. SOX10 expression is also focal to negative in high-grade MPNSTs. A complete loss of H3K27me3 staining in tumor nuclei is seen in many sporadic and radiation-induced MPNSTs and less commonly in NF1-associated MPNSTs. Factors that negatively influence survival include central location of MPNST, tumor size greater than 5 or 10 cm, subtotal resection, positive surgical margins, and MPNST recurrence or metastasis.[2]

11.6.1 Radiologic Features of MPNST

On MRI, irregular margins, heterogeneity, invasion of fat planes, and surrounding edema favor MPNST over benign peripheral nerve sheath tumors (▶ Fig. 11.10 and ▶ Fig. 11.11). FDG-PET may be useful in distinguishing MPNSTs from benign peripheral nerve sheath tumors based on a tumor's metabolic activity, with malignant tumors demonstrating moderate to high FDG accumulation.[13,14,15,16,17]

MPNSTs with perineurial differentiation are rare and are composed of spindled tumor cells arranged in whorls or in a storiform pattern. Tumor cells are positive for EMA and negative for S-100. This variant appears to be less aggressive than conventional MPNSTs.[25]

Epithelioid MPNSTs are made up of epithelioid malignant cells and may arise from pre-existing schwannoma. They are rare and unassociated with NF1, NF2, or schwannomatosis. A majority of epithelioid MPNSTs express S-100 and show membrane staining for collagen IV and laminin because tumor cells have pericellular basal lamina.

MPNSTs with divergent differentiation are rare and can exhibit rhabdomyosarcoma, chondrosarcoma, osteosarcoma, angiosarcoma, or glandular elements. There is an association with NF1 and the prognosis is poor.[2]

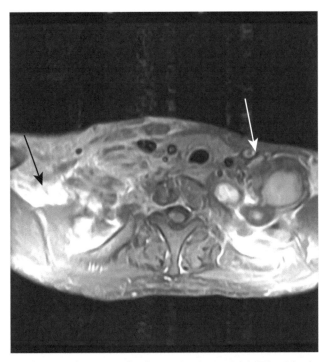

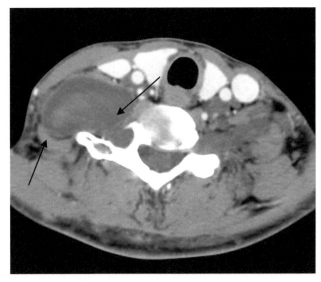

Fig. 11.11 Malignant peripheral nerve sheath tumor. Axial contrast-enhanced computed tomography (CT) shows bilateral low attenuation lesions involving and expanding the right neural foramen (*arrow*).

Fig. 11.10 Malignant peripheral nerve sheath tumor. Axial T1-weighted postcontrast magnetic resonance imaging (MRI) shows heterogeneous enhancing solid masses in the supraclavicular area (*arrows*).

11.7 Conclusion

The diagnosis of nerve sheath tumors requires a thorough understanding of how the histologic and radiographic presentation of these neoplasms may overlap, as well as their potential association with a variety of genetic disorders.

References

[1] Louis DN, Ohgaki H, Wiestler OD, Cavenee WK. World Health Organization Histological Classification of Tumours of the Central Nervous System. France: International Agency for Research on Cancer; 2016

[2] Rodriguez FJ, Giannini C, Spinner RJ, Perry A. Tumors of peripheral nerves. In: Perry A, Brat AJ, eds. Practical Surgical Pathology. A Diagnostic Approach. Philadelphia: Elsevier; 2018:323–373

[3] Antonescu C, Scheithauer BW, Woodruff JM. Tumors of the Peripheral Nervous System: AFIP Atlas of Tumor Pathology, Series 4. Silver Spring, MD: ARP Press; 2013

[4] De Luca-Johnson J, Kalof AN. Peripheral nerve sheath tumors: an update and review of diagnostic challenges. Diagn Histopathol. 2016; 22: 447–457

[5] Miettinen MM, Antonescu CR, Fletcher CDM, et al. Histopathologic evaluation of atypical neurofibromatous tumors and their transformation into malignant peripheral nerve sheath tumor in patients with neurofibromatosis 1—a consensus overview. Hum Pathol. 2017; 67: 1–10

[6] Schaefer IM, Fletcher CDM. Recent advances in the diagnosis of soft tissue tumours. Pathology. 2018; 50(1):37–48

[7] Hirbe AC, Gutmann DH. Neurofibromatosis type 1: a multidisciplinary approach to care. Lancet Neurol. 2014; 13(8):834–843

[8] Bernthal NM, Jones KB, Monument MJ, Liu T, Viskochil D, Randall RL. Lost in translation: ambiguity in nerve sheath tumor nomenclature and its resultant treatment effect. Cancers (Basel). 2013; 5(2):519–528

[9] Beert E, Brems H, Daniëls B, et al. Atypical neurofibromas in neurofibromatosis type 1 are premalignant tumors. Genes Chromosomes Cancer. 2011; 50(12):1021–1032

[10] Pilavaki M, Chourmouzi D, Kiziridou A, Skordalaki A, Zarampoukas T, Drevelengas A. Imaging of peripheral nerve sheath tumors with pathologic correlation: pictorial review. Eur J Radiol. 2004; 52(3):229–239

[11] Tagliafico AS, Isaac A, Bignotti B, Rossi F, Zaottini F, Martinoli C. Nerve tumors: what the MSK radiologist should know. Semin Musculoskelet Radiol. 2019; 23(1):76–84

[12] Chick G, Hollevoet N, Victor J, Bianchi S. The role of imaging in isolated benign peripheral nerve tumors: a practical review for surgeons. Hand Surg Rehabil. 2016; 35(5):320–329

[13] Assadi M, Velez E, Najafi MH, Matcuk G, Gholamrezanezhad A. PET imaging of peripheral nerve tumors. PET Clin. 2019; 14(1):81–89

[14] Tovmassian D, Abdul Razak M, London K. The role of [18F]FDG-PET/CT in predicting malignant transformation of plexiform neurofibromas in neurofibromatosis-1. Int J Surg Oncol. 2016; 2016:6162182

[15] Rosenkrantz AB, Friedman K, Chandarana H, et al. Current status of hybrid PET/MRI in oncologic imaging. AJR Am J Roentgenol. 2016; 206(1):162–172

[16] Broski SM, Johnson GB, Howe BM, et al. Evaluation of (18)F-FDG PET and MRI in differentiating benign and malignant peripheral nerve sheath tumors. Skeletal Radiol. 2016; 45(8):1097–1105

[17] Warbey VS, Ferner RE, Dunn JT, Calonje E, O'Doherty MJ. [18F]FDG PET/CT in the diagnosis of malignant peripheral nerve sheath tumours in neurofibromatosis type-1. Eur J Nucl Med Mol Imaging. 2009; 36(5):751–757

[18] Ardern-Holmes S, Fisher G, North K. Neurofibromatosis type 2. J Child Neurol. 2017; 32(1):9–22

[19] Schaefer IM, Fletcher CD, Hornick JL. Loss of H3K27 trimethylation distinguishes malignant peripheral nerve sheath tumors from histologic mimics. Mod Pathol. 2016; 29(1):4–13

[20] Casadei GP, Scheithauer BW, Hirose T, Manfrini M, Van Houton C, Wood MB. Cellular schwannoma. A clinicopathologic, DNA flow cytometric, and proliferation marker study of 70 patients. Cancer. 1995; 75(5):1109–1119

[21] Berg JC, Scheithauer BW, Spinner RJ, Allen CM, Koutlas IG. Plexiform schwannoma: a clinicopathologic overview with emphasis on the head and neck region. Hum Pathol. 2008; 39(5):633–640

[22] Torres-Mora J, Dry S, Li X, Binder S, Amin M, Folpe AL. Malignant melanotic schwannian tumor: a clinicopathologic, immunohistochemical, and gene expression profiling study of 40 cases, with a proposal for the reclassification of "melanotic schwannoma." Am J Surg Pathol. 2014; 38(1):94–105

[23] Fanburg-Smith JC, Meis-Kindblom JM, Fante R, Kindblom LG. Malignant granular cell tumor of soft tissue: diagnostic criteria and clinicopathologic correlation. Am J Surg Pathol. 1998; 22(7):779–794

[24] Evans DG, Baser ME, McGaughran J, Sharif S, Howard E, Moran A. Malignant peripheral nerve sheath tumours in neurofibromatosis 1. J Med Genet. 2002; 39(5):311–314

[25] Hirose T, Scheithauer BW, Sano T. Perineurial malignant peripheral nerve sheath tumor (MPNST): a clinicopathologic, immunohistochemical, and ultrastructural study of seven cases. Am J Surg Pathol. 1998; 22(11):1368–1378

12 Treatment of Peripheral Nerve and Paraspinal Tumors

Abdullah M. Abunimer, Hussam Abou-Al-Shaar, Shashank V. Gandhi, and Mark A. Mahan

Summary

Spinal nerve sheath tumors account for 25% of primary neurogenic spinal tumors, with schwannomas and neurofibromas being the most commonly encountered entities. They present with multiple signs and symptoms that depend on their size, location, and impingement on adjacent neurovascular structures. Magnetic resonance imaging remains the gold standard diagnostic modality because it offers spatial resolution of neural structures and diagnostic information that cannot be attained by other modalities. Pre-operative imaging is important in delineating tumor size, location, and involvement of adjacent anatomy, so that the optimal surgical approach can be determined. Various surgical approaches to address the lesion without jeopardizing the normal surrounding structures have been described depending on the tumor location. Resection often carries low risk of minor neurological effects. In this chapter, we review nerve sheath tumors with focus on their incidence, clinical presentation, imaging features, decision-making strategy, surgical approaches, outcomes, and potential complications.

Keywords: nerve sheath, peripheral nerve, dumbbell tumor, schwannoma, neurofibroma, paraspinal tumor, malignant peripheral nerve sheath tumor

12.1 Introduction

Spinal nerve sheath tumors make up 25% of primary neurogenic spinal tumors, with schwannomas and neurofibromas being the most commonly encountered entities, accounting for 80 and 15% of nerve sheath tumors, respectively.[1,2] The annual incidence of primary spinal tumors ranges from 1.3 to 10.0 per 100,000 individuals, and peripheral nerve sheath tumors in general represent one-third of these reported data.[2,3,4,5]

Spinal nerve sheath tumors are frequently intradural (50–83%); however, they can also occur in intradural/extradural (7–24%) or purely extradural locations (2–31%)—not including peripheral nerve sheath tumors.[6] Rarely, spinal nerve sheath tumors can occur in an intramedullary location arising from the perivascular nerve sheaths accompanying the penetrating spinal cord vessels.[7] However, it is most common to see nerve sheath tumors distal to the Redlich–Obersteiner zone, which is the transition from oligodendrocyte myelination to Schwann cell myelination that occurs a few millimeters distal to the spinal cord on the spinal rootlets. Dumbbell tumors occur from extraforaminal extension of intraspinal lesions and are seen in approximately 10 to 15% of spinal nerve sheath tumors, especially in neurofibromas.[8] While intradural schwannomas are more commonly encountered in the thoracic and lumbar regions, dumbbell tumors are primarily encountered in the cervical spine.[8,9]

Nerve sheath tumors can also originate in the peripheral nerves of the limbs or anywhere in the body where a nerve is present. These lesions are histologically identical to lesions occurring in the spinal canal; therefore, these tumors will all be addressed as one entity in the remainder of this chapter.

Histopathologically, nerve sheath tumors entail a recognized spectrum of pathological diagnoses that range from benign entities, including the aforementioned schwannomas and neurofibromas, to higher grade aggressive lesions, represented by malignant peripheral nerve sheath tumors (MPNSTs). Most schwannomas arise from the dorsal nerve roots, whereas ventral root tumors are more commonly neurofibromas.[10] These tumors are usually associated with a favorable prognosis despite having aggressive histological features.[11] In contrast, 2.5% of intradural spinal nerve sheath tumors are malignant, with at least a half of these occurring in patients with neurofibromatosis. MPNSTs carry a poor prognosis, with 5-year survival rates ranging from 35 to 52%[12,13,14] and a mortality rate of 60%.[15] Additionally, 40% of patients develop distant metastasis within a median of 12 months from their initial presentation.[12,13,14,15]

12.2 Presentation

Sporadic spinal schwannomas are most often identified in the third through seventh decades of life, with a peak incidence in the fifth or sixth decade of life. They occur at equivalent rates in men and women.[16] Spinal nerve sheath tumors present with signs and symptoms that depend on their size, location, and impingement on adjacent neurovascular structures. For the majority of dumbbell tumors, the presentation is similar to a single radiculopathy. The course is frequently insidious for benign tumors, with symptoms starting vaguely and worsening steadily as the lesion grows. Initial presentation is typically with segmental pain followed by local pain and signs of neural compression, with neurological deficits developing later in the course of the disease. Therefore, it is essential to include such lesions in the differential diagnosis of patients presenting with myelopathy, radiculopathy, or neck and back pain. Less common symptoms include gait ataxia, motor weakness, bladder paresis, and dysesthesia from spinal cord compression.[16] The average duration of symptoms before presentation ranges from 2 to 3 years. Patients with neurofibromatosis type 2 (NF2) are at increased risk to develop multiple lesions at an early age and have a greater tendency to describe pain and develop severe neurological deficits compared with those without NF2.[16]

The clinical presentation of nerve sheath tumors arising in the peripheral nerves of the body also depends on the size, location, and relationship to adjacent neurovascular elements. Such presentations include, but are not limited to, pain, swelling, weakness, and paresthesias along the involved nerve.

12.3 Differential Diagnosis

The differential diagnosis of paraspinal and peripheral nerve lesions is broad and encompasses both benign and malignant lesions, vascular anomalies, congenital malformations, and infectious entities. The differential diagnosis includes schwannoma, neurofibroma, neuroma, MPNST, solitary bone plasmacytoma, superior sulcus tumor, spine metastasis, tuberculous spondylitis, pseudomeningocele, vertebral hydatid disease, chordoma, intraforaminal synovial cyst, aneurysmal bone cyst, and extradural arachnoid cyst, among others.

12.4 Evaluation

12.4.1 History and Physical Examination

A complete and thorough history and physical examination is the first step in localizing the level of the lesion and planning the surgical intervention, if needed. It is important to identify any family history of similar lesions or family or personal history of phakomatosis (including open-ended questions on minor criteria for neurofibromatosis, such as long bone fractures or optic abnormalities) as such clues can direct the surgeon toward the diagnosis. A full neurological examination including motor and sensory tests as well as gait assessment is of paramount importance.

12.4.2 Radiographic Evaluation

Magnetic resonance imaging (MRI) with and without gadolinium contrast enhancement is the gold standard diagnostic modality for patients with nerve sheath tumors. It is important in delineating tumor size and location as well as in evaluating the degree of tumor extension and planning the optimal surgical approach. Additionally, the use of vascular studies like angiography, computed tomography angiography (CTA), or magnetic resonance angiography (MRA) may be appropriate when such tumors extend into the transverse foramen or adjacent major vessels, including the vertebral artery or abdominal vasculature.[16]

A computed tomography (CT) scan with or without myelography may also be helpful in determining the surgical approach and the degree of bony removal required to obtain adequate surgical exposure for a safe and complete resection. Furthermore, there may be significant bony destruction, particularly in dumbbell lesions, that can be delineated on CT images. This is particularly important when planning spinal instrumentation surgery, as the typical structural anatomy of the spine is remodelld by these tumors. CT myelography is a potential alternative in patients who cannot tolerate MRI or in cases where an arachnoid diverticulum is suspected.

Radiographic Features of Extramedullary Tumors

Nerve sheath tumors usually present with similar imaging features and cannot be distinguished solely on imaging. Characteristic radiological abnormalities on MRI such as cerebrospinal fluid (CSF) capping and spinal cord or cauda equina displacement are typically seen with extramedullary masses, including nerve sheath tumors. Contrast enhancement improves MRI sensitivity significantly, particularly for small tumors. Most extramedullary tumors are isointense or slightly hypointense relative to the spinal cord on T1-weighted images. With respect to the spinal cord, nerve sheath tumors are more likely

to be hyperintense on T2-weighted images. Tumors located at the cauda equina usually show increased signal intensity relative to CSF on T1- and T2-weighted sequences. Contrast uptake is typically uniform in most nerve sheath tumors, but heterogeneous enhancement from intratumoral cysts, hemorrhage, or necrosis is frequently seen on imaging studies.[17] Positron emission tomography (PET)–CT or apparent diffusion coefficient (ADC) mapping may provide valuable information in cases of MPNST. However, PET-CT is frequently elevated in schwannomas; thus, PET-CT is usually reserved for cases of known neurofibromas or neurofibromatosis. However, patients with NF1 also develop schwannomas, so care must be taken to not overinterpret an elevated SUV in the setting of NF1.

12.5 Classification Systems

Several classification systems have been proposed for the characterization of spinal nerve sheath tumors. Asazuma et al[18] characterized cervical dumbbell tumors based on radiological appearance, providing depictions of six axially determined types (▶ Table 12.1, ▶ Fig. 12.1).

A more inclusive classification system introduced by Nanda et al[19] takes into account the different imaging patterns of these tumors and also guides the surgical approach choice based on the class of the tumor. According to their classification system, tumors are classified as type A, primarily longitudinal axis tumors; type B, primarily horizontal axis tumors; or type C, giant tumors with multiple axes of involvement regardless of bone invasion.

Finally, the Klekamp–Samii[20] and Karnofsky Performance Status (KPS) scoring systems are frequently used to evaluate the clinical improvements in patients with peripheral and paraspinal nerve tumors after the surgery.

12.6 Neurophysiological Evaluation

Nerve function is usually assessed by clinical examination as well as electrodiagnostic studies including electromyography (EMG) in selected cases. Electrodiagnostic studies provide evidence of

Table 12.1 Asazuma et al[18] classification of dumbbell tumors

Type	Description
Type 1	Intradural and extradural tumors limited to the spinal canal and constricting only the dura
Type II	Epidural tumors with foramen constriction and increasingly extraforaminal involvement
Type IIa	Extradural and foraminal
Type IIb	Extradural and paravertebral
Type IIc	Foraminal and paravertebral
Type III	Both dural and foraminal tumors with resulting constriction
Type IIIa	Intradural and extradural-foraminal
Type IIIb	Intradural and extradural-paravertebral
Type IV	Extradural and intravertebral with invasion of the vertebral body
Type V	Extradural with extralaminal invasion
Type VI	Tumors with multidirectional bone invasion

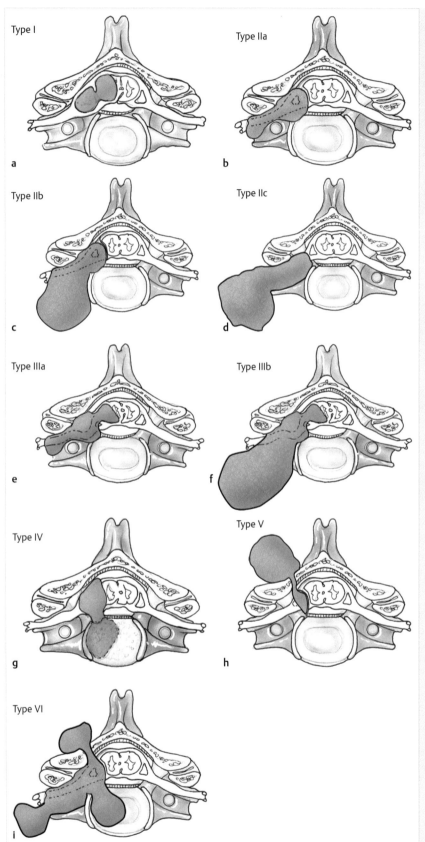

Fig. 12.1 Imaging-based anatomic classification of dumbbell tumors by Asazuma et al.[18] (a) Type I intradural and extramedullary tumors are located only in the spinal canal and constrict only the dura. (b–d) Type II epidural tumors cause foraminal narrowing and include three subtypes according to the extradural extraforaminal spread. (e, f) Type III tumors cause dural and foraminal compression and can also extend through into the paravertebral area. (g) Type IV tumors invade the vertebral body. (h) Type V tumors are extradural and involve the lamina. (i) Type VI tumors spread in several directions. (Reproduced with permission from Gragnaniello et al, Fig. 59.1.[21])

acute and chronic changes within the dermatomes and myotomes of the spinal roots. Slowly growing tumors generally show chronic remodeling of motor units, whereas rapidly growing tumors generally produce uncompensated, acute evidence of denervation (e.g., fibrillations, sharp waves, insertional activity). These findings are worrisome for a diagnosis of MPNST.

12.7 Tissue Biopsy

Since most spinal nerve sheath tumors are benign, preoperative tissue biopsy is not routinely necessary. However, in cases where malignancy is suspected, percutaneous biopsy can be attempted preoperatively to obtain tissue diagnosis and guide further therapy.[10,19,21] Radiographic characteristics of malignant nerve sheath tumors include large size, relatively irregular borders, documented rapid growth of the lesion, and involvement of bony or soft tissues. Special care must be taken in obtaining a percutaneous biopsy of the lesion to avoid seeding of the tumor. Thus, a multidisciplinary approach and proper coordination between the surgeon and interventional radiologist are essential to appropriately delineate the optimal biopsy site without jeopardizing the trajectory if further surgical removal is deemed necessary. Management of MPNSTs is beyond the scope of this chapter.

12.8 Management

The surgical management of nerve sheath tumors depends on the patient's age, symptom severity and duration, tumor location, and size of the lesion. These factors are important in formulating a plan for patients with spinal tumors. Observation is frequently recommended in cases where the lesion is small and asymptomatic or if the patient's comorbidities or general functional state do not warrant resection. Rarely, radiosurgery is a potential alternative in patients with multiple lesions or tumors not amenable to resection and in patients who cannot tolerate surgery.

Various surgical approaches to address the lesion without jeopardizing the normal surrounding structures have been described. The goal of surgery is to achieve complete resection of spinal nerve sheath tumors, as recurrence generally occurs in cases of incomplete resection, especially in tumors with extensive paraspinal involvement that are partially or subtotally resected as well as in tumors in NF2 patients.[16]

Preoperatively, blood pressure may need to be monitored closely via an arterial line, especially if significant spinal cord compression causes concern about spinal cord perfusion. Also, a Foley catheter and sequential compression devices are routinely placed. Preoperative antibiotics and steroids are given to decrease the risk of infection and reduce swelling, respectively. The steroids may be stopped or tapered off over several doses postoperatively. Blood pressure should be carefully monitored because profound hypotension may result in cord ischemia and infarction.

Intraoperative neurophysiological monitoring of both the sensory and motor tracts with somatosensory evoked potentials (SSEPs) and motor evoked potentials (MEPs) should be considered when resecting tumors that have mass effect on the spinal cord. EMG and direct nerve root stimulation are essential in identifying and preserving neural elements. However, unless specific SSEP protocols are used, direct stimulation only identifies motor

fibers. D-wave monitoring caudal and rostral to the lesion can be valuable in monitoring cortical spinal tract integrity and function.

The resected tumor should be sent for histopathological testing to confirm the diagnosis and guide further therapy.

12.9 Surgical Approaches

The subsequent sections will review some of the approaches used to resect nerve sheath tumors located in the spinal and paraspinal regions. The surgical management of nerve sheath tumors located along the peripheral nerves depends on the exact location of the lesion, tumor size, and the patient's symptomatology and functional status. Typically, local exposure of the affected area is sufficient to address such lesions, and a description of how to approach these lesions in each of the peripheral nerves is beyond the scope of this chapter. The remainder of this chapter will focus on the surgical approaches for spinal and paraspinal nerve sheath tumors.

12.9.1 Posterior Approaches

Many spinal nerve sheath tumors are located on the dorsal or lateral side of the spinal canal and can be targeted surgically through the posterior approach. Even when lesions are ventrally located, adopting a posterior approach can be feasible because nerve sheath tumors typically create a surgical corridor, allowing adequate access without substantial cord retraction. For example, ventrolateral lesions can be approached by entering through the dentate ligament with light cord retraction.[21]

After intubation, the patient is placed in a prone position on chest bolsters, a Wilson frame, or an open-frame spine table. Adequate padding of pressure points is necessary to avoid the occurrence of neuropathies. The patient's arms are placed at his or her side for cervical and thoracic lesions at or above T6; for more caudally located lesions, the shoulders are abducted 90 degrees and the arms are placed on arm boards. Access to the area of resection is achieved in whichever means the surgeon is comfortable. For example, the senior author utilizes minimally invasive spinal retractors in most tumors not requiring instrumentation, including sacral foramina and lateral lumbar foramina.

The extent of bony lamina removal depends on the degree of spinal cord compression. Often, a hemilaminotomy with sparing of the posterior tension band can reduce the need for instrumentation, which is beneficial because the metallic artifact on MRI after fusion surgery limits postoperative visualization of tumor recurrence. However, for dumbbell tumors that extend laterally, complete facetectomy may be necessary and will commonly necessitate instrumentation in the cervical and lumbar spine. Occasionally, a ventrolateral operative corridor may be required for better visualization through a facetectomy or pedicle resection. For ventrolaterally located tumors, the dentate ligament is often sectioned to obtain adequate visualization of the tumor and surrounding structures.

Intraoperative ultrasonography may be also used to aid in tumor localization before dural opening. Meticulous hemostasis must be achieved before the durotomy is performed. The dural incision is extended laterally over the nerve root sleeve to fully expose tumors extended to the foraminal and extraforaminal locations, if present. In such circumstances, the exposure usually extends up to 4 cm from the lateral dural margin. When the tumor extends beyond these limits, an anterolateral approach may be of greater value.[16]

Microscopic magnification aids in tumor resection and reduces injury to neurovascular structures. After tumor exposure, an arachnoid membrane may be found to be adherent to the tumor surface; it must be incised and reflected off. With direct electric stimulation, the nervous tissue can be identified, and the tumor is safely separated from the neural elements. Typically, a nerve root can be identified entering and exiting the tumor. In some cases, and depending on the level, it might be necessary to sacrifice the nerve root for total tumor removal, although the functioning fascicles of the nerve root can typically be preserved by releasing them circumferentially off the surface of the underlying tumor. For some proximally located lesions that are embedded in the pia, the resection of the tumor may also require mobilization of a segment of the pia.[16] The tumor and its capsule are then cauterized to shrink the tumor and reduce its vascularity. The proximal and distal nerve, fascicle, or rootlet that gives rise to the tumor is resected with the tumor. After tumor resection, the dura is closed, possibly with a dural patch.

12.9.2 Posterolateral Approaches

Posterolateral approaches facilitate exposure to tumors located ventral to the thoracic and lumbar spinal cord. The costotransversectomy approach increases ventral exposure through resection of the proximal rib, transverse process, and pedicle with lateral mobilization of the parietal pleura and thoracic contents. Additionally, the lateral extracavitary approach is an extension of the costotransversectomy approach in which a surgical window is obtained by resecting the rib at the rib angle, which is more lateral than in the standard costotransversectomy approach.[22]

In these approaches, a standard laminectomy and bony resection are performed. The focus is then shifted to resect the intradural component of the tumor. Once the posterior intradural component of the tumor is resected, a T-shaped lateral dural incision is made over the root sleeve,[16] allowing for more ventral visualization and a safe surgical corridor for tumor resection without any retraction on the spinal cord. The ventral paraspinal component is resected through the lateral portion of the exposure, and the dura and subcutaneous tissue are subsequently closed in standard fashion.

McCormick[23] noted that posterolateral approaches provide a surgical window with a wider view than the standard posterior approaches, which is needed for large dumbbell tumors. This is especially important for dumbbell tumors with intraspinal and paraspinal extension and for upper thoracic paraspinal dumbbell tumors. One of the main advantages of these approaches is their ability to provide extensive anterior compartment exposure comparable to that achieved by the transpleural and transabdominal approaches but with fewer surgical risks. Such risks may include injury to the diaphragm, pleural tear, or psoas muscle mobilization. However, given the difficulty of these approaches, a thorough understanding

of the thoracic retropleural and retroperitoneal anatomy is essential for achieving safe resection. Furthermore, because of the need for facet joint and pedicle resection, spinal instrumentation is often required because the spinal column is iatrogenically destabilized.

12.9.3 Anterolateral Approaches

Anterior Approaches to the Cervical Spine

Tumors ventral to the cord and those that have a large lateral component are often difficult to access using the standard posterior approach. Several obstacles to achieving such exposure include the risk of spinal instability as a result of extensive posterolateral bony removal, the amount of retraction exerted on the spinal cord while fully exposing the underlying tumor, and the difficulty of achieving a watertight dural closure. Therefore, ventral or ventrolateral approaches may be optimal for resecting these tumors, without requiring combined anterior and posterior approaches. However, some surgeons may avoid using the anterior approaches because they lack comfort in performing the lateral neck dissection and may seek to involve otolaryngology surgeons for assistance. Although Asazuma et al[18] advocated the use of a combined anterior and posterior approach for type IIb, IIc, and IIIb tumors (▸ Fig. 12.1), we find a combined approach unnecessary for these tumors. We routinely perform lateral neck dissections that allow removal of foraminal tumors that do not require combined approach (▸ Fig. 12.2). A combined approach is recommended for some type IV, V, and VI tumors in which gross total resection cannot be achieved with a purely anterior approach because of the large tumor size.

Hakuba et al[24] described their experience with the transuncodiscal approach to resect cervical dumbbell tumors in a single-stage operation involving anterior diskectomy, ipsilateral uncinectomy, posterolateral and posterior transverse ridge removal in the vertebral bodies at tumor level, and interbody fusion. They found that removal of a segment from the lateral part of the vertebral body might sometimes be necessary to remove large tumors in the spinal canal. The bony defect can be filled with iliac bone graft to facilitate fusions. The authors recommended this approach in cases where no more than three levels are involved with cervical dumbbell tumor.

A high lateral dissection, similar to that performed for a carotid endarterectomy, provides rich access to anteriorly based paraspinal tumors of the upper cervical spine. The supraclavicular approach affords access to pathological conditions at the anterolateral aspect of the lower cervical and cervicothoracic spine. It is similar to a retropharyngeal approach to the upper cervical spine or the transuncal approach to the midcervical spine, in which the oblique trajectory provides a unique vantage point for the management of diseases that occur on the lateral margin of the cervical spine. Thus, this approach provides the panoramic visualization of complex lesions that involve the spine and the spinal nerves. This approach is generally contraindicated if the lesion is located below the T1 level, in cases of great vessel anomaly, or if the cervical ribs may obstruct the exposure. The supraclavicular approach has many advantages, including providing adequate access to several vertebral levels

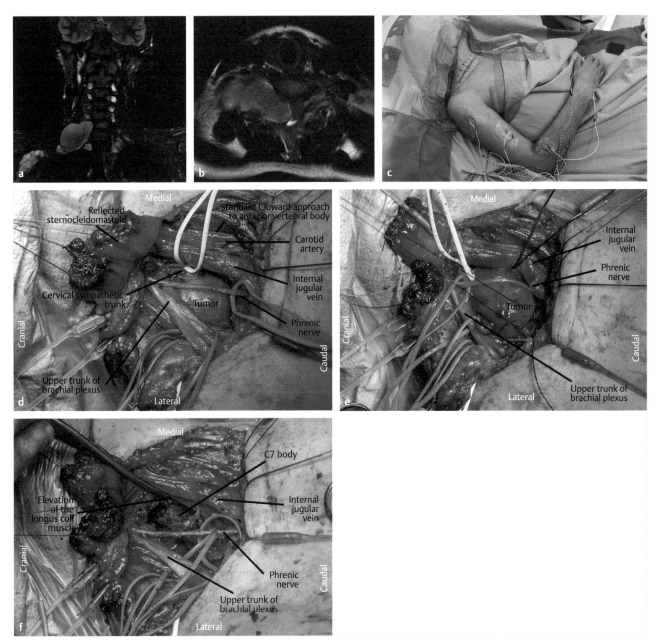

Fig. 12.2 Anterior approach to the cervical spine. **(a, b)** Preoperative T2-weighted coronal **(a)** and axial **(b)** magnetic resonance imaging (MRI) demonstrates a large dumbbell mass occupying the right C6–C7 neuroforamina with compression of the cervical spinal cord. Dural margins on the medial extent of the tumor suggested a primarily extradural tumor. Scalloping of the lateral vertebral body and widening of the neuroforamina suggested a benign tumor. **(c)** Operating room setup and patient positioning. The patient is positioned in the supine position with the operating room bed in a beach-chair, semirecumbent setting to elevate the neck above the heart and reduce venous pressure in the operative field. The arm is exposed for observation of electrical stimulation. Electromyography (EMG) wires are placed for motor-evoked monitoring. A wide transverse incision is planned to allow for medial exposure of the vertebral body as well as lateral exposure of the brachial plexus. **(d)** Intraoperative view of the tumor before resection. Wide exposure of the neural elements provides for sharp demarcation from tumor, as well as mobilization of the tumor without unnecessary traction on the nerves. The medial trajectory, similar to the Cloward approach for an anterior cervical diskectomy, is available for direct approach to the anterior face of the vertebral body. **(e)** Intraoperative view during capsular dissection of the tumor. The tumor is dissected from the C7 root along the capsular boundaries, allowing gentle traction to be applied with a suture through the tumor. **(f)** Intraoperative view after tumor removal. The tumor was removed en bloc as a single gross total specimen, away from the C7 root with preservation of the root (not visualized here). The C7 vertebral body is scalloped on the anterior margin. There was no substantial cerebrospinal fluid (CSF) leak after tumor removal, but a small amount of fibrin glue was placed at the neuroforamina as a precaution. A small bulb drain was placed at the conclusion of the case.

through a relatively bloodless plane, allowing simultaneous decompression, grafting, and internal fixation, exposing the brachial plexus as well as the anterior spine, and enabling early dissection of the vertebral artery. However, its disadvantages include the limited access below the first thoracic vertebra and the lack of access to posterior spinal column.[25,26,27]

Anterior Approaches to the Thoracic Spine

For ventrally located tumors of the thoracic spine, anterolateral approaches may have superior outcome to laminectomy.[28] Using these approaches, the stability of the posterior column remains intact. For anterolateral visualization of the thoracic vertebrae, the intercostal transthoracic approach provides an ideal surgical corridor through which vertebral body resection, anterior column instrumentation, and spinal column reconstruction are well managed. Also, anterior spinal cord tumor impingement can be directly decompressed without neural manipulation. For large and dumbbell tumors, a two-stage posterior and anterior thoracic approach can be employed to separate any attachment of the tumor to the underlying neural element, if present, and to achieve a watertight dural closure.

Recently, surgeons have started to shift gears toward video-assisted anterior thoracoscopic techniques instead of the open thoracotomy in dealing with ventral spinal tumors. Thoracoscopic approaches are considered less traumatic, which reflects many advantages over the traditional open techniques. This adequate small surgical exposure results in a lower morbidity rate, fewer complications, shorter hospitalization and recovery time, and less postoperative pain compared to traditional anterior approaches.[29] In the thoracoscopic technique, the patient is placed in the lateral decubitus position, and single-lung ventilation is used with ipsilateral lung collapse. Three trocars are usually placed to assist the thoracoscopic surgery. The first trocar is inserted at the anterior axillary line at the fifth intercostal space. For suction and irrigation, a second trocar is inserted at the middle or posterior axillary line. The third trocar is inserted close to the tumor. After the tumor is visualized, a pleural incision in performed to access the thoracic cavity. The tumor is then removed and placed in an endoscopic specimen retrieval bag to prevent contaminating the thoracic cavity with tumor seeds. Finally, a chest tube is inserted. A combination of anterior thoracoscopic and posterior approaches has been used by Konno et al,[29] who achieved a complete tumor resection in patients using a combined posterior and anterior approach to thoracic epidural (paravertebral) schwannomas, none of which developed spinal instability. Among the limitations of thoracoscopic techniques is the limited ability to dissect, and thereby preserve, neural elements. Thus, the nerve or root is often sacrificed to remove the tumor. CSF leak in the pleural space can be catastrophic in the thoracic cavity because of large volumes and negative intrapleural pressure. Therefore, thoracoscopic surgery is largely contraindicated for dural manipulation.

Anterior Approaches to the Lumbar Spine

Many nerve sheath tumors arise from the lumbar plexus and can be easily addressed with direct lateral or anterolateral paraspinal approaches (▶ Fig. 12.3). A variation of the surgical technique for direct lateral interbody fusion, for example XLIF,

provides a surgical corridor to the lumbar plexus.[30,31,32] Minimally invasive approaches can be considered for small tumors that do not involve major blood vessels. For large presacral tumors, participation of a vascular or other access surgeon comfortable with an anterior lumbar interbody fusion approach can make exposure and resection of these tumors quite manageable. Combined anterior and posterior approaches are infrequently necessary, except in cases where there is substantial tumor within the canal as well as extraforaminally[33,34] or if there is an attempt to combine minimally invasive posterior and lateral approaches.

12.9.4 Minimally Invasive Surgical Approaches

Spinal instability and deformity are a concern after laminectomy via posterior approaches, especially after multilevel laminectomy and radical facetectomy.[35,36,37] This concern has led surgeons to propose mini-open and minimally invasive approaches to resect paraspinal tumors while minimizing paraspinal tissue destruction and preserving spinal stability. The potential advantages of these techniques also include avoidance of fusion surgery, which could result in reduced postoperative pain and narcotic use. Adopting the techniques of minimally invasive surgery (MIS) in the management of paraspinal tumors yields several other advantages, which have demonstrated less blood loss and shorter hospitalization and recovery times.[38,39,40]

When considering applying the MIS approaches for the treatment of paraspinal tumors, tumor size and characteristics are important determinants for the optimal tumor resection by these approaches. Lee et al[41] reported two different techniques for hemilaminectomy in 31 patients: muscle splitting using a tubular retractor system and standard unilateral muscle retraction with contralateral paraspinal muscle preservation. The authors identified that MIS approaches are safe for tumors with an axial diameter of ≤ 16 mm.

MIS Tubular Approach

Under fluoroscopic guidance and after confirmation of the level of the tumor, a 2.5-cm paramedian incision is made and the paraspinal muscle is split with the aid of a series of dilators. A nonexpandable tubular retractor with a diameter of 18 mm is then placed, and a hemilaminectomy or complete laminectomy can be performed. The dura is then incised, and the tumor is dissected away from the surrounding neurovascular structures with the aid of intraoperative stimulation. Finally, the dura is closed, and the retractors are removed.

Limitations and Contraindication of MIS Approaches

Although MIS approaches have reduced the rate of spinal instability and complications, they are associated with inherent limitations and contraindications. Relative contraindications that preclude the use of MIS approaches include extensive extraforaminal tumors, tumors involving two or more levels, hemorrhagic tumors (e.g., paragangliomas), and obesity (because of the limited viewing angle around instruments from long tubular retractors). Additionally, there are practical challenges to the

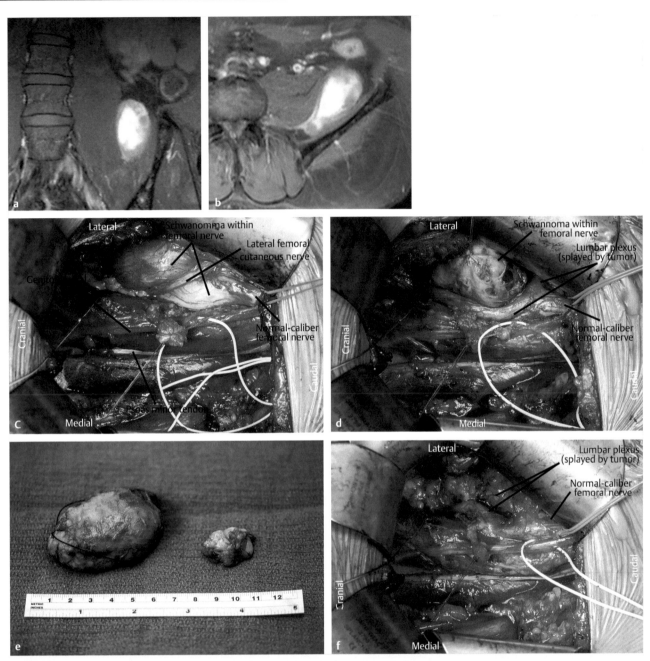

Fig. 12.3 Anterior approach to the lumbar spine. **(a, b)** T1-weighted contrast-enhanced magnetic resonance imaging (MRI) of the abdomen demonstrated a heterogeneously enhancing mass between the lateral margin of the psoas and medial margin of the iliacus in a patient with neurofibromatosis type 1 (NF1). The mass measured 6.5 ×6.7 ×3.0 cm and had no evidence of peritumoral edema, denervation atrophy, or other features of malignancy. Due to the size and enhancement pattern, a positron emission tomography–computed tomography (PET-CT) scan was ordered which demonstrated increased uptake for a neurofibroma. Preoperative needle biopsy was consistent with a schwannoma. **(c)** Intraoperative view before the tumor resection. Due to the location below the pelvic brim, a minimally invasive approach was not feasible. The tumor is exposed and the proximal lumbar plexus and distal femoral nerve are positively identified. **(d)** Intraoperative view during tumor resection. The tumor is carefully dissected along the capsular borders, allowing mobilization of the tumor away from the lumbar plexus, which was split by the tumor. **(e)** Gross specimens after tumor removal. The tumor had a second, smaller nodule arising from the neuroforamina, seen on the right. **(f)** Intraoperative view after tumor removal, showing the lumbar plexus shifted posteriorly to a normal anatomical position, in relation to the psoas muscle.

MIS approaches that must be considered. Optimal anatomic visualization and identification through a narrow surgical corridor can be difficult and requires a significant learning curve when adopting these approaches. Dural closure is challenging through a small surgical field; however, dural clips and other devices may be used.[42]

12.10 Postoperative Management

Depending upon surgeon's comfort with the dural closure, patients may be kept flat in bed for 48 to 72 hours, with deployment of sequential compression devices and a Foley catheter. Pain should be addressed and controlled well with appropriate regimens. If a CSF-diverting lumbar drain has been placed, it is generally removed before the patient is mobilized. Early mobilization and physical therapy are started on the first day after the procedure and tailored to the patient's needs. The neurological status of the patient must be checked frequently.

12.11 Complications

The most frequent complications encountered are generally related to wound healing and CSF leakage. Lumbar drainage can be used to manage CSF leak conservatively. CSF leaks in the thoracic cavity can be life threatening and frequently require complex closures.

12.11.1 Neurological Injury

Permanent injury to the cord or the nerves is uncommon with small benign tumors and technical precision. Larger tumors that require mobilization of a compressed spinal cord or aggressive tumors that may parasitize blood flow to the spinal cord are more likely to produce prolonged neurologic injury. Use of intraoperative neurophysiological monitoring is recommended in these cases. If there is any evidence of spinal cord injury after surgery, either CT or MRI must be performed urgently to confirm that there is no postoperative hematoma at the operative site. Many surgeons elect to use high-dose steroids for several days. To optimize tissue perfusion and prevent ischemia, blood pressure should be maintained in the high normal range for several days as well.

Motor and sensory deficits associated with manipulation of the nerve root or plexus typically improve postoperatively. Mild manipulation of a nerve may lead to neurapraxia, which generally resolves in hours to days. More severe manipulation of the nerve may lead to axonal loss and muscle atrophy, which may require months to years for full recovery. The duration and severity of the existing deficit and the age of the patient are important factors to determine the degree of recovery. Delayed neurologic deficits, which may occur 2 weeks after surgery, are usually neuroinflammatory disorders, such as Parsonage–Turner's syndrome. Use of high-dose steroids may reduce the degree of neurologic insult in these cases.[43]

For patients with symptomatic nerve root or plexus injuries, initial management involves evaluation for postoperative compression, if there is concern for acute worsening in the postoperative period. Most injuries from manipulation can be managed conservatively, with aggressive rehabilitation and mobilization.

Ankle and wrist splints may be applied to support function; however, joint range of motion needs to be maintained. The patient should be monitored closely for clinical and/or electrophysiological evidence of regeneration. All cases of severe weakness that last more than 3 months should be referred to a surgeon comfortable with performing nerve transfers. Substantial recovery is possible with appropriately timed interventions and patients should be counseled appropriately.[44]

12.11.2 Pleural Tear

In most instances, placement of a chest tube is not necessary if the pleura is breached with thoracic spinal approaches. A red rubber catheter can be inserted into the pleural defect, and the lung should be fully expanded and held with a Valsalva maneuver, forcing out the majority of air within the thoracic cavity. The red rubber catheter is then removed, and the pleurotomy is sutured closed. The pleurotomy site can then be flooded with irrigation and observed for any bubbles or drainage of irrigation, indicating an incomplete pleural closure. A chest tube can be placed during closure for patients who sustain an intraoperative pleural laceration where an optimal pleural repair cannot be achieved. These patients can usually be weaned off the chest tube over 3 to 4 days.

12.12 Spinal Stability

Spinal stability and the need for instrumentation must be assessed when planning the surgical approach for spinal nerve sheath tumors. Typically, a simple laminectomy does not require instrumentation. However, if more aggressive bone resection is needed, such as in the costotransversectomy and lateral extracavitary approaches, the spine becomes destabilized and requires stabilization and instrumentation.

The structures that provide the support for the spine can be divided into three stabilizing columns from anterior to posterior. As a general rule, the spine becomes unstable when at least two of the three stability columns have been compromised. The anterior column comprises the anterior half or two-thirds of the vertebral body and the intervertebral disk along with the anterior longitudinal ligament. Similarly, the middle column comprises the posterior half or one-third of the vertebral body and the intervertebral disk along with the posterior longitudinal ligament. Finally, the posterior column includes the structures posterior to the posterior longitudinal ligament: the paired facets, the transverse and spinous processes, the paired laminae, the intertransverse and interspinous ligaments, and the ligamentum flavum.

Spinal stability can be preserved even if there is disruption of the posterior neural arch (lamina) as long as the facets are preserved and there is no pre-existing abnormal kyphosis. Laminoplasty is performed in younger patients to preserve spinal stability after laminectomy; however, for bilateral laminectomy or laminoplasty of three or more levels, spinal fixation and fusion should be considered.[45] Additionally, the facet joints are considered major players in maintaining the stability of the spinal column.[35,46] Medial or partial facetectomy does not seem to affect spinal stability but total unilateral or bilateral facetectomy significantly affects the spinal stability.[47] Cusick et al[48] noted that there is an average loss of segmental strength of nearly one-third after unilateral cervical facetectomy. The loss of the segmental strength is primarily due to the delayed instability resulting from repetitive loading rather than an acute spinal instability event. Additionally, the risk of instability is proportional to the laminar and ligamentous disruption. Cusick et al[48] also pointed out several other independent factors of spinal stability that should be taken into consideration, which include the patient's age, individualized spinal mobility and loading patterns, and spinal level. Therefore, serial follow-up assessments with serial X-rays are required to identify the development of deformity (e.g., proximal junctional kyphosis) and intervene in a timely fashion.

12.13 Outcomes of Tumor Resection of Relevant Nerve Roots

Postoperative neurologic outcome is predicted by preoperative function of the nerve root. The presence of normal clinical and neurophysiological functions indicates that the affected nerve is either normal or its function is compensated by adjacent nerve roots. In cases where there is evidence of compensation by adjacent nerve roots, resection of the tumor-involved nerve root is associated with low risk of postoperative deficit. Improvement of subnormal nerve function can also be seen after resection of the tumor, especially if the root is impinged by the tumor.[49] In a series of 187 patients with spinal schwannomas, Seppälä et al[9] noted that 78% of the patients demonstrated neurological improvement postoperatively, 15% remained stable, and 7% got worse. The ability to walk was regained in 81% of patients who could not walk preoperatively, with bladder function improvement in 63% of patients. In another study, 3/52 patients had skin numbness after resection of affected nerve roots, which improved significantly over the following year, without any permanent sensory impairments.[50]

Generally, resection of spinal nerve sheath tumors does not require nerve root resection. Functioning nerve fascicles can often be preserved with meticulous microsurgical techniques. Conversely, fascicles involved in nerve sheath tumors have to be resected with the tumor, but this rarely results in a functional deficit because the nerve is either nonfunctional or compensated by an adjacent root.

12.14 Postoperative Adjuvant Therapy

Although the role of radiation therapy in the treatment of spinal nerve sheath tumors is not well defined, most authors agree that radiation is not indicated in completely resected benign lesions; however, radiation therapy is the typical standard of care for MPNST.[51] The role of radiotherapy for partially resected or unresectable benign tumors remains controversial because these tumors are generally slow growing and in most cases amenable to further resection, if necessary. Some surgeons suggest monitoring these tumors with serial MRI studies to evaluate their growth without any further intervention. Radiation therapy may be the only effective management modality among patients with multiple spinal nerve root tumors that are not amenable to surgery, although this excludes patients with neurofibromatosis because of the high risk of malignant degeneration secondary to radiation in the setting of genetic predisposition to neoplasms.

With the introduction of frameless stereotactic spinal radiosurgery systems such as the CyberKnife, radiosurgery is rapidly becoming accepted for the management of spinal and peripheral nerve sheath tumors.[52] The role of chemotherapy is usually limited to recurrent or metastatic MPNSTs, and the treatment regimens are generally similar to those for other soft tissue sarcomas.[51,53] Interestingly, neoadjuvant therapy may be used to shrink the tumor size and extension, especially in giant lesions, changing what is initially an unresectable tumor into a tumor that can be resected in an en bloc fashion.

12.15 Conclusion

Most nerve sheath tumors are located on the dorsal or lateral side of the spinal canal and, therefore, the posterior approach is considered the standard approach for such lesions. However, some tumors cannot be addressed through this approach and may require modified or other alternative approaches. The surgeon must select the most appropriate approach based on the clinical status of the patient as well as the size and location of the tumor as delineated by the preoperative imaging. Resecting paraspinal tumors rarely results in a new motor deficit. Therefore, the lowered risk of recurrence as a result of complete tumor resection validates resecting the attached and probably nonfunctional nerve fascicles. Clinical and radiological follow-up and surveillance are essential in the management of patients with nerve sheath tumors.

Acknowledgments

Portions of this chapter were based on the article by Gottfried et al.[16] We thank Kristin Kraus, MSc, for editorial assistance with this chapter.

References

[1] Nittner K. Spinal meningiomas, neuromas and neurofibromas, and hourglass tumors. In: Vinken P, Bruyn G, eds. Handbook of Clinical Neurology. New York: Elsevier; 1976:177–322

[2] Seppälä MT, Haltia MJ, Sankila RJ, Jääskeläinen JE, Heiskanen O. Long-term outcome after removal of spinal neurofibroma. J Neurosurg. 1995; 82(4): 572–577

[3] Safavi-Abbasi S, Senoglu M, Theodore N, et al. Microsurgical management of spinal schwannomas: evaluation of 128 cases. J Neurosurg Spine. 2008; 9(1): 40–47

[4] Albanese V, Platania N. Spinal intradural extramedullary tumors. Personal experience. J Neurosurg Sci. 2002; 46(1):18–24

[5] Kim P, Ebersold MJ, Onofrio BM, Quast LM. Surgery of spinal nerve schwannoma. Risk of neurological deficit after resection of involved root. J Neurosurg. 1989; 71(6):810–814

[6] Celli P, Trillò G, Ferrante L. Spinal extradural schwannoma. J Neurosurg Spine. 2005; 2(4):447–456

[7] Deruaz JP, Janzer RC, Costa J. Cellular schwannomas of the intracranial and intraspinal compartment: morphological and immunological characteristics compared with classical benign schwannomas. J Neuropathol Exp Neurol. 1993; 52(2):114–118

[8] Conti P, Pansini G, Mouchaty H, Capuano C, Conti R. Spinal neurinomas: retrospective analysis and long-term outcome of 179 consecutively operated cases and review of the literature. Surg Neurol. 2004; 61(1):34–43, discussion 44

[9] Seppälä MT, Haltia MJ, Sankila RJ, Jääskeläinen JE, Heiskanen O. Long-term outcome after removal of spinal schwannoma: a clinicopathological study of 187 cases. J Neurosurg. 1995; 83(4):621–626

[10] Parsa AT, Lee J, Parney IF, Weinstein P, McCormick PC, Ames C. Spinal cord and intradural-extraparenchymal spinal tumors: current best care practices and strategies. J Neurooncol. 2004; 69(1–3):291–318

[11] Seppälä MT, Haltia MJ. Spinal malignant nerve-sheath tumor or cellular schwannoma? A striking difference in prognosis. J Neurosurg. 1993; 79(4): 528–532

[12] Zou C, Smith KD, Liu J, et al. Clinical, pathological, and molecular variables predictive of malignant peripheral nerve sheath tumor outcome. Ann Surg. 2009; 249(6):1014–1022

[13] Fan Q, Yang J, Wang G. Clinical and molecular prognostic predictors of malignant peripheral nerve sheath tumor. Clin Transl Oncol. 2014; 16(2):191–199

[14] Kolberg M, Høland M, Agesen TH, et al. Survival meta-analyses for >1800 malignant peripheral nerve sheath tumor patients with and without neurofibromatosis type 1. Neuro-oncol. 2013; 15(2):135–147

[15] Mertens F, Lothe R. Nervous system: peripheral nerve sheath tumors. Atlas Genet Cytogenet Oncol Haematol. 2001; 5(3):210–212

[16] Gottfried ON, Binning MJ, Schmidt MH. Surgical approaches to spinal schwannomas. Contemp Neurosurg. 2005; 27(4):1–9

[17] Li MH, Holtås S, Larsson EM. MR imaging of intradural extramedullary tumors. Acta Radiol. 1992; 33(3):207–212

[18] Asazuma T, Toyama Y, Maruiwa H, Fujimura Y, Hirabayashi K. Surgical strategy for cervical dumbbell tumors based on a three-dimensional classification. Spine. 2004; 29(1):E10–E14

[19] Nanda A, Kukreja S, Ambekar S, Bollam P, Sin AH. Surgical strategies in the management of spinal nerve sheath tumors. World Neurosurg. 2015; 83(6): 886–899

[20] Klekamp J, Samii M. Surgery of spinal nerve sheath tumors with special reference to neurofibromatosis. Neurosurgery. 1998; 42(2):279–289, discussion 289–290

[21] Gragnaniello C, Costa F, Nader R, Cardia A, Lasio G, Fomari M. Intramedullary extramedullary tumors: spinal schwannomas. In: Nader R, Berta S, Gragnaniello C, Sabbagh A, Levy M, eds. Neurosurgery Tricks of the Trade: Spine and Peripheral Nerves. New York: Thieme; 2014:275–279

[22] Larson SJ, Holst RA, Hemmy DC, Sances A , Jr. Lateral extracavitary approach to traumatic lesions of the thoracic and lumbar spine. J Neurosurg. 1976; 45 (6):628–637

[23] McCormick PC. Surgical management of dumbbell and paraspinal tumors of the thoracic and lumbar spine. Neurosurgery. 1996; 38(1):67–74, discussion 74–75

[24] Hakuba A, Komiyama M, Tsujimoto T, et al. Transuncodiscal approach to dumbbell tumors of the cervical spinal canal. J Neurosurg. 1984; 61(6):1100–1106

[25] Barrey C, Saint-Pierre G, Frappaz D, Hermier M, Mottolese C. Complete removal of an intraspinal and extraspinal cervical chordoma in one stage using the lateral approach. Technical note. J Neurosurg Spine. 2006; 5(5):471–475

[26] George B, Gauthier N, Lot G. Multisegmental cervical spondylotic myelopathy and radiculopathy treated by multilevel oblique corpectomies without fusion. Neurosurgery. 1999; 44(1):81–90

[27] George B, Zerah M, Lot G, Hurth M. Oblique transcorporeal approach to anteriorly located lesions in the cervical spinal canal. Acta Neurochir (Wien). 1993; 121(3–4):187–190

[28] Cooper PR, Errico TJ, Martin R, Crawford B, DiBartolo T. A systematic approach to spinal reconstruction after anterior decompression for neoplastic disease of the thoracic and lumbar spine. Neurosurgery. 1993; 32(1):1–8

[29] Konno S, Yabuki S, Kinoshita T, Kikuchi S. Combined laminectomy and thoracoscopic resection of dumbbell-type thoracic cord tumor. Spine. 2001; 26(6):E130–E134

[30] Arnold PM, Anderson KK, McGuire RA , Jr. The lateral transpsoas approach to the lumbar and thoracic spine: a review. Surg Neurol Int. 2012; 3 Suppl 3: S198–S215

[31] Boah AO, Perin NI. Lateral access to paravertebral tumors. J Neurosurg Spine. 2016; 24(5):824–828

[32] Safaee MM, Ames CP, Deviren V, Clark AJ. Minimally invasive lateral retroperitoneal approach for resection of extraforaminal lumbar plexus schwannomas: operative techniques and literature review. Oper Neurosurg (Hagerstown). 2018; 15(5):516–521

[33] Pollo C, Richard A, De Preux J. [Resection of a retroperitoneal schwannoma by a combined approach]. Neurochirurgie. 2004; 50(1):53–56

[34] Jankowski R, Szmeja J, Nowak S, Sokół B, Blok T. Giant schwannoma of the lumbar spine. A case report. Neurol Neurochir Pol. 2010; 44(1):91–95

[35] Alexander E Jr. Postlaminectomy kyphosis. In: Wilkins R, Rengachary S, eds. Neurosurgery. New York: McGraw-Hill; 1985:2293–2297

[36] Bresnahan L, Ogden AT, Natarajan RN, Fessler RG. A biomechanical evaluation of graded posterior element removal for treatment of lumbar stenosis: comparison of a minimally invasive approach with two standard laminectomy techniques. Spine. 2009; 34(1):17–23

[37] Ogden AT, Bresnahan L, Smith JS, Natarajan R, Fessler RG. Biomechanical comparison of traditional and minimally invasive intradural tumor exposures using finite element analysis. Clin Biomech (Bristol, Avon). 2009; 24(2):143–147

[38] Haji FA, Cenic A, Crevier L, Murty N, Reddy K. Minimally invasive approach for the resection of spinal neoplasm. Spine. 2011; 36(15):E1018–E1026

[39] Mannion RJ, Nowitzke AM, Efendy J, Wood MJ. Safety and efficacy of intradural extramedullary spinal tumor removal using a minimally invasive approach. Neurosurgery. 2011; 68(1) Suppl Operative:208–216, discussion 216

[40] Tredway TL, Santiago P, Hrubes MR, Song JK, Christie SD, Fessler RG. Minimally invasive resection of intradural-extramedullary spinal neoplasms. Neurosurgery. 2006; 58(1) Suppl:ONS52–ONS58, discussion ONS52–ONS58

[41] Lee SE, Jahng TA, Kim HJ. Different surgical approaches for spinal schwannoma: a single surgeon's experience with 49 consecutive cases. World Neurosurg. 2015; 84(6):1894–1902

[42] Nzokou A, Weil AG, Shedid D. Minimally invasive removal of thoracic and lumbar spinal tumors using a nonexpandable tubular retractor. J Neurosurg Spine. 2013; 19(6):708–715

[43] van Alfen N, van Engelen BG. The clinical spectrum of neuralgic amyotrophy in 246 cases. Brain. 2006; 129(Pt 2):438–450

[44] Brown JM, Yee A, Ivens RA, Dribben W, Mackinnon SE. Post-cervical decompression parsonage-turner syndrome represents a subset of C5 palsy: six cases and a review of the literature: case report. Neurosurgery. 2010; 67 (6):E1831–E1843, discussion E1843–E1844

[45] McCormick PC. Surgical management of dumbbell tumors of the cervical spine. Neurosurgery. 1996; 38(2):294–300

[46] Lonstein JE. Post-laminectomy kyphosis. Clin Orthop Relat Res. 1977(128): 93–100

[47] Abumi K, Panjabi MM, Kramer KM, Duranceau J, Oxland T, Crisco JJ. Biomechanical evaluation of lumbar spinal stability after graded facetectomies. Spine. 1990; 15(11):1142–1147

[48] Cusick JF, Yoganandan N, Pintar F, Myklebust J, Hussain H. Biomechanics of cervical spine facetectomy and fixation techniques. Spine. 1988; 13(7): 808–812

[49] Celli P. Treatment of relevant nerve roots involved in nerve sheath tumors: removal or preservation? Neurosurgery. 2002; 51(3):684–692, discussion 692

[50] Deng Q, Tian Z, Sheng W, Guo H, Dan ME. Surgical methods and efficacies for cervicothoracolumbar spinal schwannoma. Exp Ther Med. 2015; 10(6):2023–2028

[51] Hruban RH, Shiu MH, Senie RT, Woodruff JM. Malignant peripheral nerve sheath tumors of the buttock and lower extremity. A study of 43 cases. Cancer. 1990; 66(6):1253–1265

[52] Ryu SI, Chang SD, Kim DH, et al. Image-guided hypo-fractionated stereotactic radiosurgery to spinal lesions. Neurosurgery. 2001; 49(4):838–846

[53] Merimsky O, Lepechoux C, Terrier P, Vanel D, Delord JP, LeCesne A. Primary sarcomas of the central nervous system. Oncology. 2000; 58(3):210–214

13 Peripheral Nerve and Paraspinal Tumors: Future Directions of Therapy

Clayton L. Rosinski, Rown Parola, Srjan Sreepathy, Anisse N. Chaker, and Ankit I. Mehta

Summary

The current management of peripheral nerve tumors mainly involves localized surgical interventions and radiation therapy. However, as will be discussed in the following chapter, advances in chemotherapeutics, drug delivery platforms, and radiotherapy are reshaping the therapeutic landscape of peripheral nerve tumors.

Keywords: peripheral nerve tumors, malignant peripheral nerve sheath tumors, chemotherapy, radiation therapy, therapeutic delivery platforms

13.1 Introduction

Peripheral nerve and paraspinal tumors provide unique operative and treatment challenges. As shown in the previous chapter, treatment of these pathologies ranges from predominantly surgical intervention to radiation therapy and chemotherapeutic avenues. However, the shortcomings of these treatment algorithms need to be addressed primarily in malignant plexiform neurofibromas and malignant peripheral nerve sheath tumors (MPNSTs) through future avenues of therapy. In this chapter, future avenues are described through targeted chemotherapeutics, viral therapies, and radiation therapies. Each of these future modalities are attempting to treat these aggressive cancers effectively while mitigating the side effects associated with these therapies.

13.2 Chemotherapeutics

13.2.1 Signal Transduction Pathways Implicated in NF1-Associated PNF and MPNST

Before beginning the discussion of future chemotherapeutics used in the treatment of malignant plexiform neurofibromas (PNFs) and malignant peripheral nerve sheath tumors (MPNSTs), it is important to understand the signaling pathways involved in their etiology. These two tumor types occur often in patients with neurofibromatosis type 1, with 30 to 50% of individuals developing PNFs, and 5 to 10% developing MPNSTs, most of which arise from existing PNFs.

Neurofibromatosis type 1 is genetically characterized by a dominant loss of function mutation in *neurofibromin 1 (NF1)*. The pathways described below are outlined in ▶ Fig. 13.1. *NF1*, a negative regulator of RAS small GTPases, functions by promoting cleavage of GTP to GDP on RAS by interacting with RAS with its GTPase activating domain. The loss of RAS inhibition by a second hit to somatic *NF1* results in constitutive activation of two pathways under control of RAS, the AKT/mTOR pathway and the RAF/MEK/ERK (MAPK) pathway.

Cell growth, proliferation, and survival are regulated by the mTOR kinase, which exists in the multiprotein complexes mTORC1 and mTORC2. Activation of mTORC1 results from a pathway in which RAS-GTP first activates phosphoinositide 3-kinase (PI3K). PI3K eventually activates PDK1 and AKT/PKB, which go on to activate mTORC1. One role of mTORC1 is to regulate protein synthesis, which it promotes through activation of S6 kinase (P70S6K), a ribosomal protein, and inhibition of eukaryotic initiation factor 4E binding proteins (4E-BPs) which sequester initiation factor 4e. The role of mTORC2 appears to be activation of AKT through phosphorylation, which leads to further increases in mTORC1 activity. AKT/PKB provide important survival signals by phosphorylation of many targets which ultimately results in an antiapoptotic effect.

The MAPK pathway is activated upon the binding of RAF kinase to RAS-GTP which results in RAF activation. In turn, RAF initiates a phosphorylation cascade when it activates MEK1 and MEK2 through phosphorylation. MEK1 and MEK2 then activate ERK1 and ERK2 (MAPKs) via phosphorylation, which eventually leads to proliferation and growth. One mechanism through which proliferation is activated by ERK is through its ability to activate transcription factor ELK1 and c-JUN (activates AP1 transcription factor) which leads to upregulated expression of cell cycle regulatory proteins and thus progression through the cell cycle. In the case of *NF1* heterogeneous cells, constitutive activation of this pathway promotes uncontrolled growth. Additionally, the two aforementioned downstream pathways of RAS are not independent of each other as crosstalk between the two occurs, making complete pharmacological inhibition of these pathways difficult with a single agent.

Although biallelic loss of *NF1* is sufficient to cause benign PNF, progression to MPNST requires additional mutations in other genes. For example, transformation to MPNST from PNF is often dependent on tumor suppressor genes *CDKN2A* and *TP53*. Loss of p53 has been associated with progression to MPNST due to its role as a regulator of cellular growth, apoptosis, and DNA damage response. P16INK4A and P14ARF encoded by *CDKN2A* have been associated with malignant transformation of PNF because they regulate retinoblastoma and p53 transduction pathways. Despite the inadequacy of complete loss of *NF1* to cause MPNST, many promising chemotherapeutics target components of the downstream pathways of the *NF1*-regulated RAS.

Ultimately, the majority of peripheral nerve tumors occur in patients through *NF1*. This occurs due to the loss of RAS inhibition, leading to unregulated mTOR and MAPK signaling, both of which promote cell survival, proliferation, and PNF formation. The progression of PNF to MPNST is dependent on further mutation to proteins involved in regulation of the cell cycle and apoptosis.

13.2.2 Pharmacological Agents Targeting RAS

Due to its downstream effectors which regulate cell cycle progression, growth, and survival among other aspects of cellular proliferation, RAS is an ideal target for chemotherapeutics. However, inhibition of RAS has proven elusive, despite promising preclinical trials. Many of these potential therapies target lipid

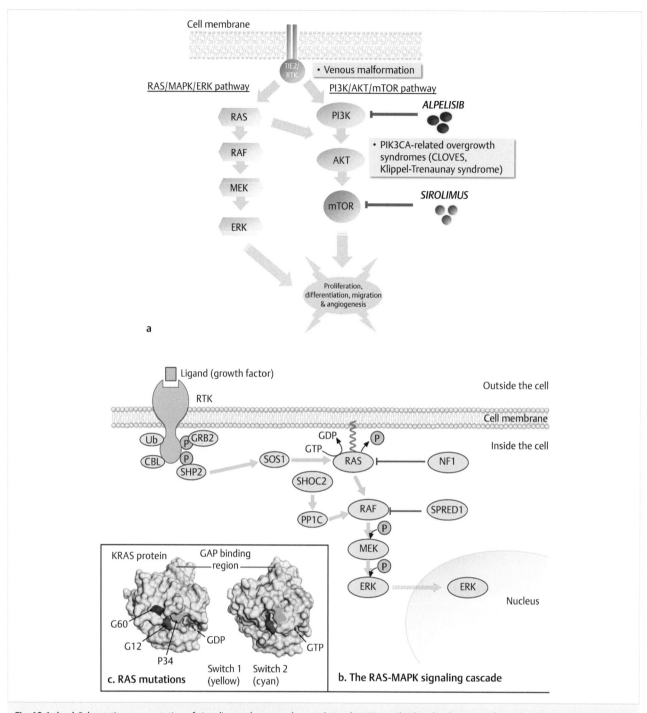

Fig. 13.1 (a-c) Schematic representation of signaling pathways under regulation by NF1 involved in development of peripheral nerve sheath tumors. ([a] Reproduced with permission from Acord M, Srinivasan A. Management of venous malformations. Seminars in Interventional Radiology. 2021; 38(2): 215–225. [b-c] Passarge E. Color Atlas of Genetics. Fifth Edition. Stuttgart: Thieme; 2018. p. 253)

modification of RAS proteins as their activities are dependent on interaction with the membrane. However, the issue was in the fact that the potential therapies did not successfully prevent membrane associations. Prevention of RAS association with membranes remains a promising potential mechanism of inhibition, and future drugs which successfully prevent this association hold much promise in the treatment of many cancers in addition to MPNST. For now, the downstream pathways of RAS hold great promise for potential treatments in the near future.

13.2.3 Pharmacological Agents Targeting the mTOR Cascade

Traditionally, rapamycin has been considered an inhibitor of mTOR, whose name actually derives from this property (mammalian target of rapamycin). Initial data demonstrated potential for rapamycin (sirolimus) to treat NF1-related tumors, as it suppressed their growth in a mouse model. However, this activity is modest as resistance to rapamycin is exhibited due to induced PI3K activity, rapamycin only affecting mTORC1, and incomplete mTORC1 inhibition. Agents used to inhibit mTOR signaling in the future will likely improve on the limitations of rapamycin.

AZD8055 is one of many mTOR inhibitors with potential to treat NF1-associated PNF and MPNST. Unlike rapamycin which only partially inhibits mTORC1, AZD8055, a dual mTOR inhibitor, inhibits both mTORC1 and mTORC2 via its ATP-competitive "active-site" inhibition of mTOR catalytic activity. AZD8055 exhibits greater inhibition of mTORC1 than rapamycin, indicated by significantly greater decrease of phosphorylated 4EBP (p-4EBP) in human MPNST cell lines. Its effect on mTORC2 is evident in the reduced phosphorylation of AKT S473, where rapamycin actually results in increased phosphorylation after 48 hours. As expected, AZD8055 caused reduced tumor growth and proliferation of NF1-associated MPNST, sporadic MPNST (to a lesser extent), and PNF cell lines that was of greater effect than rapamycin. AZD8055's antiproliferative properties stem from its ability to induce G0/G1 arrest. The mTOR pathway represents just one of the significant pathways promoting growth and survival downstream of RAS; thus, combination treatment of AZD8055 and an MAPK pathway inhibitor (PD0325901) resulted in a synergistic effect that was effective on all MPNST and PNF lines it was tested on.

AZD8055 represents just one potential treatment of MPNST that targets the mTOR pathway cascade. A preclinical trial demonstrated the ability of XL765, another dual mTOR inhibitor, to counteract human MPNST growth in a xenograft mouse model. Encouragingly, this compound caused marked autophagy and thus significant MPNST cell death which was enhanced by the addition of chloroquine, an autophagy inhibitor. Success in preclinical trials of mTOR inhibitors in combination with agents of different targets has led to clinical trials of these compounds. Barring any setbacks which cannot be overcome, mTOR inhibitors will likely play an active role in PNF and MPNST treatment in the near future.

13.2.4 Pharmacological Agents Targeting the MAPK Cascade

PD0325901 is an MEK1-specific allosteric inhibitor with demonstrated MPNST therapeutic potential. The MEK1 inhibitor reduced the number of proliferating cells in PNF and MPNST cell lines. PD0325901 has antitumor effects in vivo, as it was able to prolong the survival time of a human NF1-associated MPNST mouse xenograft model and shrink the size of PNF tumors. Another potential benefit of using PD0325901 as an MPNST treatment is its ability to decrease VEGFα expression in tumor cells leading to a reduction in microvessel density of the tumor. Additionally, PD0325901 enhances the cytotoxicity of all trans retinoic acid (ATRA) against MPNST cell lines expressing RXRG. This is of importance to note, as many of the new potential therapeutics which target downstream targets of RAS have cytostatic effects only. In addition to inducing apoptosis, the combination of ATRA and PD0325901 induces differentiation and reduces migration resulting in a viability of 53% for MPNST cells.

Due to the difficulties associated with treating these types of tumors, there is a desperate need for new therapies as well as more effective versions of existing treatments. In a study by Brosius et al,[1] a new combinatorial therapy was utilized in xenografts of MPNST cells to decrease survival and proliferation of tumor cells. It has been found that MPNST tissue expresses estrogen receptor beta as well as G-protein coupled receptor-1 (GPER). In this study, a metabolite of the selective estrogen receptor modulator tamoxifen, known as 4-hydroxytamoxifen, was found to inhibit human MPNST cell proliferation in vitro in small doses (10–100 nM), and induce cell death in MPNST tissue at higher doses (1–5 uM). It was also found that in mice with MPNST xenografts, implanting a 25 mg pellet of tamoxifen resulted in a 50% reduction in graft mass when compared to control animals not implanted with tamoxifen.

Trifluoperazine, a calmodulin inhibitor, was found to phenocopy the effects of tamoxifen on MPNST cultures. In mice with orthotopic MPNST xenografts, it was found that animals intraperitoneally injected with a pre-established maximum tolerated dose (MTD) of 20 mg/kg of trifluoperazine for 30 days straight yielded tumors that were roughly 40% smaller than mice that were injected with an intraperitoneal vehicle for the same duration of time. A third group of mice injected with a pre-established MTD of 30 mg/kg tamoxifen for the same duration of time yielded tumors that were roughly 50% smaller than the control group that received the intraperitoneal vehicle.

With the possibility that certain proteins are targeted by both tamoxifen and trifluoperazine, while others are only targeted by one or the other, the idea of combining the two compounds into a combinatorial therapy in an attempt to maximize targeting of MPNST proteins and molecules is worth investigating. In a similar test utilizing intraperitoneal injection, it was found that animals injected with a slightly smaller dose of tamoxifen (25 mg/kg) or trifluoperazine (15 mg/kg) individually exhibited an approximate tumor size reduction of 40%, while animals injected with a combination of the two drugs exhibited an approximate tumor size reduction of 73.6%.

To determine whether combinatorial therapy was more effective in reducing MPNST cell proliferation than individual administration of tamoxifen or trifluoperazine, tumors from each group were stained with Ki67, a cellular marker associated with cell proliferation, and TUNEL, which uses terminal deoxynucleotidyl transferase (Tdt) to identify apoptotic cells that have experienced late-stage apoptosis DNA degradation. Tamoxifen was found to reduce tumor proliferation by 3.9% as compared to the vehicle control group tumors, while trifluoperazine was found to reduce tumor proliferation by 7.3% as compared to the same vehicle tumors. Tumors from the combinatorial group experienced a 12.5% reduction in proliferation against the same control tumors, displaying the improved outcomes associated with combinatorial treatment.

13.2.5 Pharmacological Agents Targeting Other Pathways

PLX3397 is a selective inhibitor of the tyrosine kinases c-Fms and c-Kit. There exists a clinical trial to investigate whether the effects of PLX3397 and sirolimus in combination demonstrated in early phase clinical trials exists in human MPNST patients. PLX3397 was shown to result in significantly greater tumor volume reduction and macrophage depletion than imatinib (c-Kit and PDGFR inhibitor approved for gastrointestinal stromal tumor [GIST] treatment) in MPNST and PNF mouse models. The macrophage depletion is important, as they correlate with

Table 13.1 Potential chemotherapeutic agents for PNF and MPNST

Compound	Target	Trial type	Notes
AZD8055	mTORC1, mTORC2	Preclinical	Reduces growth and proliferation of NF1-associated MPNST, sporadic MPNST, and PNF cell lines by causing G0/G1 arrest
XL675	mTORC1, mTORC2	Preclinical	Causes autophagy and cell death of MPNST cells in combination with chloroquine
PD0325901	MEK1	Preclinical	Prolongs survival time of MPNST xenograft model, reduces PNF size, inhibits VEGFα, increases efficacy of ATRA
Trifluoperazine + tamoxifen	Calmodulin inhibitor + selective estrogen receptor modulator	Preclinical	Have a synergistic effect resulting in improved tumor size and proliferation reduction than single therapy
PLX3397 + sirolimus	c-Fms, c-Kit inhibitor + mTORC1 inhibitor	Clinical	Proapoptotic effect when combined; PLX3397 reduces tumor volume and macrophage depletion; sirolimus causes G1 arrest
PCI-34051 (PCI3), PCI-48012 (PCI4)	HDAC8 inhibitors	Preclinical	Reduce MPNST tumor size in xenograft models; cause S phase arrest and apoptosis

Abbreviations: ATRA, all trans retinoic acid; MPNST, peripheral nerve sheath tumor; NF1, neurofibromatosis 1; PNF, plexiform neurofibroma.

MPNST progression and are permissive of the established tumor. The antiproliferative effects of PLX3397 are enhanced when given in combination with rapamycin via G1 cell cycle arrest, and even demonstrate a proapoptotic effect. As previously mentioned, sirolimus (rapamycin) is not the most effective mTOR inhibitor, and it is speculated that combination with a dual mTOR inhibitor would produce even greater results when given with PLX3397.

Histone deacetylase 8 (HDAC8), a protein which can deacetylate histone 3 and 4 in some cell types, expression is prognostic for unfavorable outcome in neuroblastoma. Although the exact role of HDAC8 in MPNST pathogenesis is unknown, it may be related to its effect on its targets of deacetylation (estrogen related receptor alpha, inv-16 fusion protein, CREB). Regardless of the exact mechanism, inhibitors of HDAC8 such as PCI-34051 (PCI3) and PCI-48012 (PCI4) reduce the growth of MPNST cell lines via S phase cell cycle arrest and induction of apoptosis. These effects in cell lines translated to reduced tumor volume of a mouse MPNST xenograft model when treated with PCI4 (▶ Table 13.1).

The aforementioned compounds are just a selection of pharmacologic agents which demonstrate exciting MPNST therapeutic potential. As investigation into such compounds continues with preclinical and clinical trials, greatly needed MPNST therapies should be discovered. It is likely that therapy for PNF and MPNST in the not-so-distant future will involve multiple chemotherapeutics all targeting different pathways involved in regulation of the cell cycle, growth, proliferation, and survival of tumor cells. The therapeutics of tomorrow will be accompanied by target delivery methods which are in development today.

13.3 Targeted Chemotherapeutic Delivery Platforms

13.3.1 Interleukin-13 Receptor Alpha 2 (IL13Rα2) Targeted Drug Delivery System

Several cancers including glioblastoma and certain carcinomas express IL13Rα2. In addition to signifying the malignancy and predicting the invasiveness of such tumors, it also proves to be

a therapeutic target for toxins or chemotherapeutics fused with IL13. This IL13 receptor is expressed at greater levels on both MPNST and benign nerve sheath tumor tissues derived from human patients than normal sciatic nerves, with MPNST demonstrating greater IL13Rα2 expression. It appears as this receptor can be used to target antitumor agents to MPNST and benign nerve sheath tumors as, as IL13 conjugated liposomal doxorubicin not only was readily taken up by NF1-associated MPNST cells in culture and localized to the nucleus as well. This is an important feat, as this mechanism of doxorubicin has cytotoxic potential in MPNST cell lines. In vivo experiments are equally promising, where treatment of an MPNST mouse model with IL13 conjugated liposomal doxorubicin resulted in a greater decrease in tumor progression than mice treated with unconjugated liposomal doxorubicin, both of which showed reduced tumor progression compared to untreated animals.

The discovery that MPNST and related benign nerve sheath tumors strongly express IL13Rα2 and that liposomes conjugated to IL13 can be targeted to these cells holds great promise for the potential of this chemotherapeutic delivery method. This platform has the added benefit of versatility, as many therapeutics could be loaded into the liposomes, allowing for multiple compounds to be targeted specifically to the malignancy at the same time, or for switching of the therapeutic agent. One potential drawback to this proposed chemotherapeutic delivery platform is that if IL13Rα2 is not expressed on a patient's tumor, or a subpopulation within the tumor arose that did not express IL13Rα2, the platform would offer no benefit over standard systemic delivery methods.

13.3.2 Magnetic Targeting of Systemically Delivered Magnetic Nanoparticles (MNPs)

Unlike the previously described mechanism of using specific receptors preferentially expressed on tumor cells, this chemotherapeutic delivery platform relies on the use of magnetic field to localize drug ladened with magnetic nanoparticles (MNPs). The MNPs have an iron oxide core which is responsive to external magnetic fields. This not only localizes the systemically delivered MNPs to the site of the magnetic field, but enhances the uptake of MNPs into cells within the magnetic field. Neodymium-iron-boron magnets are surgically placed near the tumor in order to provide the magnetic field that will localize the MNPs to the tumor site. An additional option for localizing the magnetic field to the tumor would be to place a magnetic stent like cage around the tumor. This delivery platform is also able to deliver MNPs to anatomical locations that are poorly perfused, such as vertebral bodies of the spinal column. Unlike the IL13 receptor targeting system, magnetic delivery of MNPs does not rely on any inherent characteristics of the tumor to localize chemotherapeutics, making it a slightly more robust potential delivery platform.

Another beneficial property of MNPs is their ability to be carriers of many different compounds, having been used to deliver chemotherapeutics and nucleic acids to tumors. Thus, the magnetic delivery of MNPs would also allow for the use of multiple therapeutics when treating MPNST or PNF. This not only allows for increased treatment efficacy through synergistic effects of multiple therapeutics, but also prevents the rise of chemoresistant tumor subpopulations. In addition to increased concentration of therapeutics at the tumor site, the magnetic delivery platform reduces systemic drug toxicity. The one drawback to this methodology is that it requires surgical implantation of magnets, although magnets above the skin may be used for superficial tumors.

13.3.3 Polymer-Based Local Chemotherapeutic Delivery Platforms

Many novel drug delivery platforms attempt to minimize the systemic side effects of the drug being delivered by concentrating said drug at the desired site of action. Rather than attempting to localize a systemically delivered drug, an alternative approach is to only deliver the drug at the desired location. One such option to achieve this is through the deployment of a drug-laden polymer at the desired site, which in this case is the peripheral nerve tumor. Loading of the polymer with the chemotherapeutic agent allows for a prolonged release of the agent at the desired site. The rate of release can be further tailored based on the needs of the proposed treatment through varying the composition of the polymer. For instance, a fibrin hydrogel, currently used in the operating room as a sealant, can be loaded with the desired drug, and based on alterations in the ratio of fibrin to the chemotherapeutic, the rate of drug releasing from the gel can be altered.

The primary strengths of a polymer-based delivery system are that there is no need for systemic administration of the desired chemotherapeutic, greatly limiting adverse effects. Additionally, as many of the potential polymers used for such platforms come from liquid components, which when mixed form a gel-like substance, the entire platform can be delivered in a minimally invasive fashion whether it be through a needle or a very small incision. The major limitation of such a potential delivery platform is that the drug will eventually stop eluting from the polymer gel, requiring multiple implantations of such a delivery system.

In total, there are multiple promising methods for improved targeting of chemotherapeutics to peripheral nerve tumors.

These potential avenues include utilizing unique molecular aspects of the tumors to target chemotherapeutics, using magnets to concentrate systemically delivered, drug-laden magnetic nanoparticles to the site of the tumor, and local delivery of chemotherapeutics in a polymer-based gel that allows for sustained, peripheral drug release.

13.4 Oncolytic Virus Therapy for PNSTs

The most common currently accepted path of treatment for peripheral nerve sheath tumors (PNSTs) in general is surgical excision combined with therapy to reduce the likelihood of recurrence. Although this method of treatment can be effective, surgical resection does not always result in complete tumor removal and has the potential to create some loss of function for the patient. One potential avenue being investigated is the use of oncolytic viruses to kill tumors. These viruses can be weakened forms of vaccines (i.e., measles), genetically engineered viruses designed to target tumor cell receptors and avoid replicating within normal tissue (i.e., adenovirus or herpes simplex virus [HSV]), or viruses with a natural predisposition toward targeting and replicating within tumor cells (i.e., myxoma). With the ability to induce controlled cell death in tumor tissue and avoid damage to noncancerous local tissue, advances in this type of therapy could result in a new minimally invasive or potentially noninvasive means of intervention for patients with PNSTs.

There are several designer viruses that are being investigated as potential oncolytic treatments. HSV is an example of a virus that can be modified through viral gene deletions and/or mutations in order to reduce its own neurovirulence and consequently lessen the pathogenic effects of the virus itself, as well as selectively inhibit tumor growth while allowing other nearby tissue to go unharmed. HSV is a natural choice for investigation due to its neurotropic qualities, allowing it to infect the nervous system. Currently, oncolytic variants of HSV, or oHSVs, are being used in preclinical trials with human xenografts and modified mouse strains to test their efficacy in treating a few different types of tumor. In one study, schwannoma tissue from human patients suffering from either NF2 or schwannomatosis was implanted subcutaneously in a strain of immunocompromised mice. After two doses of an oHSV, tumor size reduction was noted in experimental animals in contrast to control vehicle-treated animals, whose tumors continued to grow.

oHSVs have also been investigated for potential usage in the treatment of MPNSTs. In one study, mouse NF1 MPNST cell lines were placed in the sciatic nerves of immunocompetent mice, while a human NF1 analog known as MSLCs, or MPNST stem-like cells, were placed in the sciatic nerves of immunodeficient mice. After being treated with a single dose of oHSV, one-third of the experimental MSLC-infected mouse group survived in the long term with limited neurological deficits and no evidence of remaining tumor. In contrast, none of the control group mock treated MSLC-infected mice survived their tumors.

Measles virus, or MV, is another potential candidate for use as an oncolytic virus. Wild-type MV contains signaling lymphocyte activation molecule, or SLAM, a receptor used for cellular entry which is generally not expressed in tumor cells. Weakened strains such as the Edmonston variant of MV are often better suited to serve as oncolytic viruses than their wild-type counterparts due to the addition of CD46, which is a cellular receptor that is generally expressed highly in human tumors and allows for easier entry into tumor cells. With the addition of human sodium iodide transporter (NIS), MV can be monitored in a noninvasive fashion to determine the rate of virus spread. This highly modified strain of MV, known as MV-NIS, is being tested in clinical trials for different types of tumors such as mesothelioma and ovarian cancer. MV-NIS has been noted as being highly cytotoxic to MPNST cell lines while generally not affecting normal Schwann cells. This observation lends itself to the potential modified MV strains have in improving MPNST outcomes.

13.5 Paraspinal and Peripheral Nerve Tumor Research Areas and Future Therapies in Radiotherapy

Surgical resection in combination with radiation therapy (RT) should be the standard approach for the primary tumor in patients presenting with MPNST without obvious metastatic disease. In a foundational study[2] RT combined with surgical excision improved the 5-year local control rate compared to surgery from 34 to 65%, p <0.001, and achieved 5- and 10-year survival rates of 52 and 34%, respectively. That study found radiation doses greater than 60 Gy and intraoperative RT to be significant prognostic factors for local control.

Improvements in RT including image-guided radiotherapy (IGRT), target delineation, and dose delivery may allow for further advances in treating paraspinal and peripheral nerve tumors.

One promising area of research is in reduction of the area receiving radiation to limit toxicity while delivering a tumoricidal radiation dose. Wang et al found preoperative IGRT treatment for patients with extremity soft tissue sarcomas resulted in a significant reduction of late toxicities that suggests that the reduced target volumes used in the Radiation Therapy Oncology Group (RTOG) 0630 are appropriate for preoperative IGRT.[3] The reduced target volumes used in the RTOG 0630 protocol include:

- Gross target volume (GTV) containing the gross tumor defined by T1-weighted magnetic resonance imaging (MRI) plus contrast. The protocol recommends fusion of MRI and computed tomography (CT) to delineate the GTV for RT planning.
- Clinical target volume (CTV) expansion from the GTV that envelopes the GTV and suspicious edema (defined by T2-weighted MRI images) plus 2 cm longitudinal and 1 cm radial margins.
- Planning target volume (PTV) expansion to include CTV and error of setup and organ motion. Typically, PTV includes CTV plus 5 mm.

These smaller margins were reasonable due to repositioning shifts that could be applied based on pretreatment images of bony anatomy. In the RTOG 0630 study, six imaging modalities were used to obtain pretreatment images including kilovoltage orthogonal images (KVorth), megavoltage orthogonal images (MVorth), KV fan-beam CT (KVCT), KV cone beam CT (KVCB), MV fan-beam CT (MVCT), and MV cone beam CT (MVCB). An analysis of the daily repositioning data including shifts and rotations conducted by Li et al[4] determined that had the image guidance not been used, a CTV-to-PTV margin of 1.5 cm would be required to account for daily setup variations. The means and standard deviations of daily repositioning shifts in x, y, and z directions for all patients treated with each of the six image modalities are reproduced in ▶ Table 13.2.

Magnetic resonance (MR)-guided radiotherapy, a new treatment modality, may also be useful for treatment of peripheral nerve tumors. MR-guided radiotherapy has demonstrated dosimetric equivalency for treating soft tissue sarcomas of the extremities. A future area of improvement may include further reduction of the target volume and more accurate positioning from MR-guided radiotherapy. MR-guided radiotherapy would increase accuracy in GTV definition by avoiding fusion inaccuracies between MRI and CT as a CT would no longer be needed for RT planning. Target positioning could also be improved by applying repositioning shifts on MR images of soft tissue target anatomy rather than X-ray images of bony anatomy. MR-guided radiotherapy may also be helpful in guiding treatment decision as diffusion weighted MRI obtained once or twice a week has been proposed as an early assessment of treatment response for sarcoma patients receiving preoperative RT.

Table 13.2 Mean and standard deviation of daily repositioning shifts due to setup variations prior to treatment stratified by image guidance modality. Had image guidance not been used, a CTV to PTV expansion margin of 1.5 cm would be required to account for daily setup variations.

Modality	Right–Left (x) [mm]	Superior–Inferior (y) [mm]	Anterior–Posterior (z) [mm]
KVCT	0.5 ± 4.2	1.7 ± 5.2	−1.9 ± 4.3
KVCB	0.35 ± 3.5	−0.4 ± 1.8	2.5 ± 5.6
MVCT	1.0 ± 4.0	−0.4 ± 1.8	2.5 ± 5.6
MVCB	1.1 ± 8.0	1.2 ±1.3	−0.9 ± 4.4
KVorth	−0.5 ± 4.0	0.0 ± 2.3	−0.5 ± 3.2
MVorth	1.0 ± 2.7	3.7 ± 6.5	0.1 ± 4.0

Abbreviations: CTV, clinical target volume; KVCB, KV cone beam CT; KVCT, KV fan-beam CT; KVorth, kilovoltage orthogonal images; MVCB, MV cone beam CT; MVCT, MV fan-beam CT; MVorth, megavoltage orthogonal images; PTV, planning target volume.

13.6 Conclusion

The landscape of peripheral nerve tumor treatment is rapidly changing, embracing many modalities which aim to limit the need for surgical intervention. There are many promising chemotherapeutics which target the cell survival and proliferative signaling cascades which run aberrant in NF1 patients. Other advancements in treatment have been in the platforms which are used to achieve a more localized delivery of these chemotherapeutic agents to the peripheral tumors. The delivery platforms of the future will reduce systemic side effects by concentrating the drug at the tumor by binding to unique molecular markers of the tumor, magnetism, or polymer gels. Another exciting potential treatment utilizes viruses targeted to tumor cells which can induce apoptosis. Lastly, there have been many advances in radiotherapy options which again aim to limit the harmful side effects of such therapies.

References

[1] Brosius SN, Turk AN, Byer SJ, Longo JF, Kappes JC, Roth KA, Carroll SL. Combinatorial therapy with tamoxifen and trifluoperazine effectively inhibits malignant peripheral nerve sheath tumor growth by targeting complementary signaling cascades. J Neuropathol Exp Neurol. 2014;73(11): 1078–90

[2] Wong WW, Hirose T, Scheithauer BW, Schild SE, Gunderson LL. Malignant peripheral nerve sheath tumor: analysis of treatment outcome. Int J Radiat Oncol Biol Phys. 1998;42(2):351–360

[3] Wang D, Zhang Q, Eisenberg BL, et al. Significant Reduction of Late Toxicities in Patients With Extremity Sarcoma Treated With Image-Guided Radiation Therapy to a Reduced Target Volume: Results of Radiation Therapy Oncology Group RTOG-0630 Trial. Journal of Clinical Oncology: Official Journal of the American Society of Clinical Oncology. 2015;33(20)

[4] Li XA, Chen X, Zhang Q, et al. Margin reduction from image guided radiation therapy for soft tissue sarcoma: Secondary analysis of Radiation Therapy Oncology Group 0630 results. Pract Radiat Oncol. 2016;6(4): e135–e140

Index

Note: Page numbers set **bold** or *italic* indicate headings or figures, respectively.